Clinician's Guide to
Chronic Headache and Facial Pain

Clinician's Guide to
Chronic Headache
and Facial Pain

Edited by

Gary W. Jay

Pfizer, Inc.
New London, Connecticut, USA

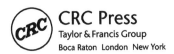

CRC Press
Taylor & Francis Group
Boca Raton London New York

CRC Press is an imprint of the
Taylor & Francis Group, an **informa** business

CRC Press
Taylor & Francis Group
6000 Broken Sound Parkway NW, Suite 300
Boca Raton, FL 33487-2742

First issued in paperback 2017

ISBN-13: 978-1-4398-2487-0 (hbk)
ISBN-13: 978-1-138-11673-3 (pbk)

A CIP record for this book is available from the British Library.

Library of Congress Cataloging-in-Publication Data available on application.

Visit the Taylor & Francis Web site at
http://www.taylorandfrancis.com

and the CRC Press Web site at
http://www.crcpress.com

Foreword

Pain specialists, noninterventionalists, primary care physicians, medical specialists, fellows, residents, and medical students all want to make clinical decisions about pain efficiently, often with an incomplete knowledge of underlying pathophysiology, while addressing global needs of their patients. Pain management is not part of the routine training for most physicians, yet the majority of patients seek medical attention because they have pain. Pain is typically addressed by primary care practitioners on an acute, time-limited basis, but when first- and second-level strategies fail, patients are referred to pain specialists and/or disease or body system specialists for more thorough evaluation and management. Primary care physicians, typically the first stopping point for patients in pain, as well as specialists from anesthesiology, internal medicine subspecialties, neurology, physical medicine, and psychiatry must be prepared to help people suffering with chronic headache and pain disorders.

Headache specialists and other medical specialists as well as primary care physicians managing patients having chronic headache and pain know that usual acute pain management strategies do not address complex needs of people having many years of continuous pain. Interventionalists focus on performing procedures intended to interrupt pain processing, while medically oriented practitioners skillfully blend multiple medications, many of which primary care physicians are not comfortable prescribing (especially methadone). The field of modern pain management has become highly procedural, often relying upon opioids, involving the use of polypharmacy and the management of patients within multidisciplinary pain clinics.

Dr. Gary Jay and contributors to this book, *Clinician's Guide to Chronic Headache and Facial Pain*, have collectively demystified chronic headache and facial pain treatment bringing the management of people with persisting pain into the understanding of pain medicine and other specialists. The chapter authors have prepared essential reviews focusing on the information most needed by specialists, fellows, residents, and medical students to confidently and competently manage complex people in pain. In the first section, chapters focus on common, but potentially vexing headache disorders: migraine, tension-type, posttraumatic, cervicogenic, cluster, trigeminal neuralgia, idiopathic, and orofacial pain syndromes. In the second section, pharmacologic therapeutics are discussed: nonopioid analgesics and adjuvants, opioids, antidepressants, and anticonvulsants, drugs used for the treatment of acute migraine, with special attention to the legal aspects of prescribing controlled substances. The third section covers other treatments addressing the psychological and neuropsychological aspects of pain as well as role for interdisciplinary models, interventional options, acupuncture, and complimentary/alternative medicine.

Today's specialists evaluating and treating people in pain are medical detectives. They make sense out of painful complaints by following clues, seeing patterns, laying their hands upon their patients, using scientific methods, while balancing clinical suspicion, intuition, and compassion. People living with chronic headaches and pain may wish for absolute pain relief, but they are grateful for any pain relief and the opportunity to receive care from clinicians demonstrating concern and ability.

Clinician's Guide to Chronic Headache and Facial Pain is a "go to" book when information is needed concisely about some aspect of headache or chronic pain. This book focuses on what matters most for busy clinicians: presentation of headache and facial pain syndromes, common causes and underlying pathophysiologic mechanisms, differential diagnosis, diagnostic assessment methods (e.g., laboratory studies, imaging, and electrodiagnostic testing), and recommended treatments. While much is said about the importance of evidence-based treatment, for some headaches and facial pain syndromes there are limited well-controlled and randomized studies. The contributors have taken care to keep their messages practical, and readers are sure to find this book one they will keep close at hand.

B. Eliot Cole, MD, MPA
Montclair, New Jersey, U.S.A.

Preface

Headache and facial pain are two of the most common medical complaints of mankind. Patients with headache and facial pain often fill the emergency, outpatient, and ambulatory settings. It has been estimated that more than 40 million Americans have headaches severe enough to require medical care. The World Health Organization ranks migraine 19th among the world's leading causes of disability. Just migraine headache is the cause of an estimated 400,000 days lost from work or school every year per million of the population in developed countries, with other headache disorders being collectively responsible for greater losses. (www.l-t-b.org, a partnership in action between the World Health Organization, World Headache Alliance, International Headache Society, and European Headache Federation.)

This book, *Clinician's Guide to Chronic Headache and Facial Pain*, is a practical, easy to use guide created for the headache specialist and other related physicians since they typically spend most of their time specifically treating headache and facial pain to the exclusion of general pain problems.

The book details the most prevalent maladies and syndromes associated with headache and facial pain. All of the headache or facial pain syndrome chapters have information on the disorder in question, the pathophysiology, the treatment, any evidence-based medicine issues and, of course, up-to-date references.

This book continues with a section dealing with other common pain treatment modalities, from psychological care to acupuncture and CAM treatments. The neuropsychological evaluation is discussed, as this may help shed some light on patients with other issues such as posttraumatic headache. Up-to-date evidence-based medicine chapters detailing interdisciplinary as well as interventional pain management treatment are also included. This section should be very useful to clinicians who treat headache, facial pain, and/or pain of any type. The book concludes with chapters on the most common medications used to treat headache and facial pain, as well as other pain problems.

In addition to headache specialists, this book is also of value to the neurologist, anesthesiologist, general pain management specialist, internists, physiatrists, general practitioners, and others dealing with headache and facial pain. In addition residents and fellows learning the ropes and other clinical specialties such as neurophysiologists, psychologists, nurses, and physical therapists may also find this information useful.

I wish to thank the many superb, patient focused, and generally wonderful contributors to this textbook!

It is my hope and expectation that the book is, in the end, helpful to our patients most of all.

Gary W. Jay, MD

Acknowledgments

First, as always, I want to thank my wonderful wife Suzanne and my incredible daughter Samantha for their love and patience with me during the extended period of time I spent working on this book. Many thanks also go to Byron Scott, R.Ph., my brother by choice, and one of the smartest and best people in the world to talk to; David Longmire, MD, another brother by choice, for his rather droll wit and strange ability to look just like my doppelganger with neither ability getting in the way of his amazing knowledge of neurology (with, of course, special attention to the Autonomic Nervous System); to my new friends at Pfizer (you know who you are) and, of course, to the thousands of patients I had the good fortune to meet, diagnose and treat- you were all my best teachers. After 25 years of clinical practice, when I made the choice to go into Pharma, I knew I would miss you all and I do.

Finally, this book is dedicated to Jim Kapp, who left us all too soon.

Contents

Contributors

Jennifer Bolen   The Legal Side of Pain®, The J. Bolen Group, LLC, Knoxville, Tennessee, U.S.A.

Roger K. Cady   Headache Care Center, Springfield, Missouri, U.S.A.

Richard H. Cox   Private Practice, Chapel Hill; Duke University Medical Center, Durham, North Carolina; Georgetown University Medical Center, Washington DC, U.S.A.

Peter T. Dorsher   Mayo College of Medicine, Jacksonville, Florida, U.S.A.

Kathleen Farmer   Headache Care Center, Springfield, Missouri, U.S.A.

Frederick G. Freitag   Diamond Headache Clinic, Chicago, Illinois, U.S.A.

Alan K. Halperin   Division of General Internal Medicine, Department of Medicine, University of Florida College of Medicine Jacksonville, Jacksonville, Florida, U.S.A.

Bernadette Jaeger   Section of Oral Medicine and Orofacial Pain, UCLA School of Dentistry, Los Angeles, California, U.S.A.

Gary W. Jay   Clinical Disease Area Expert-Pain, Pfizer, Inc., New London, Connecticut, U.S.A.

Gary D. Klasser   Department of Oral Medicine and Diagnostic Sciences, University of Illinois at Chicago, College of Dentistry, Chicago, Illinois, U.S.A.

Paul Mathew   Department of Neurology, Mayo Clinic, Rochester, Minnesota, U.S.A.

B. Lee Peterlin   Departments of Neurology and Pharmacology & Physiology, Drexel University College of Medicine, Philadelphia, Pennsylvania, U.S.A.

Frederick R. Taylor   University of Minnesota School of Medicine and Park Nicollet Health Services, Minneapolis, Minnesota, U.S.A.

1 Migraine

Roger K. Cady and Kathleen Farmer
Headache Care Center, Springfield, Missouri, U.S.A.

Migraine is difficult to conceptualize. On one hand migraine is a self-limited episodic pain disorder, while on the other, it is a chronic progressive disease. Ironically, this could even describe the same person at two different stages of life. Clearly, genetic factors are involved in migraine. This genetic predisposition through complex interactions with the environment generates repeated periods of neurological disruption that typically reoccur over a decade of a person's life. Migraine is the quintessential example of how biology and environment can interact to produce a disease. In this chapter, we will review the diagnostic criteria of migraine, pathophysiology as it is understood today, and management concepts that can lead to improved care of a migraine patient.

EPIDEMIOLOGICAL CONSIDERATIONS

Migraine is the most common neurological disease affecting humans. It is estimated that 12% of the North American population suffer from migraine (1). The prevalence in Japan is 6% (2), and in Brazil, 13% (3). Migraine is prevalent worldwide. There is a strong gender bias for migraine with females being afflicted approximately three times more often than males in the general population (4). This gender bias both in terms of prevalence and impact is even more pronounced in the population of consumers who seek medical services (5).

The onset of migraine typically begins in early life. The prevalence in children ranges from 1% to 4% without a significant gender bias being observed until puberty when menarche dramatically increases the prevalence in women (6). This gender bias remains throughout adulthood but is particularly evident during a woman's reproductive and perimenopausal years.

Migraine is also associated with significant morbidity and disability. This is due to the severity of individual acute attacks as well as the frequency and pattern of attacks over time. As migraine becomes more frequent, the time between attacks shortens and other physical and emotional symptoms complicate the person's life, significantly impacting the ability to function normally (7,8). The World Health Organization has placed migraine in the 20 most disabling medical conditions, ranked 6th for women and 18th for men (9).

Migraine like other chronic diseases such as asthma or epilepsy has the potential to be both chronic and progressive. When occurring infrequently, migraine is an unfortunate disruption of life, like a severe case of the flu, but as it transforms from episodic to chronic disorder, a wide range of associated symptoms in conjunction with headache produces functional limitations and disability that clearly define migraine as a serious chronic disease (7,10,11).

DIAGNOSIS OF MIGRAINE

Because there are no diagnostic tests for migraine, it is defined as a syndrome or collection of related symptoms. As such, diagnosing migraine requires that the clinician has both clinical knowledge of migraine and the ability to effectively communicate with the patient. The importance of these clinical skills cannot be overstated. Because the majority of migraineurs do not seek medical consultation, those who do, often bring years of experience at attempting yet failing to control migraine. They often harbor misconceptions and biases about the cause of their headaches and their clinical needs. Health care professionals also bring their own set of biases into a clinical encounter with the patient presenting with headache, which may lead to patients feeling misunderstood, alienated, and frustrated with the medical system. The American Migraine Study conducted in 1990 found that approximately 50% of migraine patients were undiagnosed (12). A follow-up American Migraine Study conducted a decade later saw little improvement in this statistic (4). The most important tool for migraine diagnosis is clinical history. A useful method for obtaining a clinical history from a patient presenting with recurrent headaches is to begin with a neutral, open-ended question, such as: "Describe your headache" or "Help me understand the headaches you experience" (13). This allows patients to tell their story, effectively establishes rapport, and in the process quickly elicits relevant historical information. Specific close-ended questions can supplement the patient's history to provide specific symptoms required to establish a formal medical diagnosis. Key information embedded in the patient's narrative often provides an understanding of the impact and pattern of headaches over time, as well as key diagnostic symptoms. Even though health care providers may assume that open-ended questions consume too much time, a recent study found that open-ended history taking actually took less time and provided a much better alignment between the patient and health care professional (13). In addition, providers and patients both rated the clinical encounter as being more satisfying.

The formal diagnosis of migraine is based on the criteria established by the International Headache Society (IHS) (Tables 1 to 3). These criteria were first established in 1988 and revised in 2004 (14,15), and since their inception have been accepted worldwide as the diagnostic criteria utilized in clinical drug

---

TABLE 1   IHS Criteria for Migraine without Aura

Migraine without aura accounts for approximately 75% of migraine attacks (28). It is formally diagnosed as follows:
At least five lifetime attacks of headache that fulfill the following:
The headache must have two of the following four characteristics:

1.   Moderate-to-severe intensity
2.   Throbbing quality
3.   Unilateral
4.   Aggravated by activity

In addition, at least one of the following two:

1.   Nausea and/or vomiting
2.   Photophobia and phonophobia

No association with an underlying disease as an etiology for the headaches.

TABLE 2 IHS Criteria for Migraine with Aura

Migraine with aura accounts for approximately 15–20% of migraine attacks and is differentiated from migraine without aura by the presence of a period of focal neurological symptoms preceding the headache, such as visual, sensory, or speech symptoms. Visual symptoms may include scotoma or seeing zig-zag lines; sensory auras may be numbness or tingling in the face or fingers; there also may be difficulties with speech

trials. The IHS divides migraine into two subcategories: migraine without aura and migraine with aura. In the 2004 revision, migraine was further divided into episodic and chronic based on the frequency of migraine attacks.

Even though the IHS criteria are specific enough to ensure that subjects enrolled in a clinical trial do indeed have migraine, their sensitivity in clinical practice is less impressive, primarily because migraine is a far more complex process than is portrayed by the symptom checklist developed by the IHS. Further, clinical treatment paradigms do not support waiting for migraine to progress and become severe enough that all IHS symptoms occur before treatment can begin (16–18). Essentially, the IHS criteria reflect a "symptom biopsy" that occurs when the process of migraine is fully developed and at its zenith. In most instances, an attack of migraine can be recognized before this point is reached. In clinical practice, IHS criteria are utilized in the diagnostic process through retrospective analysis of attacks of headache the patient has experienced. This can be better confirmed by diary analysis if needed. However, it should not be inferred that once the diagnosis is established, every subsequent attack of migraine needs to completely fulfill criteria for IHS migraine before migraine can be recognized or treated by the patient.

Chronic Migraine

Arguably, the most important addition to the revised IHS criteria of 2004 is the new diagnosis of chronic migraine. Initially, these criteria defined chronic migraine simply and consistent with the earlier classification, as greater than 15 episodes of IHS migraine per month for at least the previous three months (14). The impracticality of this definition was addressed by Bigal et al. as being academically restrictive and a barrier to clinical trials of chronic migraine (19). Consequently, an appendix definition was proposed by the IHS nomenclature committee (20) (Table 3).

The appendix criteria for chronic migraine are a clear departure from the 1988 criteria that mandated each clinical presentation of headache be classified

TABLE 3 New Appendix Criteria for Chronic Migraine

1. Headache (tension-type and/or migraine) on 15 or more days/month for at least three months
2. Headache occurring in a patient who has had at least five IHS migraine attacks (1.1)
3. On eight or more days/month, if the headaches have fulfilled
   a. IHS criteria for migraine, or are
   b. treated and relieved by triptan/ergot before the expected development of symptoms fulfilling IHS migraine criteria
4. No medication overuse headache (MOH) as defined by IHS 8.2
5. Describe the patient, not headache attack

as separate diagnoses. Instead these criteria acknowledge that episodic migraine may evolve into chronic migraine but that the specificity of each attack may be altered by natural progression of the disease or treatment. They are an effort to describe patients rather than individual attacks of headache. This is an important step forward for migraine classification.

Medication Overuse Headache

Perhaps one of the most unique concepts accepted by headache specialists is headache attributable to medication overuse. Conceptually, medication overuse headache (MOH) is a chronic headache pattern that etiologically is related to the frequent use of medication used to treat acute episodes of migraine. In the 1988 definition of medication overuse headache, the criteria indicated that the headache improved after withdrawal of the daily medication. However in 2004, this stipulation was abandoned. Instead, arbitrarily defined quantities of medication taken by the patient are listed which may suggest the diagnosis of MOH (Table 4). No clear mechanism to understand MOH exists and numerous debates abound as to whether patients do indeed improve after withdrawal of acute medication. However, third-party payers have quickly adapted limitations of acute migraine medication based on IHS criteria, thus making this a critical issue for the practicing health care professional. However, it is important to understand the concept of MOH and whenever possible prevent rather than treat this devastating disease. This can be accomplished through education and initiation of preventive strategies before rather than after the process is established.

Simplified Diagnostic Schemes

Despite the IHS criteria and millions of dollars spent on education of physicians, almost half of patients with migraine remain undiagnosed and thus many receive ineffective treatment (21). Contrary to older diagnostic approaches, migraine should not necessarily be a diagnosis of exclusion (22). In fact, those patients with a stable established pattern of disabling headache should be considered to have migraine until proven otherwise (28). This hypothesis was indirectly validated by a study of headache sufferers seeking treatment in primary care practices; 97% of them did in fact have migraine (23).

TABLE 4   New Appendix Criteria for Medication Overuse Headache (MOH)

---

1. Headache present on 15 or more days/month
2. Regular overuse for three months or more of acute medication as defined in IHS 8.2
3. Headache has developed or markedly worsened during medication overuse
4. MOH duration definition
   a. Intake on a regular basis for three months or more
   b. On 10 or more days/month, the patient takes
      i.   opiates
      ii. combination analgesics
      iii. triptans
      iv. ergots
   c. On 15 or more days/month, the patient takes simple analgesics

---

PATHOPHYSIOLOGY OF MIGRAINE

Migraine Brain

The concept that the brain of a migraineur is physiologically unique is supported by recent scientific study (24,25). In brief, the brain of the migraineur is genetically more excitable, more vigilant than the brain of an individual without migraine. In addition, the brain of a migraineur does not extinguish sensory stimuli as rapidly or as completely as the brain of those without migraine (26,27). The consequence of these two facts is that the migraineurs' brain is susceptible to "sensory overload." While sensory overload can likely occur in all humans (as all parents witness), it is far more likely to occur in people predisposed to migraine. In other words, the threshold for migraine is lower for those with a genetic predisposition to migraine than for those without this family trait.

Acute Attack

Migraine is a process more than an event. During a typical attack of migraine, there may be as many as five different phases—premonitory symptoms or prodrome, aura, headache, resolution, and postdrome. While not every attack or every patient may experience all phases of migraine, it is fair to say that for most attacks there is predictability to the pattern of an acute attack of migraine. A variety of different clinical presentations or clinical phenotypes of migraine may be observed in the migraine patient and these often become a source of diagnostic confusion. The key to understanding the diagnosis of migraine is to understand that the physiological process can resolve at any point in its evolution. Thus recognition of the phases of migraine is critical to understanding and interpreting to the patient the enigma of migraine.

Premonitory Symptoms or Prodrome

Up to 80% of migraineurs note the presence of a *prodrome* beginning 24 hours in advance of their headache (22). Premonitory symptoms include fatigue, yawning, change in appetite, increased energy, frequent urination, difficulty with memory, cold hands, irritability, and loss of concentration. If appropriately recognized, these symptoms are a physiological warning that the process of migraine has started. If migraine progresses, the headache and associated symptoms of migraine will follow. Patients who can recognize their prodromes understand that the migraine process has begun and can treat soon after the onset of headache and abort or minimize the subsequent headache (29).

Aura

Approximately 25% of migraineurs experience an *aura* prior to the headache (23). Auras typically last 5 to 60 minutes and usually terminate before the onset of headache. Auras represent focal neurological symptoms that develop as a result of a spreading wave of cortical depression moving from the occipital area of the brain forward at the rate of 2–3 mm/sec. The most common auras are visual such as scotomata (absent spots in the visual field) and teichopsia (zig-zag lines). Sensory auras also occur and can be worrisome to the patient. Dysarthria (difficulty with speech) may also occur as an aura. Auras that warrant a diagnostic workup include those that are prolonged (more than 60 minutes); associated with paralysis or syncope; and occur for the first time in a patient over 50 years of age or

TABLE 5 Migraine with Worrisome Aura: Symptoms Indicating Need for Complete Neurological Evaluation

1. Motor symptoms: hemiplegic aura
2. Brain symptoms: severe dysarthria, vertigo, syncope, bilateral sensory definition
3. Prolonged aura, greater than 60 minutes
4. Atypical aura:
    a. Alice in Wonderland: hallucinatory, changes in perception of space and time
    b. Migrilepsy: seizure associated with migraine

after initiation of oral contraceptives. Patients may experience an aura without headache (Table 5) (30).

Headache
The headache phase of migraine generally lasts 4 to 72 hours in adults. During the early headache phase, pain may be mild, diffuse, and nondescript. As migraine progresses, the intensity of the headache typically progresses to moderate-to-severe levels. Associated symptoms (nausea, vomiting, and light and sound sensitivity) also generally begin subtly but with the progression of migraine increase in severity adding to the disability of the attack. Ideally, acute therapy should be initiated when the headache is mild rather than waiting until the headache is moderate to severe (26,31).

As the headache phase reaches its full potential and pain becomes severe, patients may develop allodynia, defined as a painful response to a nonpainful stimulus. Lightly rubbing one's head or combing one's hair can be registered by the brain as painful. The chest, extremities, and back muscles may become tender. Allodynia may develop relatively soon after the onset of headache. The presence of cutaneous allodynia is suggestive of *central sensitization*—a physiological state where central neurons transmit a noxious sensory signal independent of sensory signals from the periphery (27). In this scenario, migraine can become an allodynic pain state, meaning a normally nonpainful sensory input such as touch becomes painful. At this point, migraine is at its zenith fulfilling all symptoms for an IHS diagnosis and the patient experiences profound disability. The goal of acute therapy should be to prevent this stage of migraine as triptans are considerably less effective when administered after the central nervous system is sensitized. Acute management of migraine at this phase may require the use of rescue medications and result in headache recurrence.

Postdrome
After the headache pain has resolved, many patients experience a postdrome. Although headache free, patients may experience hangover-type symptoms, such as cognitive difficulty, dizziness, fatigue, and a concern that the headache may recur. Patients feel that they must be very careful not to aggravate their system and bring back the attack. Postdrome may last 24 to 48 hours (32).

Several key messages can be understood in recognizing the process of migraine. First, although the headache of migraine typically lasts 4 to 72 hours, an attack of migraine can last 4 to 5 days. Secondly, diagnostic variability is often dependent on where in the process is the migraine terminated or resolved. Thus, migraine terminating after the mild headache may clinically appear as a tension-type headache or migraine resolving after the aura may appear as aura without headache. Finally, successful treatment is ultimately about restoring normal neurological function as quickly and completely as possible after the attack has begun.

MEDICATION FOR THE MIGRAINE PATIENT

Before prescribing medication, the pattern of a patient's migraine should be assessed. This can be understood as an assessment of where on the continuum from infrequent, episodic migraine to chronic migraine this patient's pattern of headache is currently positioned. This staging process can be used to effectively plan appropriate education and pharmacological intervention. A staging assessment is provided in Table 6.

Treatment is directed both by the attack and the pattern. A patient with only one migraine a month which forces him or her to stay home from work or alter his or her daily routine requires an aggressive acute intervention. By comparison, a pattern of more frequent, moderately severe migraine attacks needs acute as well as preventive interventions.

Another important assessment is the treatability of a patient's migraine which highlights the patient's strategy of using acute treatment medications. For example, a patient may have frequent, low-impact migraines that are controlled with over-the-counter (OTC) medications. In the exam room, though, the person describes only the few migraines that escape self-treatment efforts. On the surface, it appears that the problem is infrequent migraine but in reality there may be overuse of acute medications.

TABLE 6   Staging Questions

1. How many days per month do you have headaches?
   Stage 1: 2 or less
   Stage 2: 3 to 7
   Stage 3: 8 to 14
   Stage 4: 15 or more
2. Does the medicine you take for headaches stop them?
   Stage 1: Yes, most of the time
   Stage 2: Rely on medicine to get through the day
   Stage 3: Takes the edge off but the headache is still there
   Stage 4: Nothing works
3. Do you have physical problems other than headaches?
   Stage 1: No, I'm healthy
   Stage 2: At times, I feel down, jittery, irritable, anxious with upset stomach
   Stage 3: Some aches and pains; bloating; and I feel depressed
   Stage 4: Yes, depression, fibromyalgia, insomnia, IBS, weight problem; I'm falling apart
4. How do your headaches interfere with your life?
   Stage 1: They're a nuisance that slows me down
   Stage 2: I struggle through them and force myself to go on
   Stage 3: I'm missing work, family and social functions a lot
   Stage 4: My life revolves around headaches
5. How many days per month do you feel normal?
   Stage 1: 25, most of the time
   Stage 2: 15, half the time
   Stage 3: 510
   Stage 4: Zero

ASSESSING THE PATTERN OF MIGRAINE: PATIENT STAGING

The pattern of migraine changes over the lifetime of a migraineur. Typically migraine begins as a self-limited episodic disorder where migraine occurs as a well-defined attack that resolves, and between migraines the patient functions normally. Over time the pattern of migraine may increase and as the pattern becomes more frequent, a patient's function between attacks is disrupted. Commonly observed disruptions are sleep disturbances, other physical pain, or psychological symptomatology. These symptoms often reach a point and intensity to be recognized as a concomitant disease, such as anxiety, fibromyalgia, or depression. In the extreme, migraine may become chronic, meaning that headaches occur on more days than not and frequently with other comorbid diseases. In the process, migraine is frequently complicated by medication misuse or overuse. This process of chronification was first described by Mathew as migraine transformation. Interestingly, chronic migraine can occasionally resolve spontaneously. Consequently, it is essential that health care professionals determine where in the transformational process their patient is and reassess this at each subsequent office evaluation. The pattern of migraine determines educational needs of the patient, acute treatment pharmacological strategies, and most of all, the need for preventive treatment strategies and consultation.

STAGE 1

In stage 1, the patient has infrequent, discreet episodes of migraine (generally one attack or less per month or fewer than two headache days per month) and normal function between episodes of migraine. Because attacks are often adequately treated with OTC medications and sleep, individuals in this stage of migraine do not seek medical care. The key therapeutic steps are to optimize acute treatment and allow the person to identify and treat migraine early in its evolution so as to minimize functional impairment. Optimizing acute treatment is the core issue with the goal being that the patient is migraine free and fully functional within two hours. Early intervention, treating when the headache is mild, is the therapeutic paradigm that should be reviewed with the patient. If the strategy is effective, follow-up can occur relatively infrequently with the attention directed to potential changes in the pattern or frequency of migraine. If individual attacks are severe, triptans should be considered and formulation issues may need to be addressed. If attacks are slower to develop or not producing significant impact, then NSAIDs or OTCs, such as a combination of acetaminophen, aspirin, and caffeine, may be considered for first-line intervention. However, whatever pharmacological intervention is considered, the outcome standard should be to terminate migraine in a timely manner that allows the person to feel confident that migraine is unlikely to return.

STAGE 2

Acute therapy remains the focus but the attacks of migraine are more frequent (generally one to three per month or less than five headache days per month). However, attacks remain discreet and self-limited. In this stage of migraine, attacks begin to be more pervasive and have a measurable impact on the individual's life. There may be occasional absenteeism from work, family, or social function but more often, there is presenteeism. Frequently, stage 2 patients exhibit some degree of anxiety or apprehension about future attacks of migraine.

In this stage, the focus remains on optimizing acute therapy but structured education about lifestyle factors that increase risk of migraine and protective factors to prevent migraine should also be discussed. Providing a calendar is a good starting point for assisting the patient to understand the migraine threshold and his or her unique susceptibility to migraine. Of special importance is recording the frequency of headaches, response to treatment, and the level of functioning between migraine episodes. Patients are encouraged to rate their health between attacks, in other words, whether the nervous system returns to baseline after an attack and functions normally.

Acute therapies need to be monitored and limits on their use defined clearly to the patient. An excepted standard is to limit acute intervention to two or less days per week. The risk for the development of medication overuse is low in this population but it is better to establish these limits early rather than late. Goals for acute treatment should be clearly defined. The use of migraine-specific acute medications such as triptans generally provides the best outcome for patients. If needed, the addition of NSAIDs such as naproxen to a triptan can improve efficacy, particularly sustained efficacy, and as such decreases the overall use of acute treatment. Also providing the patient with a rescue therapy should be considered if needed by the patient. This could be injectable sumatriptan or an analgesic. Prescribed limits of two times a month or less for the use of rescue medication should also be provided.

The use of preventive pharmacology might be considered if response to acute treatment is not optimal or the patient is under significant distress and likely to be in an early progressive transformational pattern. Continuity of care becomes critical for this patient population, and office visits should be frequent until the migraines are under adequate control.

STAGE 3

In stage 3, the patient has frequent attacks of migraine (generally 4–8 per month with less than 12 headache days per month). In this stage, the therapeutic emphasis shifts from acute to preventive pharmacological intervention. The foundation of preventive intervention relies on education and the involvement of patients in their care. These are critical to encourage adherence to treatment regimens. Behavioral interventions are also a key component to the care of this patient population. The first step is to assess patients' use of acute medication and decide if they are overusing acute medications. If acute medication is being overused, then it should be discontinued or strict limits be given for its continued use.

Concomitant with medication withdrawal, preventive medication should be initiated. If a patient is using a preventive medication, the dose should be increased or the medication switched to another therapeutic class. At times, the addition of a second preventive medication is necessary. The choice of preventive medication is frequently based on the profile of comorbidities that are present or that have occurred in the past. For example, patients with mild symptoms suggestive of depression may benefit from a tricyclic antidepressant; patients with a tendency for panic disorder may benefit from a beta blocker or an anticonvulsant. However, it is important to recognize that the dosage of these medications used to prevent migraine may not be sufficient for the treatment of the comorbid condition. If comorbidity exists and requires treatment, it is often best to consider treatment of these two conditions independently.

Follow-up visits need to be scheduled frequently until the patient's pattern comes under control and the patient has mastered his or her treatment strategies. Goals of prevention need to be clarified with the patient and limits for the use of acute medications need to be established. If the patient's migraine pattern does not come under control promptly, consider consultation.

STAGE 4

Stage 4 patients have frequent episodes of migraine with more than eight attacks per month and more than 15 days per month of headache. Migraine in stage 4 is a chronic disease often necessitating referral or consultation with a headache specialist or interdisciplinary pain center. The pharmacological emphasis in this population is clearly preventive pharmacology and concentrated behavioral therapies. The evaluation of medication overuse needs to be undertaken and if medication overuse is suspected then medication needs to be withdrawn and preventive medication optimized. Quantities of medication recommended by the IHS as suggesting MOH are listed in Table 4. Often bridging therapies can be provided to attenuate rebound headache from medication withdrawal. Common bridge therapies are naratriptan 2.5 mg (1/2 tablet) bid for five days; naproxen sodium 440 mg bid for five days; or decadron 12 mg on day 1; 8 mg on day 2; and 4 mg on day 3. With narcotic withdrawal, the use of a clonidine patch may be helpful and if a patient is being withdrawn from butalbital, a tapering schedule of phenobarbital can be provided to reduce the risk of seizures (28). In addition, the use of local therapies such as occipital nerve blocks can be utilized as rescue therapy.

The use of acute therapy needs to be judicious and in many instances, acute medications will need to be withdrawn while preventive therapy is being initiated. AEDs, especially topiramate, are frequently used first-line preventives. At times, co-pharmacy with other migraine preventives can be employed. Utilization of a psychologist to assist with pain management skills can be of significant benefit. Patients failing to improve should be considered for referral to a headache specialist or a multidisciplinary treatment program.

BEHAVIORAL INTERVENTIONS

Behavioral therapy should be part of managing migraineurs. As subtle as words of encouragement or as structured as biofeedback training sessions, behavioral therapy and education enhances the efficacy of pharmacological treatment. The first step in establishing a partnership with the patient is to validate his or her incapacitating headaches as a real neurological disorder. The patient also needs to understand the concept of the migraine threshold, which is the point between physiological balance and the initiation of migraine. This threshold is significantly influenced by genetic factors; a migraineur's nervous system is more sensitive to changes in the internal and external environment. This tends to lower the migraine threshold, making the person more headache prone.

Behavioral therapy occurs in every interaction a patient has with the health care system. Sometimes these interactions are positive and other times they are not. Headache patients are often seen by the medical profession as difficult and noncompliant, yet to be fair they have often been misdiagnosed and mistreated. The method a health care professional uses to educate and teach headache patients about their disease may in the end be the most important intervention they make. Generally, this is thought of by the health care profession as evoking the placebo response. However, as a challenge to this thinking, a recent blinded placebo-controlled study that tested face-to-face education *versus* written patient instruction showed an 11% increase in medication efficacy without altering placebo response. In other words, the efficacy of the drug increased but not the "magic" of placebo. This strongly suggests that physicians, the keepers of prescription privileges, can be more effective if they properly involve and educate their patients.

Developing a Collaborative Management Style with Migraine Patients

Pain is a very personal experience. As such, it is the patient who is the expert of his or her own painful experience. The health care professional is an expert on the medical understanding of the patient's condition but not on the individual suffering with pain. These two viewpoints need to be merged together in a collaborative effort to solve the riddle of pain.

The foundation for building this relationship is respect for patients. This does not suggest giving in to their demands but instead an understanding that they are attempting to communicate their needs. Inherent in this is validation of their concerns and an earnest effort to explain and normalize their reaction or response to pain. Thus, the first and most critical step in managing a headache patient is education.

Self-management benefits anyone suffering from debilitating headaches, especially children and women who are or plan on becoming pregnant or are nursing. These tools are vital for those who take acute treatment medication more than two days a week or who have medical contraindications for or inability to tolerate migraine-specific medications. Individuals with a history of excessive use of analgesics or acute medications also need to rely on nonpharmacological methods to gain control of headaches. Self-management is learned through a variety of ways, including educational pearls provided by physicians and nurses, books, articles, websites, support groups, or referral to a psychologist for biofeedback and relaxation training.

KEY POINTS TO SELF-MANAGED HEADACHES

1. Education about migraine and what it means to be a migraineur
2. Diary to record risk factors that precipitate disabling headaches and to document the frequency of headaches and the efficacy of medication
3. Biofeedback
4. Coping skills

The prodrome, as the first stage of the migraine process, is the most effective time to use self-management, preventive measures, such as biofeedback, relaxation, exercise, removing oneself from the stressor, deep breathing, yoga, or taking an OTC remedy that has worked before. These diversionary tactics often make the difference between stopping the process in the beginning and allowing it to proceed to a full-fledge, disabling, raging, neuroinflammatory state. This knowledge gives the patient power and control. Certainly, there are migraines that begin at a moderate-to-severe painful state. Then, an injection is required.

But there are some that can be doused before the flame develops into a four-alarm fire.

RISK FACTORS
A migraine may erupt under a certain set of factors. These are often individualistic that can be identified by keeping a diary. Common risk factors include stressful situations, such as deadlines, taking on too many projects or responsibilities; not getting enough sleep; drinking alcohol; eating food with MSG, nitrates, or nitrites; a weather front; or hormonal changes. A combination of factors is usually necessary to release the shutdown response that a migraine imposes on the body.

PROTECTIVE FACTORS
Activities that are self-nurturing appear to protect the nervous system from the disruption initiated by risk factors. These include physical exercise; enjoying a 30-minute video of a comedy; receiving a massage; affection or sexual activity; and biofeedback/relaxation. By engaging in these activities, an individual creates a protective environment that balances the nervous system and lessens the frequency of migraine.

In addition, this sensitive nervous system requires stability and routine. From a common sense viewpoint, a migraineur needs to eat breakfast everyday and have established mealtimes. Bedtime too needs to be consistent, waking up at the same time each morning, even on weekends or during vacation.

BIOFEEDBACK
Biofeedback is the process of bringing involuntary physiological functions under voluntary control. Finger temperature, for instance, is a reflection of the body's level of vigilance. The average finger temperature is 85°F. As the stress response builds in the body, the finger temperature decreases. Where the finger temperature is chronically low (below 80°F), the body is in the survival mode, usually signifying that the individual has lost the ability to relax and recreate. Biofeedback trains the nervous system to shutout stimulation and directs vigilance inward to the needs communicated by one's internal physiological demands. Instead of attempting to live up to others' expectations, the migraineur learns to recognize and meet his or her own needs before caring for others. Through biofeedback, the individual steps back from daily concerns, and focuses on returning the body to homeostasis, through calming, relaxing music, and/or visualization. As this occurs, the finger temperature rises.

COPING SKILLS
Due to the sensitivity of the migraineur's nervous system, there is alertness to the feelings of others. Often, migraine sufferers feel responsible for another's distress or apathy. Essentially, there may be a lack of boundaries; love may be defined as enmeshment with significant others, identifying with another's wants and desires. Once they understand their sensitivity, they realize that they have a choice and they can decide to shut out others' demands without feeling guilty. The coping skills that headache sufferers generally find most useful include cognitive restructuring, assertiveness training, and identifying goals.

Cognitive Restructuring

Pain is a barrier to a positive outlook. The migraineur often limits activities for fear of precipitating another attack. "What's wrong with me?" often is an example of how a person in pain condemns himself or herself. Yet at the same time, these personal insults to oneself are automatic and do not register as a deprecating remark. Once a person realizes that he or she is setting himself or herself up for failure by such thinking, the negative can be replaced by affirmations. Examples of affirmations are, "I forgive myself for being imperfect;" "I deserve health and harmony." Through this process, the individual begins to recognize the power that thinking has over healing and health.

Assertiveness Training

Assertiveness training involves a step-by-step process: (*i*) identify when a behavior is being asked that you do not want to do, which is usually signaled by feelings of guilt, anxiety, ignorance, or dread; (*ii*) practice saying "no" in unimportant situations, such as in a supermarket; (*iii*) say "no" to those who will be understanding, such as a friend; (*iv*) finally, say "no" to the person who demands that you do something you do not want to do.

Identifying Goals

Once assertive behavior is learned, the person needs to establish his or her own goals rather than rely on others to dictate behavior. Goals need to be written down and divided into a time frame, such as within one week, one month, six months, one year, and five years.

CONCLUSION

Migraine is a common and frequently perplexing medical problem. It is however one of the most treatable chronic neurological diseases. To effectively treat migraine, a health care provider needs to establish an understanding of the event of migraine and the natural history of the disease over time. Through an effective partnership with the patient, therapy can be modified and shaped to the pattern of the disease and needs of the patient. The formula for success involves education, motivation, and a thoughtful use of acute and preventive pharmacological efforts. Through these efforts, migraine patients can become rewarding and successful.

REFERENCES

1. Lipton RB, Bigal ME, Diamond M, et al. Migraine prevalence, disease burden, and the need for preventive therapy. Neurology 2007; 68:343–349.
2. Takeshima T, Ishizaki K, Fukuhara Y, et al. Population-based door-to-door Survey of migraine in Japan: the Daisen Study. Headache 2004; 44:8–19.
3. Morillo LE, Alarcon F, Aranaga N, et al. Prevalence of migraine in Latin America. Headache 2005; 45:106–117.
4. Lipton RB, Stewart WF, Diamond S, et al. Prevalence and burden of migraine in the United States: data from the American Migraine Study II. Headache 2001; 41(7): 646–657.
5. Cady RK, Maizels M, Reeves DL, et al. Predictors of adherence to triptans: factors of sustained vs lapsed users. Headache 2009, in press.

6. Marcus DA, Loder E. Migraine in female children and adolescents. In: Loder E, Marcus DA, eds. Migraine in Women. Hamilton, Ontario: BC Decker, 2004:95–101.
7. Cady RK, Schreiber CP, Farmer KU. Understanding the patient with migraine: the evolution from episodic headache to chronic neurological disease. Headache 2004; 44:426–435.
8. Lipton RB, Bigal ME, Diamond M, et al. Migraine prevalence, disease burden, and the need for preventive therapy. Neurology 2007; 68:343–349.
9. World Health Organization. Estimated total DALYs ('000), by cause and WHO Member State, 2002. Available at http://www.who.int/healthinfo/statistics/bodgbddeathdalyestimates.xls.
10. Mathew NT. Migraine transformation and chronic daily headache. In: Cady RK, Fox AW, eds. Treating the Headache Patient. New York: Marcel Dekkker, 1995:75–100.
11. Bigal ME, Lipton RB. Concepts and mechanisms of migraine chronification. Headache 2008; 48(1):7–15.
12. Stewart WF, Lipton RB, Celentano DD, et al. Prevalence of migraine headache in the United States. JAMA 1992; 267:64–69.
13. Hahn SR, Lipton RB, Sheftell FD, et al. Healthcare provider-patient communication and migraine assessment: results of the American Migraine Communication Study, phase II. Curr Med Res Opin 2008; 24(6):1711–1718.
14. Headache Classification Committee of the International Headache Society. Classification and diagnostic criteria for headache disorders, cranial neuralgias and facial pain. Cephalalgia 1988; 8(Suppl 7):1–96.
15. Headache Classification Committee of the International Headache Society. The International Classification of Headache Disorders. Cephalalgia 2004;24:1–160.
16. Cady RK, Lipton RB, Hall C, et al. Treatment of mild headache in disabled headache sufferers: results of the spectrum study. Headache 2000; 40:792–797.
17. Brandes JL, Kudrow D, Cady R, et al. Eletriptan in the early treatment of acute migraine: influence of pain intensity and time of dosing. Cephalalgia 2005; 25:735–742.
18. Cady R, Martin V, Mauskop A, et al. Symptoms of cutaneous sensitivity pre-treatment and post-treatment: results from the rizatriptan TAME studies. Cephalalgia 2007; 27Z:1055–1060.
19. Bigal ME, Rapoport AM, Lipton RB, et al. Chronic daily headache in a tertiary care population. Correlation between the International Headache Society diagnostic criteria and proposed revisions of criteria for chronic daily headache. Cephalalgia 2002; 22:432–438.
20. Olesen J, Bousser MG, Diener HC, et al. (Headache Classification Committee). New appendix criteria open for a broader concept of chronic migraine. Cephalalgia 2006; 26:742–746.
21. Lipton RB, Diamond S, Reed M, et al. Migraine diagnosis and treatment: results from the American Migraine Study II. Headache 2001; 41:638–645.
22. Cady RK. Diagnosis and treatment of migraine. Clin Cornerstone 1999; 1:21–32.
23. Tepper SJ, Dahlof CG, Dowson A, et al. Prevalence and diagnosis of migraine in patients consulting their physician with a complaint of headache: data from the Landmark Study. Headache 2004; 44(9):856–864.
24. Schoenen J. Neurophysiological features of the migrainous brain. Neurol Sci 2006; 27(Suppl 2):S77–S81.
25. Coppola G, Pierelli F, Schoenen J. Is the cerebral cortex hyperexcitable or hyperresponsive in migraine? Cephalalgia 2007; 27(12):1427–1439.
26. Schoenen J. Deficient habituation of evoked cortical potentials in migraine: a link between brain biology, behavior and trigeminovascular activation? Biomed Pharmacother 1996; 50:71–78.
27. Aurora SK, Patricia M. Barrodale PM, et al. Brainstem dysfunction in chronic migraine as evidenced by neurophysiological and positron emission tomography studies. Headache 2007; 47:996–1003.
28. Bedell AW, Cady RK, Diamond ML, et al. Patient-centered strategies for effective management of migraine. Primary Care Network, 2000.

29. Luciani R, Carter D, Mannix L, et al. Prevention of migraine during prodrome with naratriptan. Cephalalgia 2000; 20(2):122–126.
30. Olesen J. The MacDonald Critchley Lecture. The migraine aura: clinical features and genetics. Cephalalgia 2002; 22(7):568–569.
31. Lipton RB, Cady RK, Stewart WF, et al. Diagnostic lessons from the Spectrum Study. Neurology 2002; 58(Suppl 6):S27–S31.
32. Burstein R, Cutrer MF, Yarnitsky D. The development of cutaneous allodynia during a migraine attack. Clinical evidence for the sequential recruitment of spinal and supraspinal nociceptive neurons in migraine. Brain 2000; 123(Pt 8):1703–1709.

2

Tension-Type Headache

Paul Mathew

Department of Neurology, Mayo Clinic, Rochester, Minnesota, U.S.A.

B. Lee Peterlin

Departments of Neurology and Pharmacology & Physiology, Drexel University College of Medicine, Philadelphia, Pennsylvania, U.S.A.

THE DISORDER

Epidemiology

Tension-type headache (TTH) is often referred to as the "patient's normal headache" by both patients and physicians, and has a life-time prevalence of 88% in women and 69% in men (1). Although it is the most prevalent type of primary headache in the general population, it is also one of the most frequently missed headache disorders (1–4). This is likely because TTH is generally less painful and debilitating than other primary and secondary headache disorders, and thus sufferers are less likely to present to a physician. It has been demonstrated that while 56% of migraine sufferers present to a physician, only 16% of TTH sufferers seek medical advice (5). Among the patients who do present to a physician with TTH, up to 50% have been estimated to be missed on clinical interview (6).

The onset of TTH is usually between 20 to 30 years of age, with a one-year prevalence estimated at approximately 38% of the general population in the United States and globally (4,5,7). The life-time prevalence of TTH has been estimated to be about 79% to 87%, with 69% of all men and 88% of all women in a Danish study (1,2). It is slightly more prevalent in women, with a male to female ratio of 4:5. TTH has been shown to be more common in Caucasians than African Americans (4,8–10). In the United States, lower education has been reported as an increased risk factor for CTTH, while higher education level has been reported to be a risk factor for ETTH (4).

Disability

In general, TTHs are less debilitating than migraine headaches. However, TTH can cause substantial disability (5,11). In terms of productivity, 43.6% of TTH patients were less productive with daily activities at home, work, and/or school with a mean of 20.4 days being affected (4,12). In regards to missing or less productive work days, the cost to society from TTH has been estimated to be roughly four times greater than epilepsy and two times greater than migraine (13).

DIAGNOSIS

According to the International Classification of Headache Disorders (ICHD-2), in order for a headache to be classified as TTH it must have *at least two* of the following four features (Table 1).

(1) *The pain is pressing/tightening.*

In a study analyzing 488 TTH sufferers, 78% of the patients reported a "pressing" feature as part of their chief complaint and 80% to 86% reported seldom or never having headaches of a throbbing nature, which is often reported with migraine (1,2,12). Patients often describe the pain as a dull, nonpulsatile, compression feeling, as if a weight was hanging over their head and shoulders.

(2) *The pain is mild/moderate in intensity and is usually inhibitive rather than prohibitive of activity.*

Low intensity pain has been reported in 87% to 99% of episodic TTH sufferers (12).

(3) *The headache occurs in a bilateral distribution.*

In a Scandinavian study, 90% of chronic TTH sufferers reported having bilateral pain (14). This distribution is often described by patients as a "band around the head" or "cap."

(4) *The headache has no aggravation with physical activity.*

In patients with episodic TTH, one study demonstrated that 72% to 83% of the patients reported no aggravation with physical activity (9,15). Similarly, in a prospective diary study, 84% showed no aggravation with physical activity (14).

TABLE 1 Classification of Tension-Type Headache According to the ICHD-2

Diagnostic criteria:
  A. At least 10 episodes fulfilling criteria B–E. Number of days with such headache <1 day per month (episodic infrequent), from 1 to 14 (episodic frequent) or ≥15 (chronic).
  B. Headache lasting from 30 minutes to 7 days.
  C. At least two of the following pain characteristics:
      1. Pressing/tightening (nonpulsating) quality
      2. Mild or moderate intensity (may inhibit, but does not prohibit activities)
      3. Bilateral location
      4. No aggravation by walking stairs or similar routine physical activity
  D. Both of the following:
      a. No nausea or vomiting (anorexia may occur)
      b. Photophobia and phonophobia are absent, or one but not the other may be present
  E. Not attributed to another disorder
  2.X.1 Associated with pericranial tenderness

Diagnostic criteria:
  A. Fulfills criteria for 2.X
  B. Increased tenderness on pericranial manual palpation.
  2.X.2 Not associated with pericranial tenderness

Diagnostic criteria:
  A. Fulfills criteria for 2.X
  Not associated with increased pericranial tenderness.

ICHD-2 = International Classification of Headache Disorders, 2nd edition.
X means the correspondent digit of infrequent episodic (1), frequent episodic (2), or chronic (3).

Once diagnosed, TTH can be further classified based on the frequency and presence or absence of pericranial tenderness. Episodic infrequent TTH consists of fewer than 1 headache per month with at least 10 total episodes, while episodic frequent TTH consists of 1 to 14 headaches per month. Chronic TTH consists of 15 or more headaches per month. The majority of patients with TTH evolve from episodic to chronic over years (16,17), and TTH chronicity directly correlates to the intensity of the headaches.

In addition to frequency, TTH can be subdivided based upon the presence or absence of pericranial tenderness on manual palpation (18,19). The presence of pericranial tenderness correlates to greater intensity and frequency of headaches. Pericranial tenderness, when present, has also been shown to worsen during headache episodes. Unfortunately, the evaluation of pericranial tenderness utilizing electromyography or pressure algometry has shown little utility as a diagnostic/prognostic tool, largely due to intersubject variability (19).

In general, TTHs tend to last anywhere from 30 minutes to 7 days, and they are not associated with nausea. TTH can involve either photophobia or phonophobia, but it cannot have both features. Mild photophobia has been reported in 10% of ETTH sufferers, and mild phonophobia has been noted in 7% of TTH sufferers (20,21).

No specific cause/effect parameters have been established; however, stress seems to be the most frequent precipitating factor (22,23). Depression, anxiety, migraine, poor sleep, and medication overuse have been shown to be predictors of poor outcomes (16).

Past Medical History

As with any headache disorder, an extensive history should be taken. Information which should be obtained from the patient includes the quality, distribution, frequency, duration, and severity of the pain. The presence or absence of associated symptoms including photophobia, phonophobia, nausea, vomiting, aura, autonomic features, weakness, numbness, and allodynia should also be part of the review of systems. As with any headache disorder, age of onset, past medical history, surgical history, psychiatric history, stressors, medication use, history of trauma, and sleep hygiene are also important factors to consider in the evaluation and treatment of TTH.

Physical Examination

The physical exam should include a general examination, neurological examination with an ophthalmoscopic exam, and palpation of cranial and vertebral structures. When performing manual pericranial muscular palpation, the examiner should be able to appreciate the difference between tender points and trigger points. Tender points are pericranial points that illicit local pain on deep palpation, while trigger points illicit both local and referred pain to other areas (24). Some common trigger/tender points include the temporalis, lateral pterygoid, masseter, sternocleidomastoid, trapezius, and insertion points such as the mastoid (25). Cervical, thoracic, and lumbar paravertebral tenderness frequently correlate with pericranial muscle tenderness (26). In addition to muscular palpation, cervical spine examination should also be performed paying special attention to any restricted or painful movements, as contraction of shoulder and cervical musculature are commonly seen in TTH (27,28). The chronic contraction of these muscles leads to posturing with elevation of the shoulders and flexion of the neck (29).

Additional Studies

Imaging studies of the brain, cervical spine, and soft tissue structures should be ordered based on clinical suspicion from history and physical examination. Cervical spine lesions are as common in TTH as in other headache disorders (27). Additional studies such as lumbar puncture for cerebrospinal fluid analysis and measurement of the opening pressure should be considered if idiopathic intracranial hypertension is in the differential diagnosis.

Differential Diagnosis

ETTH Pretenders

The diagnosis of TTH is one of the exclusions, and there are no truly mandatory criteria. As such, TTH has a highly variable presentation with a mix of many symptoms that often lead clinicians to an incorrect diagnosis; for example, a bilateral throbbing headache that is not worse with exercise involves no nausea/ vomiting/photophonophobia, although having some migrainous elements may fit the criteria for TTH. Four major headaches that are often confused for ETTH include migraine without aura, probable migraine, sinus headache, and cervicogenic headache.

Migraine without Aura and Probable Migraine

Patients with migraine without aura often have more than one coexisting type of primary headache. In general, a headache without aura that is episodic and disabling in the presence of a normal physical and neurological examination is migraine until proven otherwise (30). Although severe TTH can involve mild photophobia or phonophobia, it never has both. The presence of both photo- and phonophobia is much more consistent with migraine. In addition, if the headache is disabling to the point that the patient seeks medical care, migraine should be the foremost consideration. The ID-migraine validation study analyzed patients who presented in a primary care setting with headaches that interfered with their lives or headaches that they wished to discuss with a physician. Among these cases, 80% of the patients were shown to have migraine when assessed by a HA specialist (30). As with migraine, probable migraine can be difficult to differentiate from TTH. Probable migraine is a subtype of migraine missing one mandatory feature for the diagnosis of migraine (31) (Tables 2 and 3). According to the Spectrum Study, 32% of patients initially diagnosed with ETTH were found to have migraine/probable migraine on diary review (32).

Although distinguishing migraine or probable migraine from ETTH is generally straightforward, there are cases where it is not clear cut. It is relatively evident that a primary headache disorder which fulfills three out of four ICHD-II criteria for migraine would be most appropriately diagnosed as probable migraine, and a headache which fulfills one or no migraine criteria would be most appropriately diagnosed as ETTH. However, when a primary headache disorder fulfills two migraine criteria, the diagnosis could be either probable migraine or ETTH. In these cases, when in doubt, ETTH is the diagnosis by default as is illustrated in Table 4.

TABLE 2 Classification of Migraine without Aura According to the ICHD-2

Diagnostic criteria:
A. At least five attacks fulfilling criteria B–D
B. Headache attacks lasting 4–72 hours (untreated or unsuccessfully treated)
C. Headache has at least two of the following characteristics:
   1. Unilateral location
   2. Pulsating quality
   3. Moderate or severe pain intensity
   4. Aggravation by or causing avoidance of routine physical activity (e.g., walking or climbing stairs)
D. During headache at least one of the following:
   1. Nausea and/or vomiting
   2. Photophobia and phonophobia
E. Not attributed to another disorder

TABLE 3 Classification of Probable Migraine without Aura According to the ICHD-2

Diagnostic criteria:
A. Attacks fulfilling all but one of criteria A–D for 1.1 Migraine without aura
B. Not attributed to another disorder

Sinus Headache

Sinus headaches occur with acute sinusitis and are regarded as relatively rare headaches that are associated with sinus pain, pressure, fever, and stuffiness (33–38). The pain is usually dull, bilateral, and often bifrontal, which is a presentation similar to TTH. However, in contrast to TTH, the ICHD criteria for sinus headaches includes (*i*) purulent nasal discharge; (*ii*) pathological sinus findings in tests including radiography, computed tomography, or magnetic resonance

TABLE 4 Differences between Chronic Tension-Type Headache and Other Chronic Daily Headaches (49)

	CTTH	TM	NDPH	HC
Severity	Usually mild or moderate	Usually mild or moderate. Exacerbations may be severe	Usually mild or moderate	Usually mild or moderate
Location	Usually bilateral	Bilateral or unilateral	Usually bilateral	Strictly unilateral
Onset	Gradual	Gradual	Abrupt	Abrupt
Relation with physical activity	Usually subjects report improvement	Usually subjects report aggravation	No	No
Muscular tenderness	Common	May happen	May happen	Not common
Associated symptoms	No	Common in the exacerbations	No	Not common
Medication overuse	No	May happen	No	No
Absolute response to indomethacin	No	No	No	Yes

imaging, and/or transillumination; (*iii*) simultaneous onset of the headache and sinusitis; and (*iv*) headache localized to specific facial and cranial areas near the sinuses (39). In addition, although the presence of autonomic symptoms in TTH is not well known, autonomic symptoms in migraine are well described and can include corneal injection, rhinorrhea, and congestion (38). In order to help distinguish sinus headache from TTH or migraine, all four of the IHS diagnostic criteria for sinus headache must be met (38).

Cervicogenic Headache

Cervicogenic headache (CGHA) is always unilateral and associated with a neck trigger point (40,41). As previously stated, the differentiation between trigger points from tender points is critical in order to distinguish CGHA from TTH (14,42). Tenderness is evident as a local pain in response to manual pressure, while a trigger point is when there is referred pain from one area to another. In the case of CGHA, the origin of the pain is from the neck and is referred to the head and face (43). The most common site of CGHA is the occipital nerve emergence. On the other hand, TTH involves bilateral pain with muscle tenderness during and between episodes in areas such as the scalp, temporal area, lateral pterygoid, masseter, sternocleidomastoid, and trapezius. Thus, the presence of neck tenderness can frequently mislead practitioners to a wrong diagnosis of CGHA. Nerve blockade is both therapeutic and diagnostic of CGHA. One study compared the pain reduction after greater occipital nerve block in cervicogenic headache, tension-type headache, and migraine without aura, which demonstrated that the patients with cervicogenic headaches had more marked reduction in pain than the other groups. An index of pain reduction was pain in the forehead, which was found to be reduced in 77% of the patients with cervicogenic headache (44). In another study that examined greater occipital nerve blocks in only chronic TTHs, the treatment was found to be minimally effective and was actually pronociceptive in some patients (45).

CTTH Primary HA Pretenders

By definition, primary chronic daily headache (CDH) is a headache disorder with headaches occurring 15 days or more of the month, lasting four or more hours per day, and with no secondary cause (46). Approximately 4% to 5% of the general population suffers with CDH (47,48). It can manifest as CTTH, transformed migraine, hemicrania continua, or new daily persistent headache.

Transformed Migraine

According to American Headache Society's new criteria, transformed migraine (TM) is a headache that occurs greater than or equal to 15 days/month, lasting greater than four hours per day, and of which 50% fulfill migraine or probable migraine criteria (49). TM tends, over months to years, to worsen in frequency and intensity. Many patients will have a combination of near daily migraine and superimposed CTTH (50). Patients can fit into one of three categories. (1) Patients with purely CTTH are treated as CTTH. (2) Patients who have greater than 50% of their CDHs manifest as migraine or probable migraine are considered to have TM. (3) Patients who have less than 50% of their CDH as migraine or probable migraine are considered to have CTTH with episodic migraine (49).

Hemicrania Continua

Hemicrania continua is a continuous headache that waxes and wanes and involves both autonomic and migrainous symptoms. Patients suffer with nausea, vomiting, photophobia, phonophobia, as well as rhinorrhea, tearing, conjunctival injection, eye discomfort, sweating, and swollen/drooping eyelids. Unlike the bilateral nature of CTTH, hemicrania continua is strictly unilateral (51–53). There may also be superimposed stabbing pain with hemicrania continua. In addition, hemicrania continua is almost always responsive to indomethacin (54).

CTTH Secondary HA Pretenders

Medication Overuse Headache (MOH)

By definition, MOHs are CDHs that occur after taking acute medications for greater than 15 days per month and preclude the diagnosis of CTTH (6). The attack frequency prognosis of the headaches depends on the cause/effect relationship of the headache and the medication overuse. If the CDH begin as a consequence of medication consumption, then there is a favorable prognosis with medication cessation. This is in contrast to acute medications that were started as a result of the CTTH, for which the prognosis is not as favorable after cessation of the medications (55).

Intracranial Tumors

Headache is a common symptom associated with intracranial tumors. Classic, intracranial, tumor-induced headaches involve nausea, vomiting, and focal abnormalities on neurologic examination. These headaches may also involve increased severity in the morning and/or after laying supine which improves or resolves in the upright position. However, headaches may occur in isolation and as the presenting symptom. In general, approximately 20% of patients with brain tumors have headache at presentation, but headache develops in the course of the disease in 60% of cases. In one study evaluating 111 patients with intracranial tumors, 48% had headaches, equally for primary and metastatic brain tumors (56). Based on history at presentation, prior to imaging studies, 77% were thought to have TTH, 9% to have migraine and 14% to have other types of headaches. Of those patients with intracranial tumor headaches, 45% of patients claimed that headache was their worst symptom, 32% stated that bending over worsened their headache, and 40% complained of nausea/vomiting (56). Thus, in patients with worsening frequency or intensity of their headaches, a change in the character of their headaches or focal findings on the neurologic examination, a diagnosis of intracranial tumors should be considered.

PATHOPHYSIOLOGY

The underlying pathophysiology of TTH is not well understood. This is likely due to its lack of mandatory criteria, which leads to a very heterogeneous population of headache sufferers. It is thought that TTH is the result of both peripheral and central mechanisms (57). The peripheral mechanisms of TTH involve increased pericranial muscle tone resulting in strain or spasm of the muscles, which can directly stimulate CNS nociceptors. This prolonged increased tone may cause hypoxia via compression of small blood vessels, which in turns leads to the retention of pain triggering metabolites, such as bradykinin, lactic acid, serotonin, and prostaglandins (58,59). These metabolites directly stimulate CNS nociception, and further potentiate the already increased pericranial muscle tonicity thereby indirectly stimulating further CNS nociception (59–61). The prolonged increased tone may also cause a depletion of local epinephrine and norepinephrine resulting in a relative "sympatheticopenia." This depletion in peripheral sympathetic neurotransmitters further perpetuates the cycle of muscle strain and nociceptor stimulation (62–64). These peripheral mechanisms can be triggered or augmented by physical stress, psychological stress, as well as non-ergonomic work positions. A common posture of TTH sufferers involves elevated shoulder(s) with an anteriorly flexed head. When held over time, this unconscious positioning, often referred to as muscular splinting, may induce further pain by perpetuating the cycle of strain (29). In addition, emotional factors may stimulate the limbic system, which, can cause further muscle tension and reduce the tone of the endogenous antinociceptive system. These peripheral mechanisms can potentiate and sensitize central nociceptive neurons by altering the descending control of second order trigeminal brainstem neurons. It is believed that the continuous nociceptive input received by the CNS is what eventually transforms ETTH into CTTH. The evolution of these centrally acting mechanisms leading to progression to CTTH have, thus far, not been linked to a specific genotype, but there has been an associated familial risk (65). It is also postulated that environmental factors may also play a role (66).

TREATMENT

Pharmacologic

Abortive
Aspirin and acetaminophen have been shown to be effective abortive therapies for ETTH in several trials. While both 500 mg and 1000 mg of aspirin have been shown to be efficacious for ETTH, only the 1000 mg dose of acetaminophen has been shown to be effective (67,68). This dosage of acetaminophen was noted to be effective, as was naproxen sodium at a dose of 350 mg when compared to placebo in a randomized, double-blind, multicenter controlled study (69). In addition, diclofenac, both at 12.5 and 25 mg, has been shown to be as effective as ibuprofen at a dose of 400 mg at relieving TTH (70) (Table 5).

Although triptans have not been shown to be consistently effective for pure ETTH (71), they may be useful for TTH in migraineurs (72,73). In one study, 43 headache patients were treated with sumatriptan 6 mg subcutaneously for 232 total headache episodes. Of the 232 headache episodes, 114 met IHS criteria for migraine, 76 met IHS criteria for TTH, and 42 fit into neither category. Among the three groups, 109 (96%) of the 114 migraines, 73 (96%) of the 76 TTH, and 40 (95%) out of 42 nonmigraine/TTH were triptan responsive (72). Thus, these results suggest there is some efficacy of triptans in abortive therapy of TTH in migraine sufferers. However, triptans are generally not a cost-effective treatment in the setting of headaches that respond well to aspirin or acetaminophen. Finally, all headache patients should be cautioned to not use any analgesic agent, whether prescription or over the counter, on more than two to three days of the week, or more than 10 to 15 days out of the month, to avoid potential medication over-use headache.

TABLE 5   Evidence-based Acute Abortive Therapy for Tension-Type Headache

Treatment	First or second line	Dose	Adverse events
Aspirin	First line	500–1000 mg PRN	Gastrointestinal dyspepsia, nausea and abdominal pain, and bleeding are possible side effects.
Acetaminophen	First line	1000 mg PRN	Nausea and rash are more common possible side effects. Hepatic and renal insufficiency or failure is serious potential adverse event, although rare. Fluid retention, blood clots, heart attacks, hypertension, and heart failure have also been associated with the use of any NSAIDs.
Diclofenac	Second line	12.5–25 mg PRN	Gastrointestinal ulcerations, abdominal pain, nausea, gastritis, and kidney and liver toxicity. Fluid retention, blood clots, heart attacks, hypertension, and heart failure have also been associated with the use of any NSAIDs.
Naproxen sodium	Second line	350 mg PRN	Gastrointestinal ulcerations, abdominal pain, nausea, gastritis, and kidney and liver toxicity. Fluid retention, blood clots, heart attacks, hypertension, and heart failure have also been associated with the use of any NSAIDs.
Ibuprofen	Second line	400 mg PRN	Gastrointestinal ulcerations, abdominal pain, nausea, gastritis, and kidney and liver toxicity. Fluid retention, blood clots, heart attacks, hypertension, and heart failure have also been associated with the use of any NSAIDs.

Prophylactic

In general, prophylactic therapy should be considered for all CTTH, frequent ETTH, and ETTH patients with significant disability from their headaches, and those who have not had a sufficient response to nonpharmacological therapy (74). Controlled studies for TTH prophylaxis are limited, and the studies that have been conducted often have failed to demonstrate significant superiority of the medication over placebo. However, tricyclic antidepressants, particularly amitriptyline, have proven to be the most widely utilized and have demonstrated efficacy in several trials (75–80) (Table 6). The mechanisms of action of TCAs include increasing serotonin via reuptake inhibition, potentiation of the effects of endogenous opioids, and possible inhibition of NMDA receptors (77,84). TCAs have also been shown to inhibit cytokines implicated in neurogenic inflammation such as tumor necrosis factor alpha (TNF-α) (78). These mechanisms likely reduce myofascial tissue pain transmission by reducing increased

TABLE 6 Evidence-Based Prophylactic Therapy Options for Tension-Type Headache

Treatment	First or second line	Dose	Adverse events
Amitriptyline[a]	First line	10–100 mg HS	Dry mouth, drowsiness and fatigue, and weight gain are common adverse events with amitriptyline as with other TCAs. In addition, as with other antidepressants, amitriptyline has a black box warning for the increased risk of suicidality in children/adolescents with major depressive or psychiatric disorders (75)
Tizanidine	First line	24 mg daily	Common side effects include drowsiness and dry mouth and are usually mild. There are no black box warnings (81,82)
Mirtazapine	Second line	15–30 mg daily	Dry mouth, drowsiness and fatigue, and weight gain are the most common adverse events. Mirtazapine does have a black box warning for the increased risk of suicidality in children/adolescents with major depressive or psychiatric disorders (83)

[a]Other tricyclic antidepressants are likely to be effective, although data proving this is limited and/or absent.

excitability in the central nervous system (75–78). Although amitriptyline is the best studied TCA for TTH, others are likely effective. Nortriptyline has not been as well studied, but has been shown to have fewer side effects than amitriptyline (66). Amitriptyline is the most sedating tricyclic and is thought to repair damage in stage 4 sleep architecture (58). Tricyclic antidepressants in the setting of TTH are initially dosed at 10 to 25 mg at night, which for many sufferers improves HA frequency, as well as sleep hygiene. However, for full benefit the average patient generally requires doses of 75 to 100 mg (85). The most significant side effects of amitriptyline were weight gain and sedation. As a group, selective serotonin reuptake inhibitors (SSRIs) have not had any proven efficacy in the prevention of TTH. One study found Paroxetine 20 to 30 mg daily to be less effective than sulpiride 200 to 400 mg daily, which is not approved for use in the United States (80). Another trial found SSRIs to be ineffective in CTTH sufferers that did not respond to TCAs (84). A third study found that citalopram showed no superiority to placebo, but rather, reinforced the efficacy of amitriptyline in TTH prophylaxis (86). In contrast, mirtazapine, which is a noradrenergic/serotonergic antidepressant, has shown some efficacy in TTH prevention and has proven to be an effective alternative in patients who failed amitriptyline (83). Tizanidine is an alpha2-adrenergic agonist that inhibits the release of norepinephrine at both the spinal cord and brain, with antinociceptive effects that are independent of the endogenous opioid system that has shown mixed efficacy in CTTH prophylaxis (81,82,87). However, one of the larger studies demonstrated advantage over placebo in an open label, multicenter trial (81). Botox has not demonstrated clear evidence for efficacy (58).

Nonpharmacologic

Nonpharmacologic interventions can be used alone or in conjunction with pharmacologic therapy. Relaxation training, electromyographic (EMG) biofeedback, and a combination of the two have demonstrated a near 50% reduction in headache activity (88). One study showed that relaxation by 50% on EMG by the fourth session was indicative of favorable outcomes (88). Although cognitive behavioral therapy, like stress management, can be time consuming for the patient and therapist, as well as costly, there has been proven efficacy. Limited contact treatment with audiovisual media and written materials may provide a cost-effective alternative to the traditional frequent direct therapist interaction. Cognitive therapy has been found to be especially useful when added to relaxation and biofeedback therapies (89). On the other hand, patients with continuous headaches or elevated scores on tests that assess depression or psychiatric disturbances tend to respond poorly to cognitive therapy (90). In one study, stress management combined with amitriptyline up to 100 mg/day or nortriptyline up to 75 mg/day was more effective than medication or therapy alone (91). Physical therapy modalities in the form of positioning, ergonomic instruction, massage, transcutaneous electrical nerve stimulation, hot/cold application, and manipulations have been utilized in the treatment of TTH (92,93). One study showed that physical treatment with multiple modalities including massage, home exercise, and relaxation had a modest 32% reduction in headache days per month in responders, with a responder rate of 29% of the study group. In addition, the study demonstrated that physical modalities had some effect on CTTH, but not on ETTH (59).

CONCLUSIONS

TTH is the most common primary headache disorder, with a life-time prevalence of 98% in women and 89% in men. Although generally less debilitating than migraine headache, TTH can be associated with substantial disability. A thorough history and examination with attention to pain characteristics as well as an evaluation of associated comorbid conditions can help the physician make an accurate diagnosis and recommend the most appropriate therapy for the patient. TTH generally responds favorably to abortive therapy such as aspirin and acetaminophen, but for those headache sufferers with CTTH, frequent ETTH, and ETTH with significant disability, nonpharmacological and prophylactic therapy should be strongly considered. By considering all these factors, the physician can help prevent disability from TTH and restore the patient to active participation in life.

REFERENCES

1. Rasmussen BK. Epidemiology of headache. Cephalalgia 1995; 15(1):45–68.
2. Rasmussen BK, Jensen R, Schroll M, et al. Epidemiology of headache in a general population—A prevalence study. J Clin Epidemiol 1991; 44(11):1147–1157.
3. Lyngberg AC, Rasmussen BK, Jorgensen T, et al. Has the prevalence of migraine and tension-type headache changed over a 12-year period? A Danish population survey. Eur J Epidemiol 2005; 20(3):243–249.
4. Schwartz BS, Stewart WF, Simon D, et al. Epidemiology of tension-type headache. JAMA 1998; 279(5):381–383.

5. Edmeads J, Findlay H, Tugwell P, et al. Impact of migraine and tension-type headache on life-style, consulting behaviour, and medication use: A Canadian population survey. Caj J Neurol Sci 1993; 20:131–137.
6. Russell MB, Rasmussen BK, Brennum J, et al. Presentation of a new instrument: The diagnostic headache diary. Cephalalgia 1992; 12(6):369–374.
7. Jensen R, Stovner LJ. Epidemiology and comorbidity of headache. Lancet Neurol 2008; 7:354–361.
8. Headache Classification Subcommittee of the International Headache Society. The International Classification of Headache Disorders: 2nd edition. Cephalalgia 2004; 24(Suppl 1):9–160.
9. Rasmussen BK, Olesen J. Epidemiology of migraine and tension-type headache. Curr Opin Neurol 1994; 7:264–271.
10. Göbel H, Petersen-Braun M, Soyka D. The epidemiology of headache in Germany: A nationwide survey of a representative sample on the basis of the headache classification of the International Headache Society. Cephalalgia 1994; 14:97–106.
11. Silva HM Jr, Garbelini RP, Teixeria SO, et al. Effect of episodic tension-type headache on the health-related quality of life in employees of a Brazilian public hospital. Arq Neuropsiquiatr 2004; 62(3B):769–773.
12. Schwartz BS, Stewart WF, Lipton RB. Lost workdays and decreased work effectiveness associated with headache in the workplace. J Occup Environ Med 1997; 39: 320–327.
13. Lavados PM, Tenhamm E. Epidemiology of tension-type headache in Santiago, Chile: A prevalence study. Cephalalgia 1998; 18(8):552–558.
14. Jensen R, Rasmussen BK, Pedersen B, et al. Muscle tenderness and pressure pain thresholds in headache. A population study. Pain 1993; 52:193–199.
15. Pascual J, Colas R, Castillo J. Epidemiology of chronic daily headache. Curr Pain Headache Rep 2001; 5(6):529–536.
16. Lyngberg AC, Rasmussen BK, Jørgensen T, et al. Favourable prognosis for the majority with migraine and tension-type headache. Neurology 2005; 65:580–585.
17. Jensen R, Olesen J. Initiating mechanisms of experimentally induced tension-type headache. Cephalalgia 1996; 16:175–182.
18. Sandrini G, Antonaci F, Pucci E, et al. Comparative study with EMG, pressure algometry and manual palpation in tension-type headache and migraine. Cephalalgia 1994; 14:451–457.
19. Jensen R, Fuglsang-Frederiksen A. Quantitative surface EMG of pericranial muscles.Relation to age and sex in a general population. Electroenceph Clin Neurophysiol 1994; 93:175–183.
20. Rasmussen BK, Jensen R, Schroll M, et al. Interrelations between migraine and tension-type headache in the general population. Arch Neurol 1992; 49(9):914–918.
21. Rasmussen BK, Jensen R, Olsen J. A population-based analysis of the diagnostic criteria of the International Headache Society. Cephalgia 1991; 11:128–134.
22. Zeeberg P, Olesen J, Jensen R. Efficacy of multidisciplinary treatment in a tertiary referral headache center. Cephalalgia 2005; 25(12):1159–1167.
23. Ylinen J, Takala EP, Nykanen M, et al. Active neck muscle training in the treatment of chronic neck pain in women: A randomized controlled trial. JAMA 2003; 289(19):2509–2516.
24. Jay GW. Chronic daily headache and myofascial pain syndromes: Pathophysiology and treatment. In: Cady RK, Fox AW, eds. Treating the Headache Patient. New York: Marcel Dekker, 1995:211–233.
25. Inan LE, Tulunay FC, Guvener A, et al. Characteristics of headache in migraine without aura and episodic tension-type headache in the Turkish population according to IHS classification. Cephalalgia 1994; 14:171–173.
26. Langemark M, Olsen J, Poulsen DP, et al. Clinical characterization of patients with chronic tension headache. Headache 1988; 28:590.
27. Jensen R. Tension-type headache. Curr Treat Options Neurol 2001; 3(2):169–180.

28. Murphy AI, Lehrer PM. Headache versus nonheadache state: A study of electrophysiological and affective changes during muscle contraction headache. Behav Med 1990; 16:23.
29. Fernandez-de-las-Penas C, Alonso-Blanco C, Cuadrado ML, et al. Forward head posture and neck mobility in chronic tension-type headache: A blinded, controlled study. Cephalgia 2006; 26(3):314–319.
30. Lipton RB, Dodick D, Sadovsky R, et al. ID Migraine validation study. A self-administered screener for migraine in primary care. Neurology 2003; 61(3): 375–382.
31. Silberstein S, Loder E, Diamond S, et al. AMPP Advisory Group. Probable migraine in the United States: Results of the American Migraine Prevalence and Prevention (AMPP) study. Cephalalgia 2007; 27(3):220–234.
32. Lipton RB, Cady RK, Stewart WF, et al. Diagnostic lessons from the spectrum study. Neurology 2002; 58(9 Suppl 6):S27–S31.
33. Cady RK, Schreiber CP, Billings C. Subjects with self-described "sinus" headache meet IHS diagnostic criteria for migraine. Cephalalgia 2001; 21:298.
34. Cady RK, Schreiber CP. Sinus headache or migraine? Considerations in making a differential diagnosis. Neurology 2002; 58(Suppl 6):S10–S14.
35. Couch JR. Sinus headache: A neurologist's viewpoint. Semin Neurol 1988; 8:298–302.
36. Schuller DE, Cadman TE, Jeffreys WH. Recurrence headaches: What every allergist should know. Ann Allergy Asthma Immunol 1996; 76:219–230.
37. Close LG, Aviv J. Headaches and disease of the nose and paranasal sinuses. Semin Neurol 1997; 17:351–354.
38. Headache Classification Committee of the International Headache Society. Classification and diagnostic criteria for headache disorders, cranial neuralgias and facial pain. Cephalalgia 1988; 8(Suppl 7):1–96.
39. Eross E, Dodick D, Eross M. The Sinus, Allergy and Migraine Study (SAMS). Headache 2007; 47(2):213–224.
40. Sjaastad O, Fredriksen TA. Cervicogenic headache: The importance of sticking to the criteria. Funct Neurol 2002; 17(1):35–36.
41. Antonaci F, Fredriksen TA, Sjaastad O. Cervicogenic headache: Clinical presentation, diagnostic criteria, and differential diagnosis. Curr Pain Headache Rep 2001; 5(4): 387–392.
42. Jensen R, Bendtsen L, Olesen J. Muscular factors are of importance in tension-type headache. Headache 1998; 38:10–17.
43. Jay GW. Post-traumatic headache: Diagnosis, pathophysiology and treatment. In: Boswell MV, Cole BE, eds. Weiner's Pain Management. 7th ed. Boca Raton, FL: CRC Press, 2006:333–360.
44. Bovim G, Sand T. Cervicogenic headache, migraine without aura and tension-type headache. Diagnostic blockade of greater occipital and supra-orbital nerves. Pain 1992; 51(1):43–48.
45. Leinisch-Dahlke E, Jürgens T, Bogdahn U, et al. Greater occipital nerve block is ineffective in chronic tension type headache. Cephalalgia 2005; 25(9):704–708.
46. Silberstein SD, Lipton RB, Sliwinski M. Classification of daily and near-daily headaches: Field trial of revised IHS criteria. Neurology 1996; 47(4):871–875.
47. Scher AI, Stewart WF, Liberman J, et al. Prevalence of frequent headache in a population sample. Headache 1998; 38:497–506.
48. Castillo J, Muñoz P, Guitera V, et al. Epidemiology of chronic daily headache in the general population. Headache 1999; 38:497–506.
49. Silberstein SD, Lipton RB, Solomon S, et al. Classification of daily and near daily headaches: proposed revisions to the IHS classification. Headache 1994; 34:1–7.
50. Peres MF, Gonçalves AL, Krymchantowski A. Migraine, tension-type headache, and transformed migraine. Curr Pain Headache Rep 2007; 11(6):449–453.
51. Sjaastad O, Spierings EL. Hemicrania continua: Another headache absolutely responsive to indomethacin. Cephalalgia 1984; 4:65–70.
52. Bordini C, Antonaci F, Stovner LJ, et al. "Hemicrania continua": A clinical review. Headache 1991; 31:20–26.

53. Pareja J, Antonaci F, Vincent M. The hemicrania continua diagnosis. Cepahalalgia 2002; 7:563–564.
54. Goadsby PJ, Lipton RB. A review of paroxysmal hemicranias, SUNCT syndrome and other short-lasting headaches with autonomic feature, including new cases. Brain 1997; 120 (Pt 1):193–209.
55. Diener HC. Medication overuse is more than just taking too much. Cephalalgia 2005; 25(7):481.
56. Forsyth PA, Posner JB. Headaches in patients with brain tumors: A study of 111 patients. Neurology 1993; 43(9):1678–1683.
57. Olsen J, Schoenen J. Tension-type headache, cluster headache, and miscellaneous headaches. Synthesis of tension-type headache mechanisms. In: Olsen J, Tfelt-Handsen P, Welch KMA, eds. The Headaches. 2nd ed. New York: Lippincott Williams & Wilkins, 1999:615–618.
58. Jay GW. Tension-type headache. In: Jay GW, ed. Chronic Pain. Informa Healthcare, 2007:193–222.
59. Dorpat TL, Holmes TH. Mechanisms of skeletal muscle pain and fatigue. Arch Neurol Psychiatry 1955; 74:628.
60. Perl S, Markle P, Katz LN. Factors involved in the production of skeletal muscle pain. Arch Intern Med 1934; 53:814.
61. Hong S, Kniffki K, Schmidt R. Pain Abstracts. Second World Congress on Pain 1978; 1:58.
62. Cailliet R. Pain: Mechanisms and Management. Philadelphia: F.A. Davis, 1993:83.
63. Jay GW. The autonomic nervous system: Anatomy and pharmacology. In: Raj P, ed. Pain Medicine-A Comprehensive Review. St. Louis: Mosby, 1996:461–465.
64. Jay GW. Sympathetic aspects of myofacial pain. Pain Digest 1995; 5:192–194.
65. Ostergaard S, Russell MB, Bendtsen L, et al. Increased familial risk of chronic tension-type headache. BMJ 1997; 314:1092–1093.
66. Goadsby T, Silberstein S, Dodick D. Chronic Daily Headache for Clinicians. Hamilton: BC Decker Inc, 2005:57–64.
67. Dahlöf CGH, Jacobs LD. Ketoprofen, paracetamol and placebo in the treatment of episodic tension-type headache. Cephalalgia 1996; 16:117–123.
68. Steiner TJ, Lange R, Voelker M. Aspirin in episodic tension-type headache: Placebo-controlled dose-ranging comparison with paracetamol. Cephalalgia 2003; 23(1):59–66.
69. Prior MJ, Cooper KM, May LG, et al. Efficacy and safety of acetaminophen and naproxen in the treatment of tension-type headache. A randomized, double-blind, placebo-controlled trial. Cephalalgia 2002; 22(9):740–748.
70. Kubitzek F, Ziegler G, Gold MS, et al. Low-dose diclofenac potassium in the treatment of episodic tension-type headache. Eur J Pain 2003; 7(2):155–162.
71. Brennum J, Brinck T, Schriver L, et al. Sumatriptan has no clinically relevant effect in the treatment of episodic tension-type headache. Eur J Neurol 1996; 3:23–28.
72. Cady RK, Gutterman D, Saiers JA, et al. Responsiveness of non-IHS migraine and tension-type headache to sumatriptan. Cephalalgia 1997; 17(5):588–590.
73. Brennum J, Kjeldsen M, Olesen J. The 5-HT1-like agonist sumatriptan has a significant effect in chronic tension-type headache. Cephalalgia 1992; 12:375–379.
74. Jensen R. Tension-type headache. Curr Treat Options Neurol 2001; 3(2):169–180.
75. Bendtsen L, Jensen R, Olesen J. Amitriptyline, a combined serotonin and nora-drenaline re-uptake inhibitor, reduces exteroceptive suppression of temporal muscle activity in patients with chronic tension-type headache. Electroencephalogr Clin Neurophysiol 1996; 101:418–422.
76. Bendtsen L, Jensen R. Amitriptyline reduces myofascial tenderness in patients with chronic tension-type headache. Cephalalgia 2000; 20(6):603–610.
77. Eisenach JC, Gebhart GF. Intrathecal amitriptyline acts as an N-methyl-D-aspartate receptor antagonist in the presence of inflammatory hyperalgesia in rats. Anesthesiology 1995; 83:1046.
78. Dredge K, Connor TJ, Kelly JP, et al. Differential effect of a single high dose of the tricyclic antidepressant imipramine on interleukin-1beta and tumor necrosis

factor-alpha secretion following an in vivo lipopolysaccharide challenge in rats. Int J Immunopharmacol 1999; 21(10):663–673.

79. Couch JR, Micieli G. Tension-type headache, cluster headache, and miscellaneous headaches: Prophylactic pharmacotherapy. In: Olsen J, Schoenen J, eds. Tension-type Headache: Classification, Mechanisms and Treatment. New York: Raven Press, 1993:275–280.

80. Langemark M, Olsen J. Sulpiride and paroxetine in the treatment of chronic tension-type headche. An explanatory double-blind trial. Headache 1994; 34:20–24.

81. Saper JR, Lake AE III, Cantrell DT, et al. Chronic daily headache prophylaxis with tizanidine: A double-blind, placebo-controlled, multicenter outcome study. Headache 2002; 42(6):470–482.

82. Fogelholm R, Murros K. Tizanidine in chronic tension-type headache: A placebo controlled double-blind cross-over study. Headache 1992; 32:509–513.

83. Bendtsen L, Jensen R. Mirtazapine is effective in the prophylactic treatment of chronic tension-type headache. Neurology 2004; 62(10):1706–1711.

84. Holroyd KA, Labus JS, O'Donnell FJ, et al. Treating tension-type headache not responding to amitriptyline hydrochloride with paroxetine hydrochloride: Evaluation. Headache 2003; 43:999–1004.

85. Boline PD, Kassak K, Bronfort G, et al. Spinal manipulation vs. amitriptyline for the treatment of chronic tension-type headaches: A randomized clinical trial. J Manipulative Physiol Ther 1995; 18:148–154.

86. Bendsten L, Jensen R, Olesen J. A non-selective (amitriptyline), but not a selective (citalopram), serotonin reuptake inhibitor is effective in the prophylactic treatment of chronic tension-type headache. J Neurol Neurosurg. Psychiatry 1996; 61:285–290.

87. Nakashima K, Tumura R, Wang Y, et al. Effects of tizanidine administration on exteroceptive suppression of the temporalis muscle in patients with chronic tension-type headache. Headache 1994; 34:455–457.

88. Schoenen J, Pholien P, Maertens de Noordhout A. EMG biofeedback in tension-type headache: Is the 4th session predictive of outcome? Cephalgia 1985; 5:132–133.

89. Holroyd KA, Penzien DB. Client variables and behavioral treatment of recurrent tension headaches: A metaanalytic review. J Behav Med 1986; 9:515–536.

90. Holroyd KA. Tension-type headache, cluster headache, and miscellaneous headaches: Psychological and behavioral techniques. In: Olsen J, Tfelt-Hansen P, Welch KMA, eds. The Headaches. New York: Raven Press, 1993:515–520.

91. Holroyd KA, O'Donnell FJ, Stensland M, et al. Management of chronic tension-type headache with tricyclic antidepressant medication, stress management therapy, and their combination: A randomized controlled trial. JAMA 2001; 285(17):2208–2215.

92. Jay GW, Brunson J, Branson SJ. The effectiveness of physical therapy in the treatment of chronic daily headaches. Headache 1989; 29:156.

93. Jay GW. Headache Handbook: Diagnosis and Treatment. Boca Raton: CRC Press, 1999:17–32.

3

Posttraumatic Headache

Gary W. Jay

Clinical Disease Area Expert-Pain, Pfizer, Inc., New London, Connecticut, U.S.A.

INTRODUCTION

Posttraumatic headache (PTHA) is a poorly understood disorder. There are 1.4 to 2 million traumatic brain injuries (TBI) each year, 500,000 of which are serious enough to require hospitalization (1,2). Another study indicates that PTHA affects over 2 million Americans each year (3).

Patients with PTHA range from 30% to 80% of patients who have had a mild head injury (4). Chronic PTHA (see below) is associated with increased headache frequency and disability compared with nontraumatic headache (5).

The ICD-10 classification system is based on the criteria that primarily concern the temporal relationship as well as pathogenicity between the relationship of PTHA with trauma, and ignore the clinical features of the PTHA (6). These criteria state that the headache onset must occur within two weeks of the traumatic event or the patient's return to consciousness. However, posttraumatic cluster headache, for example, typically does not fit this time course. Furthermore, the ICD-10 criteria for acute or chronic PTHA require one of the following: loss of consciousness (LOC), a period of anterograde amnesia of at least 10 minutes, or abnormal neurological examination/neurodiagnostic testing. The ICD-10 criteria find that acute PTHA resolves in eight weeks, while chronic PTHA lasts longer than eight weeks. This is in counter-distinction to the IHS (International Headache Society) criteria. See below (7).

These criteria are contrary to the most commonly accepted criteria, those of the Brain Injury Special Interest Group of the American Congress of Rehabilitation Medicine (8), which state that a minor traumatic brain injury (MTBI) is a "traumatically induced physiological disruption of brain function" associated with at least one of the following: any period of loss of consciousness; any memory loss for events just before or after the accident; any alteration in mental state at the time of the accident, such as feeling dazed, disoriented, or confused; and focal neurological deficits which may or may not be transient. Most importantly, there is no necessity of direct head trauma to meet the diagnosis.

Nosological problems abound, such as the synonymous use of various terminologies—concussion, minor traumatic brain injury, postconcussion syndrome/disorder, and posttrauma syndrome. For a number of specific reasons, it is felt that the postconcussion syndrome, which affects multiple organ systems, should be differentiated from an MTBI (9). Patients with PTHA do not, by medical or clinical definition have to have a coexisting MTBI.

PTHA may occur alone or as part of the postconcussion syndrome. Posttraumatic headache has been classified by the IHS as being associated with head trauma and being acute (resolving within three months after the injury) or chronic (lasting longer than three months). The IHS divided PTHAs into disorders associated with (*i*) significant head trauma and/or confirmatory signs or (*ii*) minor head trauma with no confirmatory signs. They stated that significant head trauma is defined by loss of consciousness, posttraumatic amnesia lasting more than 30 minutes, or abnormalities in at least two of the following: neurologic evaluations, skull X-ray, neuroimaging, evoked potentials, spinal fluid evaluation, vestibular functioning, or neuropsychological testing. The IHS determined that headache must occur within seven days after the injury or after a patient regains consciousness (7).

There is an inverse relationship between the occurrence of PTHA and the degree of a traumatic brain injury. One study found chronic daily posttraumatic headache in 80% of patients ($N = 54$) with an MTBI while 11% of these patients had no headache. In patients with a moderate-to-severe TBI ($N = 23$), 27% had chronic daily PTHA, 68% had no headache (10). A number of other authors also found that PTHA was the most common symptom after an MTBI as well as the most common part of the postconcussion syndrome (11–13).

By some definitions, headache after head trauma can be "postconcussive" if the patient has had a period of unconsciousness, or "posttraumatic" if there was no associated LOC. Furthermore, studies note that patients with MTBIs who had no LOC developed headaches that were more intractable to treatment (14).

The trauma-inducing PTHA has been noted in one study to be less than half (45%) secondary to motor vehicle accidents, 30% from falls, 20% from accidents at work or play (15). Typically, the neurological examination is negative, so these patients' complaints are considered inconsequential, unless the patients are in litigation, when other possibly incorrect assumptions about the patients' PTHA may be made.

Post-MTBI, or "whiplash," headaches are one of neurotraumatology's most prominent problems. One study found that out of 112 patients who experienced "whiplash," or an acceleration/deceleration injury, 42 (37%) had posttraumatic tension-type headaches, 30 patients (27%) had posttraumatic migraine headache, 20 patients (18%) had cervicogenic headache, and 20 patients (18%) had headaches that fit the nonspecific primary headache criterion (16). Of 104 patients, 93% had neck pain along with headaches (16).

Another study (17) found that a whiplash injury and minor head trauma are followed by PTHA in about 90% of patients. PTHA secondary to a whiplash injury was noted to be located occipitally in 67% of patients, with dull, pressing or dragging characteristics in 77%. Posttraumatic tension-type headache was most common and was found in 85% of patients. Eighty percent of patients with PTHA after minor head trauma or a whiplash injury had remission of their headaches within six months. Chronic PTHA lasting at least four years was found in 20% of patients.

PTHA has been found to have great variation in both nature and severity. In another study, 78% of 297 patients had either continuous or intermittent HA secondary to an MTBI (18).

A German study found that 80% of patients who had a whiplash injury recovered within a few months, while 15% to 20% developed "late whiplash injury syndrome" with many complaints of the cervicocephalic syndrome, including PTHA, vertigo, instability, nausea, tinnitus, and hearing loss (19).

As noted above, many view chronic PTHA as persisting three months or longer, including the IHS criteria (an arbitrary time frame), as the definition of chronic pain is different, three to six months or longer. Some studies indicate that the condition of PTHA patients improves or changes over six months and then plateaus. It was felt that six months was a better time period for chronicity as it was more consistent with the chronic pain literature (20).

Other estimates of persistence for six months or more are as high as 44% (12).

PTHAs can be classified as part of the PTHA syndrome, part of the postconcussive syndrome or by themselves, as an independent medical problem which may be secondary to an MTBI or a whiplash injury or a part of the postconcussive syndrome (21). If the latter, it may be associated with depression, irritability, decreased memory, fatigue, dizziness, decreased concentration and tinnitus (22). The postconcussive syndrome is associated with decreased cognitive functioning, impairment of rapid processing of information, decreased attention, and short-term memory (4,9).

The pathophysiology of chronic PTHA (CPTHA) has biological, psychological, and sociological aspects. Posttraumatic tension-type headache is the most common form of PTHA, but initiation and/or exacerbation of migraine-like headaches also occurs (9,23).

Patients with the postconcussive syndrome react differently to treatment (9). MTBI patients with posttraumatic headache or pain frequently have attentional deficits as well as psychological distress, both of which can coexist with chronic headache/pain alone. It is, therefore, important to determine all coexisting diagnoses early on, and to factor these problems into the design of treatment for headache and/or pain (9,11).

It is also important to note that after a structural lesion has been ruled out, the treatment of PTHA is very similar to the treatment of the primary headaches, vascular and tension type (23).

A closed head injury with brain concussion or contusion is the most frequent type of head injury in children. Headache is a major complaint of early and late postinjury periods. Eighty-three percent of 100 children (3–14 years of age) had headache after cerebral concussion/contusion: 56% had acute PTHA; 27% had CPTHA, tension type; and 3% had posttraumatic migraine. Twenty-one percent had headache lasting the entire year of observation (24). Another author stated that the majority of patients with headache had their symptoms clear within three to six months (25).

In another study of children 3.3 to 14.9 years of age (mean 11.2) who were followed for 5 to 29 months (average 12.5), 5 patients had posttraumatic migraine, 13 patients had posttraumatic tension-type headache, and 3 children had mixed headache. Tension-type headache was more common in children with chronic PTHA than those with no history of head injury (26).

Sakas et al. (27) felt that children who experience neurological deterioration after a trivial head injury without focal structural abnormalities (i.e., headache, confusion, vomiting, hemiparesis, cortical blindness, and seizures) may have an "unstable trigeminovascular reflex" that is activated by craniofacial trauma. They note that head trauma may be associated with noncongestive cerebral hyperemia. They further propose that head trauma activates the trigeminal nerve endings in the face, scalp, dura, or cortex and, via a reflex, causes vasodilatation and cerebral hyperemia.

The most important aspect to keep in mind is that the "type" of PTHA must be accurately diagnosed so that appropriate treatment can be prescribed.

Typically, PTHA is noted after acceleration/deceleration injuries ("whiplash") in up to 90% of patients who experience an MTBI (28). These headaches can be determined to be posttraumatic tension type, migraine, cluster or, possibly, cervicogenic headache. PTHAs may be secondary to work-related injuries, slip and fall injures, and violent altercations, aside from motor vehicle injuries. These headaches are frequently part of the postconcussive syndrome, which refers to the above-noted signs and symptoms that may follow a blow to the head or an acceleration/deceleration injury, but which may or may not induce a minor traumatic brain injury.

Acute, posttraumatic tension-type headache, the most frequently diagnosed PTHA (defined as 15 headache days or less a month) may last up to three to six months; after that it becomes "chronic." The IHS has determined that 15 headache days or more a month defines chronic headache (7). General pain management principles place pain as chronic after three to six months, after physiological healing has occurred. Up to 80% of PTHA patients will have their pain remit within six months, leaving an estimated 20% of patients with chronic PTHA, which may last years in many cases.

A simple concussion may also be associated with PTHA, as well as, in the extremes, vegetative and even psychotic difficulties (29,30).

PTHA may also be associated with dizziness, irritability, and decreased concentration, even without the additional finding of a minor traumatic brain injury.

The chronic PTHA patient frequently engenders significant difficulties for the typical general practitioner, as well as the neurological specialist. This may be especially true if there is evidence of de novo migraine or cluster headache.

Because of the emotional/affective aspects that most frequently accompany PTHA, including depression and anxiety disorders as well as problems with anger, the affective component of PTHA may contribute to the patients' perception of the degree to which their PTHAs are disabling (31,32). Patients with PTHA may also meet the diagnostic criteria from the DSM-IV for posttraumatic stress disorder (PTSD), and thus, require additional appropriate treatment (33).

It is important to note that one study of Operation Iraqi Freedom/Operation Enduring Freedom veterans with PCS found that PTSD accounted for the majority of symptoms except pain, which suggests that the pain is physiologically associated with brain injury (34).

Clinically, it has been noted that patients with PTHA who also have an MTBI may have additional treatment-related problems. It may be difficult to establish the presence of an MTBI via neuropsychological testing as long as the PTHAs persist, as the headache pain generally makes such evaluations more difficult for the patient and may have a true negative effect on the testing itself, making the differential diagnosis more difficult (9,31). Other reports indicate that there is little, if any, problem with an MTBI patient performing a neuropsychological evaluation while he or she is having significant PTHA (35), but clinically this appears to be quite unrealistic.

What can happen? A great deal of research has shown that when the head is free, rather than confined, it is more susceptible to the effects of an acceleration/deceleration injury. Six decades ago, it was shown in cats that less force was required to produce concussion when the head was free to move, as compared to when it was fixed or confined in place (36). The concept of "whiplash," essentially a legal term, medically known as acceleration/deceleration, is very important, as it involves a multitude of medical aspects. When an acceleration/deceleration injury occurs (most frequently from a rear-end automobile accident), the physical or gravitational forces of a massive object such as a car striking another automobile are passed onto the most fragile and movable object not firmly secured in the automobile that was struck: the passenger. Even when the passenger is wearing a seatbelt, the head—the ball at the end of a tether (the neck)—is first thrown forward, and then backward, when the tether can reach no farther forward and snaps back. If the head is turned at the moment of impact, the rotational forces are also very important, particularly in the etiology of a TBI.

THE DISORDER
Posttraumatic headache encompasses a number of different diagnostic entities. Specific diagnosis is needed for appropriate treatment. These diagnoses include

- Posttraumatic tension-type headache
- Posttraumatic migraine headache
- Cervicogenic headache
- Temporomandibular Joint (TMJ) related headache
- Posttraumatic cluster headache
- Neuropathic pain syndromes.

Details of several primary headache disorders in the nontraumatic form may be found in separate chapters in this textbook, while neuropathic pain information will be found in the sister textbook, *Practical Guide to Chronic Pain Syndromes* (Informa Healthcare, 2009). This chapter will dwell on the two most common types, posttraumatic tension-type headache (PTTHA) and posttraumatic migraine. This chapter will focus on PTTHA.

Posttraumatic Migraine
Trauma may be one of the triggers of migraine, and in some cases, it may be the predominant or even the sole precipitating event in the onset of migraine (37). Trauma may trigger the first attack of migraine in a susceptible patient; biochemical along with epidemiological studies/factors have implicated trauma as the main etiological factor in the onset of new migraine (37).

"Whiplash," with or without an MTBI, may decrease an individual's migraine threshold as well as exacerbate an episodic migraine pattern, which was previously under good control (15).

Posttraumatic migraine, which may begin de novo, without a previous personal or family history of migraine, may have neurochemical similarities with MTBIs, although they are not always found together. These may include increased extracellular potassium and intracellular sodium, calcium, and chloride; serotonergic changes; decreases in magnesium; excessive release of excitatory amino acids; changes in catecholamine and endogenous opioid tonus; decreased glucose utilization; changes in neuropeptides; and abnormalities in nitric oxide formation and function (38,39). Packard hypothesized that the presence of similar changes suggested PTHA associated with MTBI and migraine may share a common headache pathway (39).

Migraine, including posttraumatic migraine, may be associated with a number of neurological symptoms or phenomena. This may include transient global amnesia, vestibular dysfunction, visual and auditory changes, and possibly, an increased incidence of seizures (38,40,41).

The trigeminovascular system is of great import in migraine (38). In some children who develop posttraumatic neurological deterioration without focal lesions after minor head trauma, there may be an association with an "unstable trigeminovascular reflex," which induces the release of perivascular vasodilatory peptides that can contribute to cerebral hyperemia (27).

Transient global amnesia (TGA) was initially attributed to bilateral temporal lobe seizure phenomena, but more recently, has been attributed to migraine by some (38), and thought to be a totally separate disorder by others, possibly due to a different form of paroxysmal disorder in the brain stem (42). TGA in the pediatric population is still felt to be secondary to ischemia of the temporobasal structures induced by an MTBI and associated with a migrainous diathesis (43).

PTHA, including migraine, is commonly associated with children, adolescents, and teens who play football, and frequently goes unreported (44). Any degree of postconcussion headache in high-school athletes a week postinjury is likely associated with an incomplete recovery postconcussion (45).

Caution is needed to return high school athletes to the playing field after a concussion. On-field mental status changes appear to have some prognostic utility and should be taken into account when making return-to-play decisions after concussion. Athletes who show on-field mental status changes for more than five minutes have longer lasting postconcussion symptoms and memory decline (46).

"Roller coaster" migraine is also seen, following many short but fairly significant brain insults delivered during a roller coaster ride, and may be an important factor in triggering a patient's posttraumatic migraine headache (47).

Migraine equivalents, transient neurological symptomatology not associated with headache, are not uncommon: proper diagnosis is more difficult to the generalist, as well as the neurologist. In some possibly more susceptible individuals, minor, even trivial, head trauma can induce a migraine equivalent known as "footballer's migraine" as well as "posttraumatic cortical blindness." This particular migraine equivalent is rare; but transient, total blindness may certainly be a cause to call for a total, "full court press" work-up (48).

Still more common forms of transient neurological disturbance associated with migraine are brain stem symptoms including vestibular difficulties, including dizziness, disequilibrium, vertigo, and motion intolerance. These symptoms may also present as a migraine equivalent, between migraine headache episodes or instead of the cephalic pain. Vertigo as a migraine equivalent may occur in about 25% of migraine patients, with the diagnosis being made, typically, by history of familial migraine, as all testing is typically negative. Migraine can also mimic Meniere's disease, with "vestibular Meniere's disease" being more frequently, but still not commonly, associated with migraine (49,50). Also, one should not forget the cervical causes of vertigo and dizziness, secondary to posttraumatic cervical and/or myofascial pathophysiology.

There is also a question of the possible relationship between posttraumatic migraine and posttraumatic benign encephalopathy. In children, the latter may be associated with cortical blindness, brain stem disturbances, and seizure, lasting from 5 minutes to 48 hours (51).

A significant question then arises. Posttraumatic vertigo or dizziness is a very frequent accompaniment to MTBIs. It may be secondary to peripheral, labyrinthine disturbance, brain stem disturbance secondary to trauma, or it may be a migraine equivalent. The importance of this differential is most significant, possibly, when treatment is attempted.

As noted, trauma may induce the first migraine attack in a possibly susceptible patient or increase the frequency and possibly the severity of pre-existing migraine. The etiology of these changes may be secondary to neuronal and/or axonal abnormalities secondary to trauma as well as posttraumatic involvement of the trigeminovascular system.

Prophylactic treatment is typically with valproic acid, an anticonvulsant medication. The use of beta blockers such as propranolol may also be useful, but it may have significant side effects. The same is true for verapamil. The use of a triptan for abortive care is well tolerated, if used appropriately.

Cluster headache has also been seen secondary to head trauma, again possibly secondary to a neuronal and/or axonal injury. The incidence ranges from 6% to 10% (39,52). Many times, this is seen as a primary chronic, rather than episodic, form of cluster, or cluster-like headache. Clinically, this is one of the rarest forms of PTHA seen. Treatment, abortive or prophylactic, has been dealt with elsewhere (38).

Posttraumatic Tension-Type Headache

Posttraumatic tension-type headache (PTTHA) (with or without secondary analgesic rebound headache) is probably the most common primary headache disorder found after trauma. Diagnostically, and clinically, this entity appears to be almost, if not totally, identical to acute and chronic tension-type headache without a traumatic etiology.

According to the IHS (7), the diagnostic criteria of tension-type headache states that episodic tension-type headache is recurrent, occurring fewer than 15 days a month, lasting from 30 minutes to 7 days. The pain characteristics include two of four of the following: pain with a pressing/tightening (nonpulsating) quality; pain which is mild to moderate in intensity and may inhibit, but not prohibit, activities; pain which is always bilateral; and pain which is not aggravated by walking stairs or doing other routine physical activity. These criteria also state that both of the following are true: no nausea or vomiting, but anorexia may occur; and photophobia and phonophobia are absent, or one but not the other is present.

All other organic diagnoses must be ruled out first, as well as other primary headache diagnoses, including migraine and cluster headache.

In PTTHA, like nonposttraumatic tension-type headache, the pain is typically described as aching, pressure like, or feeling like a tight band or "like there's a vice around my head." The pain is typically bilateral, although it may be unilateral. It may include some or all of various areas such as occipitonuchal, bifrontal, bitemporal, suboccipital, at the vertex (crown) of the head, as well as extend into the neck and shoulders.

The pain intensity may wax and wane depending on a number of factors including movement, activity level, stress, and others. Even in PTTHA, emotional/psychological aspects may increase pain.

There is a female preponderance.

Unlike migraine headache patients, PTTHA patients may carry on with their activities. Most take some form of analgesic, frequently on a daily basis. Without question, PTTHA patients may also have migraine, posttraumatic or otherwise.

The chronic PTTHA patient has headache 15 or more days a month. This is also a diagnostic exercise, as most frequently, nosologically, PTTHA may be one of several headache diagnoses that are part of a chronic daily headache differential, which would include analgesic-rebound headache, at a minimum.

The PTTHA patient frequently has headache daily or every other day. The headache is typically present upon awakening, and remains until sleeping. The intensity of the pain varies, decreasing for several hours after analgesics are taken.

The majority of PTTHA patients, if seen early on, have associated pericranial muscle spasm or pain, while others do not, yet still complain of pain.

Patients with PTTHA will also endure elements of depression and anxiety. There is a "chicken and egg" aspect to this, in terms of which problem comes first. In many cases, central neurochemical changes begin concurrent with the injury and manifest as both pain and affective disturbances (see below).

Nosologically, posttraumatic headache is incident to trauma. Some problems noted in making this diagnosis are as follows: the patient may not experience direct trauma to the head, but may have an acceleration/deceleration injury (whiplash); there may not be significant physical findings on examination (conversely, there may be physical findings that are missed unless a good musculoskeletal examination is done); secondary to the lack of profound physical findings, the patient may be labeled with a psychogenic diagnosis, or worse, with the term, malingering.

THE DIAGNOSIS
The International Headache Society Headache Diagnostic Criteria (revised in 2004) (7) is the basis for most diagnoses and states:

5.1.1 Acute post-traumatic headache attributed to moderate or severe head injury
  A. Headache, no typical characteristics known, fulfilling criteria C and D
  B. Head trauma with at least one of the following:
      1. Loss of consciousness for > 30 minutes
      2. Glasgow Coma Scale (GCS) < 13
      3. Post-traumatic amnesia for > 48 hours
      4. Imaging demonstration of traumatic brain lesion (cerebral hematoma), intracerebral and/or subarachnoid hemorrhage, brain contusion, and/or skull fracture
  C. Headache develops within 7 days after head trauma or after regaining consciousness after head trauma
  D. One of the following:
      1. Headache resolves within 3 months after head trauma
      2. Headache persists but 3 months have not yet passed since head trauma
5.1.2 Acute post-traumatic headache attributed to mild head injury
  A. Headache, no typical characteristics known, fulfilling criteria C and D
  B. Head trauma with at least one of the following:
      1. Either no loss of consciousness or loss of consciousness for < 30 minutes.
      2. GCS ≥ 13
      3. Symptoms and/or signs diagnostic of concussion

    C. Headache develops within 7 days after head trauma
    D. One of the following:
        1. Headache resolves within 3 months after head trauma
        2. Headache persists but 3 months have not yet passed since head trauma

5.2.1 Chronic post-traumatic headache attributed to moderate or severe head injury
    A. Headache, no typical characteristics known, fulfilling criteria C and D
    B. Head Trauma with at least one of the following:
        1. Loss of consciousness for > 30 minutes
        2. GCS < 13
        3. Post-traumatic amnesia for > 48 hours
        4. Imaging demonstration of traumatic brain lesion (cerebral hematoma), intracerebral and/or subarachnoid hemorrhage, brain contusion, and/or skull fracture
    C. Headache develops within 7 days after head trauma or after regaining consciousness
    D. Headache persists for > 3 months after head trauma

5.2.2 Chronic post-traumatic headache attributed to mild head injury
    A. Headache, no typical characteristics known, fulfilling criteria C and D
    B. Head trauma with at least one of the following:
        1. Either no loss of consciousness or loss of consciousness for >30 minutes
        2. GCS ≥ 13
        3. Symptoms and/or signs diagnostic of concussion
    C. Headache develops within 7 days after head trauma or after regaining consciousness after head trauma
    D. Headache persists for >3 months after head trauma

5.3 Acute headache attributed to whiplash injury
    A. Headache, no typical characteristics known, fulfilling criteria C and D
    B. History of whiplash (sudden and significant acceleration/deceleration movement of neck) associated at the time with neck pain
    C. Headache develops within 7 days after whiplash injury
    D. One of the other of the following:
        1. Headache resolves within the following 3 months after whiplash injury
        2. Headache persists but 3 months have not yet passed since whiplash injury

5.4 Chronic headache attributed to whiplash injury
    A. Headache, no typical characteristics known, fulfilling criteria C and D
    B. History of whiplash (sudden and significant acceleration/deceleration movement of neck) associated at the time with neck pain
    C. Headache develops within 7 days after whiplash injury
    D. Headache persists for >3 months after whiplash injury

The headache examination should consist of, after a general examination, a neurological as well as a musculoskeletal examination. Close attention must be paid to the neck, as well as to the cervical and cranial musculature (53).

PATHOPHYSIOLOGY

The typical PTTHA begins post-acceleration/deceleration injury, which occurs most frequently during a motor vehicle accident. A slip and fall accident as well as a sports-related injury or a violent altercation or blow to the head can be the initiating event.

As described above, the head and the neck, likened to a ball on a chain, is flung forward and backward from acceleration/deceleration forces, frequently without direct trauma to the head, or following direct trauma to the head. However it occurs, the physical forces involved will cause the cervical and shoulder musculature, at a minimum, to be suddenly stretched and to sustain both microtears and strain/trauma as well as endure a reflex muscle contraction after the sudden stretching. It is obviously important to understand the myofascial pain syndrome (MPS).

Pathological changes in the musculoskeletal system may initiate, modulate, or perpetuate PTTHA. Episodic and chronic PTTHA are, at least at first, secondary to a muscle-induced pain syndrome that is typically associated with the aforementioned MPS.

The central nervous system controls muscle tone via systems that influence the gamma efferent neurons in the anterior horn cells of the spinal cord, which act on the alpha motor neurons supplying muscle spindles. The Renshaw cells, apparently via the inhibitory neurotransmitter gamma aminobutyric acid (GABA) will influence this synaptic system. There is also supraspinal control from cortical, subcortical, and limbic afferent and efferent systems. Physiological and emotional inputs interact in the maintenance or flux of muscle tone. Adverse influences from both localized or regional myofascial nociception, with or without limbic (affective) stimulation, may produce significant muscle spasm, which, if prolonged, will become tonic with the additional aspects of increased anxiety or a maintained muscle contraction–pain cycle (53–55). This helps to differentiate acute *versus* chronic PTTHA, to a degree.

Tonic or continued posttraumatic muscle contraction may induce hypoxia via compression of small blood vessels. Ischemia, the accumulation of pain-producing metabolites (bradykinin, lactic acid, serotonin, prostaglandins, etc.) may increase and potentiate muscle pain and reactive spasm. These nociception-enhancing or algetic chemicals may stimulate central mechanisms that, through continued stimulation, may induce continued reactive muscle spasm/contraction and maintenance of the myogenic nociceptive cycle (56–58).

Changes in the peripheral blood flow in muscles seen in patients with chronic tension-type headache appear to be secondary to disturbances in the regulation of peripheral mechanisms due to central sensitization. Muscle pain in tension-type headache may be secondary to microtrauma of muscle fibers and tendonous insertions, accentuated by the accumulation of algetic metabolites: serotonin, bradykinin, and potassium ions effectively stimulate skeletal muscle nociceptors (59). Combinations of endogenous substances (serotonin, bradykinin, prostaglandin E2, histamine), when slowly infused into the trapezius muscles of patients with episodic tension-type headache developed significantly more pain and muscle tenderness than healthy controls (60).

Although PTTHA may include migraine, some of Moskowitz's work (61) may be pertinent here. He has shown that when stimulated antidromically, the trigeminal nerve can release vasoactive/algetic peptides such as substance P, neurokinin A, bradykinin, neuropeptides Y, vasoactive intestinal peptide (VIP) and calcitonin-gene-related peptide (CGRP) from its afferent nerves which innervate vascular structures. This can initiate a sterile inflammation that will lower the pain threshold, causing exacerbations in pain from typically benign behavior such as movement of the head. (This is NOT allodynia—that may be most commonly associated with migraine.) It is conceivable that such a disruption of the trigeminal system may possibly help determine neurogenic pain in some patients, who may be susceptible to migraine, who develop PTHA.

The myofascial aspects of tension-type headache are clinically identical to those of PTTHA, the significant difference in diagnoses being the etiology—posttraumatic or otherwise.

The MPS was, for a long while, ignored in the pathophysiology of headache of any type. Some researchers found a causal relationship between muscle spasm and headache (62–64) while others have felt that muscle spasm associated with headache is an epiphenomenon, not the etiology of headache (65–70), but a reflexive response. Other authors have indicated that muscle activity/spasm or increased tone may be more pronounced in migraine than in tension-type headaches (71,72).

Unfortunately, this research, which was obtained via electromyographic (EMG) studies, appears to be problematic, as the various authors evaluated different groups of muscles in different types of patients, many of whom had poorly defined diagnoses (63,71,73,74). Other authors defined chronic tension-type headache as an entity with or without associated pericranial muscle disorder. The concept of muscle fatigue was not taken into consideration, metabolically spent muscles, which may become relatively flaccid, losing aspects of increased tonus or spasm.

The sympathetic nervous system interacts with the trigeminal system, and may act as an activating entity. Sympathetic fibers from the stellate ganglia innervate the cranial and cervical structures. These fibers go rostrally and form a large nerve plexus behind the origin of the vertebral artery and superiorly, with the cervical ganglia lying on the capitus longus muscle behind the carotid sheath at the base of the skull. Sympathetic fibers supply the carotid, basilar, and cerebellar circulatory vessels. Sympathetic fibers in the carotid sheath interconnect with the caudate nucleus of the trigeminal nerve, providing interactions between the two systems (75–77). Autonomic fibers surrounding the carotid do appear to be involved in the induction of significant pain in cluster headache patients (78).

Three mechanisms of muscle pain are thought to be relevant to acute, but more often chronic tension-type headache, which has the same physiological stigmata of PTTHA, in that myogenic nociception may be induced by (*i*) low-grade inflammation associated with the release of algetic, or pain-inducing substances, rather than signs of acute inflammation; (*ii*) short or long-lasting relative ischemia; and (*iii*) tearing of ligaments and tendons secondary to abnormal sustained muscle tension (79). These factors do not take into consideration the possibly more significant initial trauma from acceleration/deceleration injuries, slip and fall accidents, and other reasons for direct or indirect head trauma that induces muscle trauma, primarily or secondarily.

Increased myofascial pain sensitivity in tension-type headache as well as posttraumatic tension-type headache may be secondary to the activation or sensitization of peripheral nociceptors, most probably from a combination of mechanisms.

Part of the differential diagnosis should also include cervical spondylosis (38,39,48,80), cervicogenic headache (38,81–83), as well as temporomandibular joint dysfunction (67,84–87).

Mild Traumatic Brain injury

Briefly, the basic pathophysiologic elements found in an MTBI may include axonal shearing; marked increases in the excitotoxic neurotransmitters including acetylcholine and glutamate causing neuronal death; a lack of the cohesiveness of the blood–brain barrier, which becomes "porous" for 8 to 24 hours or more; and possible changes in the hemodynamics of the brain (9).

While others believe that axonal shearing may have an element of stretching, it results in an indiscriminate release of excitatory neurotransmitters as well as the development of uncontrolled ionic fluxes leading to a disruption of ionic gradients which the cells try to compensate for by activating ion pumps to try to restore homeostasis, and instead increasing glucose use, leading to significant increases in the local cerebral metabolic rate of glucose (88–90). The hypermetabolism is also associated with diminished cerebral blood flow. Other changes occur in oxidative metabolism, mitochondrial function, and diminished intracellular magnesium levels (91).

Headache Pathophysiology

Looking at the upper portion of Figure 1, most of the basics have been mentioned: continuous peripheral stimulation from myofascial nociceptive input from a MPS, posttraumatic or not, with or without trigger points, may effectively trigger a change in the central pain "rheostat" associated with nociceptive input, secondary to the continuous need for pain-modulating antinociceptive neurotransmitters. This increased myofascial pain sensitivity may be secondary to activation or sensitization of peripheral nociceptors. The affective aspects of pain, including depression, anxiety, and fear, which are secondary to changes in neurotransmitters such as serotonin and norepinephrine, directly influence myofascial nociception, as well as further reinforce central neurochemical changes.

After 4 to 6 and 12 weeks or so, changes in the central nervous system's central modulation of nociception can occur. Secondary to continuous peripheral nociceptive stimulation, in association with affective changes, the central modulating mechanisms will assume a primary rather than a secondary or reactive role in pain perception, as well as antinociception, shifting the initiating aspects of pain perception from the peripheral regions to the central nervous system.

As noted earlier, patients with chronic tension-type headache, posttraumatic or not, show lower pressure pain tolerance than normal controls which indicates that the CNS is sensitized at the level of the spinal cord dorsal horn and trigeminal nucleus (92,93). Sensitivity in muscles (94) as well as the skin is also noted, and the latter may indicate an expansion of receptive fields and convergence secondary to central sensitization.

This intrinsic shift may make innocuous stimuli more aggravating to the pain-modulating systems, the "irritable everything syndrome." The already dysmodulated internal feedback mechanisms may react until central neurochemical mechanisms dominate, secondary to neurotransmitter exhaustion, and receptor

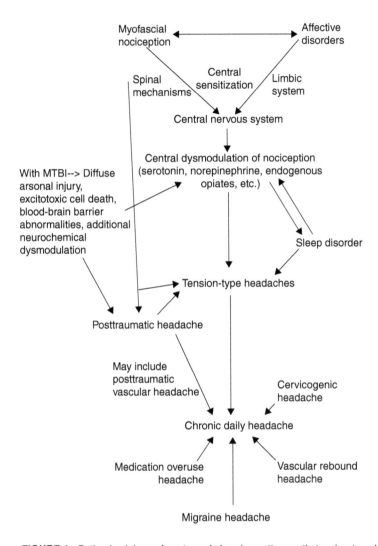

FIGURE 1 Pathophysiology of acute and chronic posttraumatic tension-type headache.

hypersensitivity and abnormal biogenic amine metabolism/exhaustion occur. These neurochemical changes may induce and/or exacerbate a sleep disorder (serotonergic in nature, from the nucleus raphe magnus), which, by itself, can perpetuate the central neurochemical dysmodulation that is primarily responsible for chronic posttraumatic tension-type headache.

Chronic posttraumatic tension-type headache, whether or not it is associated with an MTBI, has the same pathophysiological mechanisms. In the presence of an MTBI, other significant pathophysiological changes occur which can potentiate or exacerbate the mechanisms described above.

In the face of dysmodulated neurochemical systems found in chronic tension-type headache, add direct myofascial trauma as an initiating event. The effects of diffuse axonal injury from an MTBI, which also affects the neurochemistry of the brain as neuronal degeneration and death occurs, can exacerbate the neurotransmitter pathophysiology. This may also explain the initiation of de novo migraine, as brain stem trigeminovascular mechanisms may obviously be affected. Finally, an excitotoxic injury that leads to cell death from the overexuberant production of acetylcholine and glutamate may also induce significant neuropathological "holes" in the primary neurotransmitter systems and exacerbate the headache pathophysiology.

Affective changes follow, with the additional problem of possible cognitive changes resulting from the MTBI. The latter may make treatment of PTTHA more difficult.

Posttraumatic tension-type headache is the most common sequela of an MTBI. It may also be associated with iatrogenic analgesic abuse. Before treatment or even before diagnosis of cognitive deficits is attempted, inappropriate medications must be stopped and the headache ameliorated. Most commonly, for this to be done, the patient must be treated using an interdisciplinary headache treatment protocol. Please see the *Headache Handbook: Diagnosis and Treatment* for the details of this protocol (38) or *Chronic Pain* (53) for more up to date information.

Nitric oxide is found in the nociceptive neurons in the trigeminal nucleus caudalis, and possibly higher in the CNS (95). The inhibition of nitric oxide synthase (NOS), which enables the generation of nitric oxide (NO), decreases central sensitization in animal models of continuous pain. In a clinical investigation of an NOS inhibitor, both headache and pericranial myofascial tenderness and hardness in patients with chronic tension-type headache were diminished (95,96). This study supports the theory that central sensitization is involved in the pathophysiology of chronic tension-type headache

The neurochemical factors leading to the perpetuation of posttraumatic tension-type headaches appear to be further and more complexly involved than in chronic tension-type headache without an associated MTBI. Treatment is most appropriately and cost-effectively performed in an interdisciplinary headache rehabilitation program. Tricyclic medications, GABAnergic medications and NSAIDs are appropriate, while narcotics, Dilantin, barbiturates, and early generation benzodiazepines are not.

As noted above, patients with an MTBI who complain of headache do not appear to perceive their headache pain the same way a headache patient without an MTBI does. These patients know that they have headaches. On a scale of 0 (no pain) to 10 (worst pain imaginable), individual patients, when first seen, will give high numbers, e.g., 7 to 10, which is correlated with pathophysiological myofascial findings, including decreased cervical range of motion, muscle spasm, active trigger points, and more. As they go through treatment and regain appropriate physical functioning (normal cervical range of motion, amelioration of spasm, trigger points, etc., with a marked associated improvement in function), the patients' affect will be brighter; they will smile, have fewer if any pain behaviors, and resume doing the physical things they enjoy.

Yet, when asked, they will continue to state that their headache pain is at the same level of 7 to 10 as when they were first seen. Whether they are perseverating or are just unable to give an accurate subjective pain level (possible frontal lobe involvement), their stated pain levels may not change very much at all. Therefore, you must evaluate them on improvements in function, and not by self-reported subjective decrements in headache pain levels.

TREATMENT

Treatment of Acute Posttraumatic Tension-Type Headache

The medical management of acute or episodic posttraumatic tension-type headache is relatively simple. The older nomenclature titled these headaches as "acute muscle contraction headache" or "tension headache." This form of headache is the most common, as previously indicated, accounting for up to 80% of all nonorganic types of headache. It has been estimated that over 90% of Americans experience an acute tension-type headache, with or without pre-disposing trauma, at some time. The majority of these headaches are self-treated with over-the-counter medications and, therefore, never come to the attention of a physician. This indicates that the statistics are probably low, in that a fairly large number go unnoticed by physicians.

The greatest problem in the treatment of acute PTTHA is the avoidance of the development of medication overuse headache (MOS), which can easily occur if a patient is overmedicated. This is one step into the development of chronic or daily posttraumatic tension-type headache.

Physicians should be particularly familiar with the various types of medications that can be utilized for patients complaining of acute posttraumatic tension-type headache.

Many patients deal with the pain and discomfort by taking two aspirin and relaxing. Exercise is useful, as is a simple glass of wine, on an occasional basis. Any type of relaxation which distracts the patients from their headache is useful.

Dealing with the medication management, physicians have a more than ample supply to choose from. It may be tempting, therefore, to overtreat a minor headache with medications which have a significant risk of dependency.

The simple analgesics are easily chosen by the patient, if not the physician. They are inexpensive and easy to get. They include aspirin and acetaminophen. Like the nonsteroidal anti-inflammatory drugs (NSAIDs), aspirin appears to work by inhibiting the synthesis of prostaglandin by blocking the action of cyclooxygenase, an enzyme which enables the conversion of arachidonic acid to prostaglandin to occur. Prostaglandins are synthesized from cellular membrane phospholipids after activation or injury, and sensitize pain receptors.

The most frequently used medications include (see chapter 21 for details) the following:

Acetaminophen	500–100 mg Q4–6 hr, maximum 2.5–3 g/day
NSAIDs	
Aspirin	650 mg Q6 hr
Ibuprofen	400–600 mg Q4–6 hr, maximum 1200 mg/day
Naproxen sodium	275–550 mg Q6–8 hr, maximum 1375 mg/day
Ketoprofen	75 mg Q6 hr
Keterolac	IM injection of 60 mg followed by 10 mg Q8 hr for 5 days
Celecoxib	100–200 mg BID

The most significant side effect of the NSAIDs is gastrointestinal discomfort in up to 15–20% of patients, and some clinicians suggest that these medications be taken with food.

The use of some, possibly all, NSAIDs may negate the purpose of low-dose (81 mg) aspirin taken daily for cardiovascular reasons.

These medications are frequently sold in combination with other drugs such as caffeine, which exerts no specific analgesic effects, but may potentiate the analgesic effects of aspirin and acetaminophen. There are aspirin–caffeine combination drugs (Anacin®) and aspirin, and acetaminophen and caffeine combinations (Excedrin Extra-Strength®, Excedrin Migraine®, and Vanquish®). The recommended dosage is two tablets every six hours as needed.

The biggest problem is that taking aspirin, acetaminophen, or combination tablets daily or even every other day for a week or more (possibly less) can induce the problem of medication overuse headache (which will be discussed later).

There are a number of NSAIDs that are prescribed. Because of the variability in their efficacy, pharmacokinetics, and side effects, patients may need to be tried on more than one, sequentially, not in combination, to determine the best one for them.

Muscle Relaxants

Muscle relaxants are given for acute tension-type headache by some clinicians. They are probably best utilized during the first three weeks postinjury-related headache. They are useful in patients with significant muscle spasm and pain, which may be seen in acute PTTHA, but which is not usually seen with an episodic tension-type headache. They are used appropriately after the development of muscle spasm after an injury such as a slip and fall, motor vehicle accident, work and athletic injuries, or overstretching.

These medications work via the development of a therapeutic plasma level. Their exact mechanism of action is unknown, but they do not directly affect striated muscles, the myoneural junction, or motor nerves. They produce relaxation by depressing the central nerve pathways, possibly through their effects on higher CNS centers, which modifies the central perception of pain without affecting the peripheral pain reflexes or motor activity.

They are most typically given with an NSAID.

These medications include (see chapter 16 for details) the following:

Carisoprodol	350 mg Q6–8 hr
Chlorzoxazone	500 mg TID
Metaxalone	Recommended dose is 2400–3200 mg/day in divided doses (tablets are 400 mg each)
Methocarbamol	500–750 mg TID
Orphenedrine citrate	IM dose is 2 mg, IV dosage is 60 mg, oral form 100 mg Q12 hr (has anticholinergic effects, and should be contraindicated in patients with glaucoma, prostatic enlargement. or bladder outlet obstruction)

Typically these medications are given for 7 to 10 days.

Many of these medications are given in combination with other drugs, including barbiturates (butalbital and meprobamate) and narcotics (codeine, oxycodone, propoxyphene, etc.) This is probably not a good idea, as the barbiturates and narcotics can easily help develop patient dependence; also, in the MTBI patient, these medications can help induce decreased cognition.

For patients with extreme pain on an acute basis, the use of tramadol hydrochloride (50–100 mg every four to six hours) may be helpful. This medication appears to bind to the opioid receptors as well as inhibit the reuptake of serotonin and norepinephrine. Other patients may need an opioid such as codeine or Hydrocodone. These medications should be given for up to 7 to 10 days, if necessary. One published rule of thumb notes that immediate-relief analgesic medication of any kind should be taken no more than two days a week to prevent medication overuse headache (MOH).

Narcotic medications should not be used, if they can be avoided, for the patient with acute TTHA, as the risk of dependence, as well as MOH, is too great.

It may be appropriate to include a short course of physical therapy on an acute basis for patients with significant myofascial findings (97).

Simple acute posttraumatic tension-type headache is a problem that headache specialists are rarely called in to see. It is the patient's family physician or chiropractor who most frequently sees this problem.

One of the most important treatments is most often forgotten—simply educating the patient as to what exactly is going on. Patients need explanations as to what is causing their pain and what is being done to help them as well as how a particular medication or treatment helps in their particular problem. This is even more important for the patients with chronic PTHA.

Medication Management of Chronic Posttraumatic Tension-Type Headache

The medication treatment of choice is the tricyclic antidepressants (TCAs).

The TCA medication of choice is amitriptyline, a sedating tricyclic antidepressant. Like all of the tricyclics, it works in the synapse to decrease the reuptake of serotonin and (depending on the individual medication) norepinephrine. Amitriptyline, unlike the other TCAs, also works to repair the damage in stage 4 sleep architecture. It is the most sedating tricyclic. The typical dosage is between 10 and 50 mg at night. The author has found it rare to need more than 20 or 30 mg at night.

Amitriptyline appears to have prophylactic treatment ability secondary to its blockade of serotonin and noradrenergic reuptake in the central nervous system. It has been noted that amitriptyline may also act as an N-methyl-D-aspartate (NMDA) receptor antagonist (98). The analgesic effects of amitriptyline may result from this ability (99). NMDA receptor activation is prominently involved in the development of sensitization of the spinal cord dorsal horn, which appears to be found in chronic tension-type headache patients, particularly if the hypothesis of central sensitization in these patients is correct, as this clinical fact could indicate.

Treatment with amitriptyline may also be associated with a reduction in myofascial tenderness, probably secondary to segmental reduction in central sensitization along with the peripheral antinociceptive activity (100).

Doxepin® is also a very good tricyclic. Anticholinergic side effects such as sedation are reduced (but not by much) when compared to amitriptyline. It does *not* work on the sleep architecture. It is used at the same dosage levels as of amitriptyline.

Notice that the tricyclics are not used in their antidepressant dosages, anywhere from 100 to 350 mg a day. Even though the doses are low, their effectiveness in the treatment of chronic posttraumatic tension-type headache is there.

While selective serotonin reuptake inhibitor (SSRIs) have little if any antinociceptive activity, the clinician can also safely combine 10 to 40 mg of Prozac® or Paxil®, or 50 mg of Zoloft® (used for depression) with a small dose of amitriptyline or doxepin (10–30 mg) at night. Inappropriate dosages of these two forms of medications can, rarely, induce the serotonin syndrome.

SNRIs (serotonin–norepinephrine reuptake inhibitors) appear to have a more antinociceptive activity. Duloxetine is FDA approved for neuropathic pain and fibromyalgia, as well as "chronic pain." It can be used, typically, at 60 mg Qday or BID. It is not FDA approved for headache.

Do not combine these medications with the MAO inhibitors.

Muscle relaxants for chronic muscle spasm appear to work better than the acute muscle relaxants. They include Clonazepam®, a fifth-generation form of benzodiazepine. It is GABAnergic in effect. It works at the level of the internuncial neurons of the spinal cord to enhance muscle relaxation. It helps, a bit, with anxiolysis. It has a side effect of sedation. In doses of 4 to 12 mg a day, it acts as an anticonvulsant. At smaller doses, 0.5 mg to 3 mg given at night, it is very useful in the treatment of patients with chronic tension-type headache posttraumatic or otherwise. The sedation lasts for a shorter time than the sedation from tricyclics, and this, itself, is useful.

Tizanidine is a good choice of medication after the first three weeks or so have gone by and the patient is still exhibiting painful neuromuscular spasm. Tizanidine is an alpha-2 noradrenergic agonist (101,102). Dosages should be slowly increased, starting at 1 to 2 mg at night and slowly increasing to 20 to 24 mg. Maximum dosage is 36 mg in divided dosages, typically found in patients who need an antimyotonic. Interestingly, this medication appears to decrease muscle pain while providing its antimyotonic effects.

In the opinion of the author, treating patients with chronic posttraumatic tension-type headache with tricyclics, physical therapy, psychotherapy, etc., will not work if the patient is taking analgesic medications of any type daily or four times a week. In the presence of medication overuse headache, nothing will show long-lasting effectiveness until the chronic analgesics are stopped. More information regarding the appropriate use of medications can be obtained from any clinical pharmacology text (103).

Nonmedication treatments may include physical therapy (97), biofeedback-assisted relaxation (104), as well as a trial of percutaneous electrical nerve stimulation (105).

If these simple individual treatments fail, the treatment of CPTTHA is best accomplished via an interdisciplinary rehabilitation approach, the main purpose of which is NOT to "teach the patient to live with the headache," but to properly diagnose and effectively ameliorate or stop the patient's headache.

Drug detoxification is typically the necessary first step, whether the patient is overutilizing simple, over-the-counter analgesics, or narcotics or barbiturates. Chronic daily analgesics appear to prevent appropriate functioning of the endogenous opiate system (EOS) (via negative neurochemical feedback loops) and other associated antinociceptive systems, inducing analgesic-rebound headaches (now called medication overuse headaches), which are secondary problems from the medications that induce headache secondary to purely neurochemical/neurophysiological changes. Vascular rebound headaches from overutilization of vasoconstrictors may also occur and must be stopped before other treatment is applied. Clinically, an effective way to detoxify CTTHA patients is following the repetitive DHE-45 protocol described by Raskin (106). Concurrently, prophylactic medications should be started. The use of prophylactic medications, as well as physical therapy and other treatments given while a patient is enduring analgesic-rebound headaches is an ineffectual waste of time and money.

One study of 34 patients with PTHA and the postconcussion syndrome found that the repetitive use of DHE-45 and metaclopramide induced improvement in headache in 85% of patients, improved memory in 94%, improved sleep in 94%, and decreased dizziness in 88% (107). Many of the postconcussive syndrome improvements might have been secondary to the diminution of headache pain.

Another small study found the use of subcutaneous sumatritptan (6 mg) to be useful when treating PTHA that is refractory to other medication treatment (108).

The use of divalproex sodium was found to be a safe, effective treatment for patients with persistent chronic daily posttraumatic headaches in a study that did not differentiate migraine from nonmigrainous PTHA (109). Sodium valproate is a good anticonvulsant choice for the patient with TBI as it does not produce any further cognitive decline, unlike Dilantin®, Phenobarbital®, or Neurontin® (9).

Patients with posttraumatic migraine may use triptans to abort them, and topiramate (50–200 mg/day) or divalproax (250 mg BID-TID) for migraine prophylaxis. Many patients with this disorder also have acute and/or chronic PTTHA.

After detoxification, an outpatient interdisciplinary headache rehabilitation program utilizing neuropharmacological therapy (to restore neurochemical homeostasis), physical therapy (97), psychotherapy, and stress management (including biofeedback-enhanced neuromuscular reeducation and muscle relaxation) is the most time- and cost-effective treatment. Optimal psychotherapy or physical therapy regimes, by themselves, will not resolve myofascial difficulties or depression if the affective, sleep and central nervous system neurochemical dysmodulation affecting them is not concurrently and appropriately treated. The interdisciplinary treatment paradigm also enables fine-tuning of diagnosis and possible determination of a secondary or "hidden" etiology for a patient's headaches.

In patients with recalcitrant soft tissue pain problems, the use of botulinum toxin A or B to decrease muscle spasm and pain has increased significantly (110,111). However, several randomized, placebo-controlled studies do not support the effectiveness of botulinum toxin in the treatment of headache, particularly migraine (112,113). In one randomized study (114) no improvement in primary or secondary pain endpoints was found after six weeks. Similar findings were found in a study of episodic tension-type headache (115).

Future use of nitric oxide synthase inhibitors may also promise to bring headache relief (116,117). These studies indicate that the locus for nociception for CPHTA is found in the brain stem, not the peripheral nervous system.

The use of the interdisciplinary pain management paradigm to treat these patients also enables early goal setting and continued education throughout the evaluation and treatment process.

Failure to treat the chronic PTTHA patient with an interdisciplinary, whole-person approach (Fig. 1) is responsible for multiple treatment failures as well as monetary waste, as long-term response—headache remediation—is most often not achieved.

REFERENCES

1. Brown SJ, Fann SR, Grant I. Postconcussional disorder: time to acknowledge a common source of neurobehavioral comorbidity. J Neuropsychiatry Clin Neurosci 1994; 6:15–22.
2. Langlois JA, Rutland-Brown W. Thomas KE. Traumatic brain injury in the United States: emergency Department visits, hospitalizations and deaths. Atlanta, GA. Centers for Disease Control and Prevention, National Center for Injury Prevention and Control, 2004.
3. Cady RK, Farmer K. Posttraumatic headache. In: Windsor RE, Lox DM, eds. Soft Tissue Injuries: Diagnosis and Treatment. Philadelphia, PA: Hanley & Belfus, 1998: 207–224.
4. Elkind AH. Posttraumatic headache. In: Diamond S, Dalessio DJ, eds. The Practicing Physician's Approach to Headache. 5th ed. Baltimore, MD: Williams & Wilkins, 1992:146–161.
5. Marcus DA. Disability and chronic posttraumatic headache. Headache 2003; 43(2):117–121.
6. World Health Organization. ICD-10 guide for headaches. Cephalalgia 1997; 17(S19):1–82.
7. Headache Classification Subcommittee of the International Headache Society. The international classification of headache disorders. 2nd ed. Cephalalgia 2004; (Suppl 1):1–152.
8. Kay T, Harrington DE, Adams R, et al. Definition of mild traumatic brain injury. J Head Trauma Rehabil 1993; 8(3):86.
9. Jay GW. Minor Traumatic Brain Injury Handbook: Diagnosis and Treatment. Boca Raton, FL: CRC Press, 2000.
10. Couch JR, Bearss C. Chronic daily headache in the posttrauma syndrome: relation to extent of head injury. Headache 2001; 41(6):559–564.
11. Uomoto JM, Esselman PC. Traumatic brain injury and chronic pain: differential types and rates by head injury severity. Arch Phys Med Rehabil 1993; 74(1):61–64.
12. Martelli MF, Grayson RL, Zasler ND. Posttraumatic headache: neuropsychological and psychological effects and treatment implications. J Head Trauma Rehabil 1999; 14(1):49–69.
13. Packard R, Ham LP. Posttraumatic headache. J Neuropsychiatry Clin Neurosci 1994; 6(3):229–236.
14. Yagamuchi M. Incidence of headache and severity of head injury. Headache 1992; 32:427–431.
15. Jennet B, Frankowski RF. The epidemiology of head injury. In: Braakman R, ed. Handbook of Clinical Neurology. Elsevier: New York, 1990:116.
16. Radanov BP, Di Stefano G, Augustiny KF. Symptomatic approach to posttraumatic headache and its possible implications for treatment. Eur Spine J 2001; 10(5): 403–407.

17. Keidel M, Diener HC. Posttraumatic headache. Nervenarzt 1997; 68(10):769–777.
18. Jacobsen SA. The Posttraumatic Syndrome Following Head Injury. Springfield, IL: Charles C. Thomas, 1963:63–65.
19. Claussen CF, Claussen E. Neurootological contributions to the diagnostic follow-up after whiplash injuries. Acta Otolaryngol Suppl 1995; 520(Pt 1):53–56.
20. Packard RC, Ham LP. Posttraumatic headache: determining chronicity. Headache 1993; 33(3):133–134.
21. Packard RC, Weaver R, Ham LP. Cognitive symptoms in patients with posttraumatic headache. Headache 1993; 33(7):365–368.
22. Alberti A, Sarchielli P, Mazzotta G, et al. Event related potentials in posttraumatic headache. Headache 2001; 41(6):579–585.
23. Solomon S. Posttraumatic headache. Med Clin North Am 2001; 85(4):987–996.
24. Lemka M. Headache as the consequence of brain concussion and contusion in closed head injuries in children. J Neurol Neurochir Pol 1999; 33(Suppl 5):37–48.
25. Linder SL. Post-traumatic headache. Curr Pain Headache Rep 2007; 11:396–400.
26. Callaghan M, Abu Arafeh I. Chronic posttraumatic headache in children and adolescents. Dev Med Child Neurol 2001; 43(12):819–822.
27. Sakas DE, Whittaker KW, Whitwell HL, et al. Syndromes of posttraumatic neurological deterioration in children with no focal lesions revealed by cerebral imaging: evidence for a trigeminovascular pathophysiology. Neurosurgery 1997; 41(3): 661–667.
28. Keidel M, Diener HC. Post-traumatic headache. Nervenarzt 1997; 68:769–777.
29. Kojadinovic Z, Momcilovic A, Popovic L, et al. Brain concussion—a minor craniocerebral injury. Med Pregl 1998; 51:165–168.
30. Muller GE. Atypical early posttraumatic syndromes. Acta Neurol Belg 1974; 74: 163–181.
31. Duckro PN, Chibnall JT, Tomazic TJ. Anger, depression, and disability: a path analysis of relationships in a sample of chronic posttraumatic headache patients. Headache 1995; 35(1):7–9.
32. Fordyce CJ, Roueche JR, Prigatano GP. Enhanced emotional reactions in chronic head trauma patients. J Neurol, Neurosurg Psychiatry 1982; 46:62–624.
33. Hickling EJ, Blanchard EB, Schwartz SP, et al. Headaches and motor vehicle accidents: results of the psychological treatment of post-traumatic headache. Headache Q 1992; 3:285–289.
34. Hoge CW. McGurk D, Thomas JL, et al. Mild traumatic brain injury in US soldiers returning from Iraq. N Engl J Med 2008; 358(5):453–463.
35. Lake AE, Branca B, Lutz TE, et al. Headache level during neuropsychological testing and test performance in patients with chronic posttraumatic headache. J Head Trauma Rehabil 1999; 14(1):70–80.
36. Denny-Brown D, Russell WR. Experimental cerebral concussion. Brain 1941; 64:93.
37. Solomon S. John Graham Senior Clinicians Award Lecture. Posttraumatic migraine. Headache 1998; 38(10):772–778.
38. Jay GW. Headache Handbook: Diagnosis and Treatment. Boca Raton, FL: CRC Press, 1999:17–32.
39. Packard RC, Ham LP. Pathogenesis of posttraumatic headache and migraine: a common headache pathway? Headache 1997; 37:42–52.
40. Buchholz DW, Reich SG. The menagerie of migraine. Semin Neurol 1996; 16: 83–93.
41. Leisman G. Lateralized effects of migraine and ANS seizures after closed head injury. Int J Neurosci 1990; 54:63–82.
42. Schmidtke K, Ehmsen L. Transient global amnesia and migraine. A case control study. Eur Neurol 1998; 40:9–14.
43. Vohanka S, Zouhar A. Transient global amnesia after mild head injury in childhood. Act Nerv Super (Praha) 1988; 30:68–74.
44. Sallis RE, Jones K. Prevalence of headaches in football players. Med Sci Sports Exerc 2000; 32(11):1820–1824.

45. Collins MW, Field M, Iverson, et al. Relationship between postconcussion headache and neuropsychological test performance in high school athletes. Am J Sports Med 2003; 31(2):168–173.

46. Lovell MR, Collins MW, Iverson GL, et al. Recovery from mild concussion in high school athletes. J Neurosurg 2003; 98(2):296–301.

47. McBeath JG, Nanda A. Roller coaster migraine: an underreported injury? Headache 2000; 40(9):745–747.

48. Harrison DW, Walls RM. Blindness following minor head trauma in children: a report of two cases with a review of the literature. J Emerg Med 1990; 8:21–24.

49. Harker LA, Rassekh C. Migraine equivalent as a cause of episodic vertigo. Laryngoscope 1988; 98:160–164.

50. Baloh RW. Neurotology of migraine. Headache 1997; 37:615–621.

51. Vohanka S, Zouhar A. Benign posttraumatic encephalopathy. Act Nerv Super (Praha) 1990; 32:179–183.

52. Duckro PN, Greenberg M, Schultz KT, et al. Clinical factors of chronic post-traumatic headache. Headache Q 1992; 3:295–308.

53. Jay GW. Chronic Pain. New York: Informa Healthcare, 2007:193–222.

54. Speed WG. Muscle contraction headaches. In: Saper JR, ed. Headache Disorders. Boston: John Wright, 1983:115.

55. Diamond S, Dalessio DJ. The Practicing Physicians Approach to Headache. 3rd ed. Baltimore, MD: Williams and Wilkins, 1980.

56. Dorpat TL, Holmes TH. Mechanisms of skeletal muscle pain and fatigue. Arch Neurol Psychiatry 1955; 74:628.

57. Perl S, Markle P, Katz LN. Factors involved in the production of skeletal muscle pain. Arch Intern Med 1934; 53:814.

58. Hong S, Kniffki K, Schmidt R. Pain abstracts. Second World Congress on Pain, 1978; 1:58.

59. Mense S. Nociception from skeletal muscle in relation to clinical muscle pain. Pain 1993; 54:241–289.

60. Mork H, Ashina M, Bendtsen L, et al. Induction of prolonged tenderness in patients with tension-type headache by means of a new experimental model of myofascial pain. Eur J Neurol 2003; 10:249–256.

61. Moskowitz MA, Cutrer FM. Sumatriptan: a receptor-targeted treatment for migraine. Ann Rev Med 1993; 44:145–154.

62. Rodbard S. Pain associated with muscle contraction. Headache 1970; 10:105.

63. Martin PR, Mathews AM. Tension headaches: psychophysiological investigation and treatment. J Psychosom Res 1978; 22:389.

64. Sakuta M. Significance of flexed posture and neck instability as a cause of chronic muscle contraction headache. Rinsho Shinkeigato 1990; 30:254.

65. Riley TL. Muscle-contraction headache. Neurol Clin 1983; 1:489.

66. Philips C. Tension headache: theoretical problems. Behav Res Ther 1978; 16:249.

67. Philips C, Hunter MS. A psychophysiological investigation of tension headache. Headache 1982; 22:173.

68. Simons DJ, Day E, Goodell H, et al. Experimental studies on headache: muscles of the scalp and neck as sources of pain. Assoc Res Nerv Ment Dis Proc 1943; 23:228.

69. Robinson CA. Cervical spondylosis and muscle contraction headaches. In: Dalessio DJ, ed. Wolff's Headache and Other Head Pain. 4th ed. New York: Oxford University Press, 1980:362.

70. Haynes SN, Cuevas J, Gannon LR. The psychophysiological etiology of muscle-contraction headache. Headache 1982; 22:122.

71. Bakal DA, Kaganov JA. Muscle contraction and migraine headache: psychophysiologic comparison. Headache 1977; 17:208.

72. Cohen MJ. Psychological studies of headache: is there a similarity between migraine and muscle contraction headaches? Headache 1978; 18:189.

73. Anderson CD, Franks RD. Migraine and tension headache: is there a physiological difference? Headache 1981; 21:63.

74. Pozniak-Patewicz E. Cephalgic spasm of head and neck muscles. Headache 1976; 15:261.
75. Jay GW. The autonomic nervous system: anatomy and pharmacology. In Raj P, ed. Pain Medicine—A Comprehensive Review. St. Louis, MO: Mosby, 1996: 461–465.
76. Jay GW. Sympathetic aspects of myofascial pain. Pain Digest 1995; 5:192–194.
77. Shealy CN. Spinally mediated headache. In: Cady RK, Fox AW, eds. Treating the Headache Patient. New York: Marcel Dekker, 1995:235–256.
78. Jay GW. Cluster headache. Encyclopedia of Life Sciences. London: Elsevier, 2001.
79. Langemark M, Jensen K. Myofascial mechanisms of pain. In: Olesen J, Edvinsson L, eds. Basic Mechanisms of Headache. Amsterdam: Elsevier, 1988:321.
80. Iansek R, Heywood J, Karnaghan J, et al. Cervical spondylosis and headaches. Clin Exp Neurol 1987; 23e:175.
81. Sjaastad O, Fredriksen TA, Pfaffenrath V. Cervicogenic headache diagnostic criterion. Headache 1990; 30:725–726.
82. Bogduk N. The anatomical basis for cervicogenic headache. J Manipulative Physiol Ther 1992; 15:67–70.
83. Blume HG. Diagnosis and treatment modalities of cervicogenic headaches. Head and Neck Pain, Newsletter of the Cervicogenic Headache International Study Group, 1997; 4:1–2.
84. Forsell H. Mandibular dysfunction and headache. Proc Finn Dent Soc suppl II 1985; 81:591.
85. Mikail M, Rosen H. History and etiology of myofascial pain-dysfunction syndrome. J Prosthet Dent 1980; 44:438.
86. Magnusson T, Carlsson GE. Comparison between two groups of patients in respect to headache and mandibular dysfunction. Swed Dent J 1978; 2:85.
87. Magnusson T, Carlsson GE. Recurrent headaches in relation to temporomandibular joint pain-dysfunction. Acta Odontol Scand 1978; 36:333.
88. Packard RC. Chronic post-traumatic headache: associations with mild traumatic brain injury, concussion and post-concussive disorder. Curr Pain Headache Rep 2008; 12:67–73.
89. Povlishock JT, Becker DP, Cheng CL, et al. Axonal change in minor head injury. J Neuropathol Exp Neurol 1983; 42:225–242.
90. Nevin NC. Neuropathological changes in the white matter following head injury. J Neuropathol Exp Neurol 1967; 26:77–84.
91. Iverson GL, Lange RT, Gaetz M, et al. Mild TBI. In: Zasler ND, Katz KI, Zafonte RD, eds. Brain Injury Medicine. New York: Demos, 2007:333–372.
92. Langemark M, Jensen K, Jensen TS, et al. Pressure pain thresholds and thermal nociceptive thresholds in chronic tension-type headache. Pain 1989; 38:203.
93. Bendtsen L. Central sensitization in tension-type headache: possible pathophysiologic mechanisms. Cephalalgia 2000; 20:486–508.
94. Bendtsen L, Jensen R, Olesen J. Qualitatively altered nociception in chronic myofascial pain. Pain 1996; 65:259–264.
95. Ashina M, Lassen LH, Bendtsen L, et al. Effect of inhibition of nitric oxide synthase on chronic tension-type headache: a randomized crossover trial. Lancet 1999; 353:287.
96. Ashina M, Bendtsen L, Jensen R, et al. Possible mechanisms of action of nitric oxide synthase inhibitors in chronic tension-type headache. Brain 1999; 122:1629.
97. Jay GW, Brunson J, Branson SJ. The effectiveness of physical therapy in the treatment of chronic daily headaches. Headache 1989; 29:156.
98. Olesen J. Clinical and pathophysiologic observations in migraine and tension-type headache explained by integration of vascular, supraspinal and myofascial inputs. Pain 1991; 46:125–132.
99. Watanabe Y, Saito H, Abe K. Tricyclic antidepressants block NMDA receptor-mediated synaptic responses and induction of long-term potentiation in rat hippocampal slices. Neuropharmacology 1993; 32:479–486.

100. Eisenach JC, Gebhart GF. Intrathecal amitriptyline acts as an *N*-methyl-D-aspartate receptor antagonist in the presence of inflammatory hyperalgesia in rats. Anesthesiology 1995; 83:1046–1054.
101. Bendtsen L, Jensen R. Amitriptyline reduces myofascial tenderness in patients with chronic tension-type headache. Cephalalgia 2000; 20:603–610.
102. Sayers AC, Burki HR, Eichenberger E. The pharmacology of 5-chloro-4-(2-imidazolin-2gamma-1-amino)-2,1,3-benzothiadiazole (DS 103 282), a novel myotonic agent. Arzneimittelforschung 1980; 30:793–803.
103. Koch P, Hirst DR, von Wartburg BR. Biological fate of sirdalud in animals and man. Xenobiotica 1989; 19:1255–1265.
104. Professional's Handbook of Drug Therapy for Pain. Pennsylvania: Springhouse, 2001.
105. Ham LP, Packard RC. A retrospective, follow-up study of biofeedback-assisted relaxation therapy in patients with posttraumatic headache. Biofeedback Self Regul 1996; 21(2):93–104.
106. Raskin NH. Headache. 2nd ed. New York: Churchill Livingstone, 1988.
107. Ahmed HE, White PF, Craig WF, et al. Use of percutaneous electrical nerve stimulation (PENS) in the short-term management of headache. Headache 2000; 40(4): 311–315.
108. McBeath JG, Manda A. Use of dihydroergotamine in patients with postconcussion syndrome. Headache 1994; 34(3):148–151.
109. Gawel MG, Rothbart P, Jacobs H. Subcutaneous sumatriptan in the treatment of acute episodes of posttraumatic headache. Headache 1993; 33(2):96–97.
110. Gobel H, Heinze A, Heinze-Kuhnk A, et al. Evidence-based medicine: botulinum toxin A in migraine and tension-type headache. J Neurol 2001; 248(Suppl 1):34–38.
111. Argoff C. successful treatment of chronic daily headache with Myobloc. Poster presented at the 21st Annual Scientific Meeting of the American Pain Society, Baltimore, MD, March 14–17, 2002.
112. Smuts JA, Baker MK, Smuts HM, et al. Botulinum toxin-type A as prophylactic treatment in chronic tension-type headache. Cephalalgia 1999; 19:454.
113. Gobel H, Lindner V, Krack P, et al. Treatment of chronic tension-type headache with botulinum toxin. Cephalalgia 1999; 19:455.
114. Rollnik JD, Tanneberger O, Schubert M, et al. Treatment of tension-type headache with botulinum toxin-type A: a double-blind, placebo-controlled study. Headache 2000; 40:300.
115. Eros EJ, Doric DW. The effects of botulinum toxin-type A on disability in episodic and chronic migraine [abstract]. Presented at the American Headache Society Meeting, June 21–23, 2002. Seattle, WA.
116. Keidel M, Rieschke P, Juptner M, et al. Pathological jaw opening reflex after whiplash injury. Nervenarzt 1994; 65(4):241–249.
117. Keidel M, Rieschke P, Stude P, et al. Antinociceptive reflex alteration in acute posttraumatic headache following whiplash injury. Pain 2001; 92(3):319–326.

4   Cervicogenic Headache

Frederick R. Taylor

University of Minnesota School of Medicine and Park Nicollet Health Services,
Minneapolis, Minnesota, U.S.A.

THE DISORDER

Neck pain and cervical muscle tenderness are common and prominent symptoms of primary headache disorders (1,2). Less commonly, head pain may actually arise from bony structures or soft tissues of the neck, a condition known as cervicogenic headache (CeH) (2,3). While the source of the abnormality in CeH resides in the cervical area, the nature and localization of the lesion seem to vary from case to case. CeH, accordingly, is a syndrome, not a disease (4,5). CeH syndrome as described by Sjaastad presents clinically as (*i*) unilateral referred headache of fluctuating intensity triggered by movement of the head/neck or posture; (*ii*) unilateral headache triggered by pressure on the neck; (*iii*) unilateral headache spreading to the neck and ipsilateral shoulder/arm, all originating from either structural cervical bones and/or soft tissue damage (6).

Upper neck pain and cervical muscle tenderness and tightness are common and often prominent in primary headache disorders, especially tension-type and migraine headaches, and are not CeH merely because of occipital or posterior location. It is insufficient to label posterior headache with neck pain as cervicogenic because such complaints can be found in virtually all ages (7). It is also insufficient to label posterior headache in the presence of degenerative C-spine disease as cervicogenic because such changes can be found in virtually all people over 40 years of age and 67% of 17 year olds with headache with or without neck pain (7–9). Strictly anterior/temporal or ocular pain is not CeH while posteriorly predominant, strictly unilateral head pain may or may not be CeH. When pain originates from, i.e., the source of the pain is from, either cervical boney structures or soft tissues, the condition is known as CeH. Typically, this pain is strictly unilateral and posteriorly predominant. In 97% of cases in the Vaga study of CeH, pain exacerbations began in the neck/occipital region; yet pain may radiate anteriorly to the ipsilateral temple/eye or contralateral occipital region. While cervicogenic traits (mechanical precipitation, etc.) are frequently present in CeH, "migraine traits," like nausea, vomiting, and throbbing, are rarely present (10). These major and systematic differences indicate that CeH has a different nature than primary headaches: tension-type headache (TTH)/migraine without aura (MwoA) are unlikely to be CeH variants. Equally, CeH is unlikely to be a TTH or an MwoA variant (10). While the source for CeH pain is in the neck, much debate still exists regarding its pathophysiology.

Prevalence

Authors on CeH do not all use the same criteria perhaps explaining the reported variation in the frequency of CeH in the population. Prevalence estimates range from 0.4% to 2.5% of the general population to 15–20% of patients with chronic headaches (11). Patients' mean age is 42.9 years with a 4:1 female predisposition with chronic tendency (11). In the most recent prevalence data published, Sjaastad from the Vågå study reported a prevalence of 4.1% (10). The prevalence data define CeH as one of the three large, recurrent headaches.

DIAGNOSIS

Diagnostic criteria have been established for CeH. The first preliminary "criteria" were based on 11 patients and published in 1987 but ignored by the International Classification of Headache Disorders (ICHD)-I published in 1988 (12). 1990 brought the release of finalized criteria (6), which were supported by the International Association for the Study of Pain in 1994 under section VII-2 with latest revision in 1998 (13,14). Suijlekom has validated these CeH criteria and found that, generally, they function (15). The ICHD-2004 adopted its first set of criteria encoded as 11.2.1 CeH (16).

Occasionally, CeH presenting characteristics may be difficult to distinguish from primary headache disorders such as migraine, tension-type headache, or hemicrania continua (2). To the clinician, CeH is a headache related to structural problems in the neck and is most probable to definite when the patient presents with unilateral, side-locked, nonthrobbing pain that starts in the neck, spreads to the ipsilateral temple, forehead or eye without contralateral spread, and may be aggravated or exaggerated by neck movements or tender points in the neck. The Cervicogenic Headache International Study Group diagnostic criteria provide a detailed, clinically useful description and diagnostic methodology for the condition (Fig. 1) (2,6,14). The 1990 criteria listed unilaterality as the first major criteria. Three studies challenged this criterion by looking at unilaterality without side shift and found this characteristic in between 17% and 30% of migraineurs (17–19). Zwart reported that CeH showed significant differences for rotation and flexion/extension, but not for lateral neck movement compared to migraine, tension-type headache, or control subjects, which did not differ between one another (20). The 1998 criteria now feature cervical involvement with provocation of pain, or shoulder and arm pain, as the first major criteria. Anesthetic blockade became the second major criteria in 1998 while it was listed as an "other" criteria in 1990. Sjaastad and colleagues suggest that patients with CeH report a fairly uniform profile of characteristics that point to the neck as the source for the headache (6,21–24). This believed diagnostic profile includes (*i*) intermittent or continuous, nonthrobbing, moderate pain (unless migraine is another superimposed headache disorder) provoked by neck movements or sustained awkward head postures or neck/occiput pressure; (*ii*) unilateral side-locked pain beginning in the neck and spreading anteriorly where it may be maximal; (*iii*) transient relief by anesthetic blockade of the major occipital nerve or the upper cervical roots C2–C3–C4; (*iv*) nonradicular shoulder or arm pain with reduced neck range of motion; (*v*) female gender, especially with a history of neck or head trauma. Sjaastad and colleagues carefully stipulate that CeH is a reaction pattern disorder which may emanate from several structures or processes in the neck including soft tissues. These stipulations are important

—Point I—Symptoms and Signs of Neck Involvement
  (*listed in a surmised sequence of importance; obligatory that
  one or more of phenomena are present*)
—Precipitation of head pain, similar to the usually occurring
  (*suffices as the sole criterion for positivity*)*:
—by neck movement and/or sustained awkward head positioning
  (suffices as the sole criterion for positivity within group, and/or:
—by external pressure over the upper cervical or occipital region on
  the symptomatic side
  (*Provisionally, the combination of the following two points has been
  set forth as a satisfactory combination within Point 1*)
—Restriction of the range of motion (ROM) in the neck*
—Ipsilateral neck, shoulder, or arm pain of a rather vague
  nonradicular nature or, occasionally, arm pain of a radicular nature*
**—Point II—Confirmatory Evidence
  by Diagnostic Anesthetic Blockades**
  (*This is an obligatory point in scientific works.*)
—Point III—Unilaterality of the Head Pain, Without Sideshift
  (*For scientific work, Point III should preferably be adhered to.*)
  HEAD PAIN CHARACTERISTICS
—Point IV
  (*None of the following points is obligatory*)
—Moderate to severe, nonthrobbing, and nonlancinating pain,
  usually starting in the neck
—Episodes of varying duration, or
—Fluctuating, continuous pain
  OTHER CHARACTERISTICS OF SOME IMPORTANCE
—Point V
  (*None of the following points is obligatory*)
—Only marginal effect or lack of effect of indomethacin
—Only marginal effect or lack of effect of ergotamine and
  sumatriptan succinate
  (c) female sex
  (d) not infrequent occurrence of head or indirect neck trauma
  by history, usually of more than only medium severity
  OTHER FEATURES OF LESSER IMPORTANCE
—Point VI
—Various attack-related phenomena, only occasionally present:
—nausea
—phonophobia and photophobia
—dizziness
—ipsilateral "blurred vision"
—difficulties on swallowing
—ipsilateral edema, mostly in the periocular area

*The presence of all three points indicated with asterisk fortifies the diagnosis
(but still Point II is an additional obligatory point for scientific work

FIGURE 1 Major criteria.

in considering both the differential diagnoses and the ultimate best management of this disorder. These original authors created a controversy when they concluded that CeH is extremely common and may be misclassified as migraine without aura.

Common symptoms of a migraine attack include neck pain and muscle tension (1,25,26). Tfelt–Hansen studied 50 patients with typical common migraine during the attack. Eighteen regions of the head and neck were recorded for pain followed by systematic palpation of 26 cranial and neck muscles and tendon insertions. All 50 patients were tender during the attack and tenderness corresponded to pain in all but two cases. The most frequent sites of tenderness were: sternocleidomastoid, anterior temporal, neck and shoulder muscles, the coronoid process, and occipital insertions. Referred pain was found in 73% of patients with sternocleidomastoid referring to temporofrontal area or occiput, occiput to vertex or temporofrontal area, neck to vertex or brow. The tenderest spots were infiltrated with lidocaine 1.5% or saline double blindly. Of a total 48 patients, 26 patients were symptom free after 70 minutes, which was significantly better than with medical treatment ($p < 0.01$) with no difference between lidocaine and saline (25). In another small study by Blau of 50 patients diagnosed with migraine, 64% reported neck pain or stiffness with their attack, 31% with prodrome, 93% during the headache phase, and 31% during recovery. Seven of these subjects reported referred ipsilateral shoulder pain to headache and one patient reported pain referred into the low back region (1). In a larger, more recent study by Kaniecki of 144 patients diagnosed with migraine, 69% described neck pain as "tightness," 17% as "stiffness," and 5% as "throbbing." Fifty-seven percent reported unilateral neck pain with 98% ipsilateral to headache pain. Sixty-one percent reported prodrome neck pain, 92% during the headache phase, and 41% in recovery (26). All of these studies are headache clinic-based with uncertainty to differential consideration of migraine from cervicogenic headache, as the oldest are pre-recognition of CeH with the newest focusing particular attention on differentiating migraine from tension-type headache.

Shoulder and arm pain are considered under the first major criteria in the 1998 CeH revised criteria. Conventional wisdom relates these symptoms to dysfunction at C2–4. Diener reported the first prospective study of cervical disk prolapse involving levels C5–6 through C7-Th1 in 50 patients matched for age and sex to 50 patients with lumbar disk prolapse (27). Computed tomography, myelography, or magnetic resonance imaging proved the cervical disk prolapses. Patients were asked at different time points about headache and neck pain by questionnaires and structured interviews. These data were collected on three occasions: prior to and 7 and 90 days after surgery for the disk prolapse. Twelve of 50 patients with cervical disk prolapse reported new headache and neck pain presurgery. Seven patients (58%) fulfilled the 2004 IHS criteria for CeH. One week after surgery, 8 of 12 patients with cervical disk prolapse and new headache reported to be pain free. One patient was improved and three were unchanged. Three months after cervical prolapse surgery, seven patients were pain free, three improved, and two were unchanged. This prospective study shows an association of low cervical disk prolapse with CeH: headache and neck pain improves or disappears in 80% of patients after surgery for the cervical disk prolapse. These results may change the conventional wisdom that only C2–4 contribute to CeH, as they seem to indicate that pain afferents from the lower cervical roots can converge on the cervical trigeminal nucleus and the nucleus caudalis to cause CeH (27). Caveats include no objective headache calendar data (only retrospective report) with patient surgical selection prior to study lacking specified criteria for the intervention.

Manual Examination
No manual examination findings have been validated as clinically defining CeH. Furthermore, neither the current CeH nor the ICHD-2004 criteria contain recommendations regarding quantitative assessment. Sjaastad et al., in an "entirely tentative approach," grouped five separate factors pertaining to the neck under the umbrella: "features indicative of cervical abnormality." These include tenderness of (*i*) neck muscles, (*ii*) nerves/tendons in the neck/occiput, (*iii*) facet joints, (*iv*) rotation range of motion in the neck, and (*v*) skin-roll test (28).

Diagnostic Testing
Testing, other than by manual examination, is nearly always normal in cases of CeH when the source is accepted as the upper cervical spine segments. Positive diagnostic blockade of cervical structures or its nerve supply is not specific for CeH (29). Nerve blockade is used diagnostically as well as therapeutically (30).

Imaging
Diagnostic imaging such as radiography, magnetic resonance imaging (MRI), and computed tomography (CT) myelography is typically normal at C3 and higher levels of generally agreed upon pathophysiological interest. When abnormal at these levels, imaging does not confirm the diagnosis of CeH but can lend support to its diagnosis (31,32). One study reported no demonstrable differences in the appearance of cervical spine structures on MRI scans when 24 patients with clinical features of CeH were compared with 20 control subjects. Cervical disk bulging was reported equally in both groups (45.5% vs. 45.0%, respectively) (33).

While studied systematically in only several dozen patients, radiological investigative methods, such as standard X-ray of the cervical spine, functional radiographs in flexion and extension, cerebral and cervical CT scans, cerebral angiography, and cervical myelography, did not contribute to the diagnostic work-up of individuals with CH (31,32).

Diagnostic Blocks
According to the ICHD-II diagnostic criteria, evidence that the pain can be attributed to the neck disorder or lesion can be based on abolition of headache following positive diagnostic blockade using placebo or other adequate controls (Criterion C2) (16). The Cervicogenic Headache International Study Group considers anesthetic blockade as the second major criteria for the diagnosis of CeH and obligatory for scientific works (14). An essential feature of a confirmatory diagnosis of CeH is a positive response, i.e., a transient, pain-free period following an appropriate diagnostic nerve block. These diagnostic blocks should be directed to the nerve(s) or anatomical structure(s) suspected of mediating or causing the pain. Appropriate blocks include the greater occipital nerve, the minor occipital nerve, zygapophyseal joints (facet joints), segmental nerves, and intervertebral disks (34,35).

Greater occipital nerve (GON) blockade

In one early study, response at 30 minutes to a GON blockade was significantly more marked in the CeH group [54% (13 of 24 patients)] than in migraine without aura [6% (1 of 14 patients)] or tension-type headache [14% (2 of 14 patients)] (36). Pain reduction in the forehead was generally only found in the CeH patients (77%). Pain reduction (in %) was significantly more marked following the GON than supra-orbital nerve blockade (36). The specificity of GON diagnostic blockade for CeH as well as primary headaches is called into question by several additional studies suggesting limited significance diagnostically. CeH proponents could argue against the validity of subject diagnosis in at least some of these series. Anthony studied 383 migraine subjects with 48% "arrested" for up to four weeks with GON depomedrol injections or several months with surgical division. He wrote that this is "not typical migraine but headache due to neural irritation" or "occipital neuralgia" (37). The same year another smaller series revealed that the GON block was effective in 54% (52 of 97 patients) of migraine and 71% (62 of 87 patients) of post-traumatic headaches (38). In a large clinical survey, D'Amico categorized CeH as "probable" in the absence of diagnostic blockade and "confirmed" with positive response to blockade. Five patients met a "probable" diagnosis of CeH, and three out of five patients responded to blockade and were, therefore, "confirmed" (39). Twenty-seven migraine subjects, "unresponsive to several combinations of pharmacological treatments," were given GON blocks by Caputi "only if such nerves were conspicuously pain sensitive to pressure" and reported significant improvement in 85% (23/27) (40).

Cervical blocks

Bovin et al. evaluated the diagnostic potential of GON, C2–5 nerve, and C2/C3 facet joint blocks in a series of 14 patients with CeH (41). In this study, the GON blockade was completely effective in four of the five responders to C2 nerve blockade; and six of the nine CeH patients had partial pain relief following the C3 nerve block. No patients experienced complete pain relief following the isolated blockade of the C3, C4, or C5 nerves. The C2/C3 facet joint injection gave relief from pain in only two out of nine patients. They argued that the GON is composed of the medial fibers from the dorsal ramus of the C2 nerve and that a blockade of the C2 nerve should relieve the pain in all patients who experience relief following a GON blockade. The C2 blockade should also be effective whether the pain is mediated through the lesser occipital nerve (ventral ramus of C2) or originates from deeper structures innervated by C2 fibers (periosteum of the occiput, vertebrae, etc.) or from the C2 nerve itself. Their results (with the complete effect of the GON blockade in four of the five patients showing the same response to the C2 blockade) suggest that the simpler GON blockade may be sufficient in many patients with CeH (41,42). Inan published a comparative study in 28 patients, 14 with a C2/C3 blockade compared to 14 patients with a GON blockade and reported no significant differences (42).

Differential Diagnosis

The differential diagnosis in cases of suspected CeH is large and could include posterior fossa tumor, Arnold–Chiari malformation, cervical spondylosis or arthropathy, herniated intervertebral disk, spinal nerve compression or tumor, arteriovenous malformation, vertebral artery dissection, and intramedullary or extramedullary spinal tumors.

PATHOPHYSIOLOGY
CeH pathophysiology and source of pain have been debated (2,9,34,43), but the pain is likely referred from one or more osseous, articular, muscular, neurogenic, or vascular structures in the neck (9,44).

Edmeads requires disease or dysfunction of the neck, which causes headache to meet three conditions: (*i*) implicated cervical structures are pain sensitive, (*ii*) the referral pain pattern from neck to head is physiologically based, and (*iii*) the disease or dysfunction is identifiable and verifiable (4,9). Implicated nociceptive cervical structures include vertebral column apophyseal and atlantal–occipital condylar joints, annulus fibrosus and spinal ligaments, and vertebral periosteum; cervical muscles around the spine; cervical nerve roots and nerves; and vertebral arteries (9). The referral pattern from cervical structures to the head can be achieved via C2 sensory roots and extensions, which include the greater and lesser occipital nerves; possibly the C1 sensory root allowing pain referral to the vertex or frontal region; posterior fossa branches of C2 connections to tentorial branches of the trigeminal nerve ophthalmic division allowing referral to the front of the head; and the descending spinal track of the trigeminal nucleus in the upper cervical cord, which intermingle impulses from cervical segments C4 and above with trigeminal cranial nerve V allowing referral from these cervical segments to appropriate, uncrossed locations in the head (4,45,46). This functional convergence of the upper cervical root and trigeminal sensory pathways in the trigeminocervical nucleus allows the bidirectional referral of painful sensations between the neck and trigeminal sensory receptive fields of the face and head (47). A functional convergence of sensorimotor fibers in the spinal accessory nerve (CN XI) and upper cervical nerve roots which ultimately converge with the descending tract of the trigeminal nerve might also be responsible for the referral of cervical pain to the head. Given the generic importance of trigeminal cervical complex neurons in primary headache, the interplay between brainstem modulatory systems and the TCC is likely to play an important role in the expression of many headache phenotypes (47). Numerous developmental anomalies and acquired lesions of the craniovertebral junction and upper cervical spine fulfill Edmeads third requirement of "identifiable and verifiable." These disorders make up the differential diagnosis for suspected CeH as discussed previously under the section "Diagnosis."

Biological Markers
Neurophysiological investigations give some insight into the pathophysiological mechanisms of CeH but are not diagnostic (29).

Calcitonin Gene-Related Peptide
In CeH, calcitonin gene-related peptide levels do not differ between the symptomatic and the asymptomatic side, between the jugular and the cubital blood, and between days with and without headache (48). Unlike migraine, there is no evidence for activation of the trigeminovascular system in CeH. It can be concluded that CeH is not just a migraine variant triggered by neck dysfunction but is different biologically (29).

Cytokines
Cytokine patterns in CeH patients, like those seen in cluster headache, tend toward an inflammatory status. Interleukin-1 beta (IL-1β) and tumor necrosis factor-alpha (TNF-α) exert multifunctional biological effects by promoting and increasing the molecular events of cellular inflammation. Higher levels of both IL-1β and TNF-α were detected in the sera of 15 CeH subjects, both during the natural course of a painful attack and during a phase of mechanically worsened pain, than in that of 15 subjects with migraine without aura during or outside an attack and 15 historically healthy controls. Differences also emerged in CeH between spontaneous and mechanically worsened pain phases (49,50). Although the role of these pro-inflammatory cytokines remains unknown, both IL-1β and TNF-α may promote hyperalgesia in CeH. While not relevant in clinical laboratory testing, this discovery may lead to a potential therapeutic treatment modality (35).

Nitric Oxide
CeH patients exhibit a marked activation of the NO pathway compared with patients with migraine or cluster headache (36). However, NO release resulting from a spontaneous CeH attack and CeH pain elicited by NO donors (NOD) was unchanged. The upregulation of the NO-ergic system cannot be attributed to cerebrovascular dysfunction, but it may be possible that in the presence of reactive oxygen species NO may combine with IL-1β and TNF-α to produce deleterious, proinflammatory, pain producing effects (49–51).

Role of Trauma
Reports are numerous that subjects with CeH very often have a preceding whiplash or other neck or head injury. The validity of acute and chronic whiplash has never been analyzed (52). Stovner in a prospective cohort study of 210 rear-end collision victims with headache reports that headache after this collision lacks specificity both for headache features and prognosis whether or not they fulfilled ICHD-2004 criteria for whiplash. Previous headache was a major risk factor for headache both in the acute and chronic stage (52). This confirmed a prior historical cohort analysis drawing the same conclusion (53). In a retrospective chart review of 2771 Vincent reports, 93 patients suffered from occipital/neck pain either fulfilling or not fulfilling CeH Sjaastad criteria, but not migraine tension-type headache. Previous trauma, not definitely whiplash, was reported in 1.3% of individuals with migraine, 1.5% with TTH, and 15% with neck/CEH (54).

In 587 whiplash victims that were followed up for a year after emergency service consultation, de novo unilateral CeH seemed to be present in 8% ($n = 48$) at six weeks and 3% ($n = 20$) at one year. Previous car accidents, pre-existing headache, and neck pain were more frequent among individuals with chronic CeH than in those without CeH at one year. Those with CeH characteristics were followed up for five more years with 35% ($n = 7$) still having headache, although the frequency had been reduced appreciably. Generally, pain could still generally be precipitated from areas along the occipital tendons ipsilaterally, but interestingly, increased tenderness in these areas could also be found on the previously symptomatic side in now asymptomatic individuals (55,56). The authors conclude that whiplash-related CEH seems similar to, but probably not identical to, non-whiplash CEH, although the natural course seems favorable for unilateral CEH during the first postinjury years (57).

Hormonal Influences

Hormonal influences in CeH are largely unstudied. No peer-reviewed literature exists on hormones, in general or specifically. In the only study available, hormonal influence appears less likely in CeH than in migraine. Approximately 80% of 14 CeH patients during 25 pregnancies had no change in headache pattern while 80% of a control group of 49 migraine women during 116 pregnancies experienced headache improvement (58).

TREATMENT

An important first management step in CeH is to identify any symptomatic forms and treat the underlying cause(s), if possible (4). Medications alone are often ineffective or provide only modest benefit for CeH (2). Successful treatment according to Martelletti usually requires a multifaceted approach using pharmacologic, behavioral, manipulative, anesthetic blockade, and occasionally surgical interventions (35). To these, Grgić specifically adds acupuncture, neural therapy, local botulinum toxin injection, cervical epidural corticosteroid injection, massage, kinesiotherapy, and traction, suggesting that the best results are achieved by a combination of manual therapy, physical therapy, and kinesiotherapy (59). Determining patient beliefs and preferences enhances success since integration of this multifaceted approach demands individualized treatment with patient input. Individualized treatment of CeH is mandatory, while conservative multifaceted-integrated management is preferred in the initial stage and in mild cases, invasive therapy may be the treatment of choice in severe, chronic cases (5).

Pharmaoclogical Treatment

Choices are neither evidence based from double-blind placebo-controlled trials nor package insert based by any governmental agency worldwide. Options are largely anecdotally clinician based, mirroring preventive or palliative treatments used for migraine, tension-type headache, and "neuropathic" pain syndromes.

Acute Treatments

Given that treatment is common to other headache or pain treatment types, individual agent or class agents will not be discussed in detail. The reader is referred to chapters in Section II on either individual or class of agents for specifics. As in other headache syndromes, particularly episodic and chronic migraine, overuse of acute analgesics with development of physical or psychological dependence and medication overuse headache must be an overriding concern. However, since acute medications are often much less effective in CeH, particularly if descriptive migraine characteristics are absent, this may be less frequent in this population. Despite these necessary concerns, the judicious use of acute medications may provide enough pain relief to allow greater patient participation in a physical therapy and rehabilitation programs (2). Analgesics with psychotropic effects, particularly butalbital compounds and opioids, are not recommended for the long-term management of CeH. They may be cautiously prescribed for a very limited time period if they provide temporary pain relief to expedite the advancement of manual modes of therapy or improve tolerance for anesthetic interventions (2,60). Extra special caution is warranted regarding use in those with significant anxiety disorder. Emphasis on medications must be on preventative treatments.

Preventative Treatments

As with recommendations for other headache syndromes, prevention should be started, in a patient naïve to that therapy, at the lowest dose with increments no more rapidly than every one to two weeks over four to eight weeks or even longer. Increments should be individualized to increase patient adherence. Increments should also be based on side effects and dosage needed for 50% or greater improvement in intensity, duration, or frequency or on a quality of headache disability measurement (MIDAS, HIT-6, HDI, MSQ-12) or until a maximum physiologic dosage is achieved. Final dosage should be maintained, ideally, for a minimum of two months prior to determination of failure. Consider that the proof of therapeutic efficacy of preventatives is generally lacking in CeH and that chronic pain syndromes, anecdotally in this practitioner's experience, may respond to multi-drug regimens better than single drug therapy (i.e., multimechanistic approach). If the patient is not responding to monotherapy, the options include higher doses of the single agent or the addition of a second agent while maintaining the initial agent at some dose. The cautious combination of medications from different drug classes, including complementary or alternative medications, or with complementary pharmacologic mechanisms may provide greater efficacy than using individual drugs alone (e.g., an antiepileptic drug combined with a beta-blocker), although the proof of this specific to CeH remains unproven (2,5,61). Duration of preventative treatment is also unknown in CeH. In migraine guidelines, reconsideration for taper or withdrawal is often suggested at three to six months posttherapy initiation, but in a study of this recommendation nearly 50% (38 of 80) of the patients attending a specialized clinic in Spain due to frequent headache needed preventive treatment for more than one year to prevent relapse (62). Follow-up visits will need to be no farther apart than two months, ideally. Initially, we adjust drug dosages and consider determination of the value of serum drug levels or other monitoring, such as EKG in the elderly who are on TCAs or acid–base balance for topiramate or evidence for drug-related toxicities and interactions (particularly serotonin syndrome for those on multiple psychotropics).

Tricyclic Antidepressants (TCAs)

The TCAs have long been used for management of various neuropathic, musculoskeletal, headache, and face pain syndromes. In a Cochrane Review, TCAs had a number needed to treat (NNT) of approximately three for neuropathic pain syndromes (63). Analgesic dosages are typically lower than those required for the treatment of patients with depression (2). The TCAs are the only drug class proven to be effective in tension-type headache, with amitriptyline being the only agent in the class shown to be effective in several controlled trials (64). The literature is without proven trials in CeH, with limited literature addressing its use (65). Treatment recommendations are similar to those previously published for other conditions.

Serotonin Reuptake Inhibitors

There is not a single controlled study in the peer-reviewed, published literature regarding use of this class of agents in CeH. The selective serotonin reuptake inhibitors (SSRIs) are generally ineffective for pain control (2). In a Cochrane Review, the serotonin and norepinephrine reuptake inhibitor (SNRI), venlafaxine hydrochloride, had an NNT of approximately 3 for neuropathic pain syndromes similar to amitriptyline, but with a larger number needed to harm indicating better tolerance (63). Inadequate date exists for any other drug in this class. Venlafaxine is reported efficacious in several open-label and or retrospective studies and one controlled trial for migraine (66). Similar observations are reported for venlafaxine in the treatment of painful diabetic neuropathy, fibromyalgia, and regional myofascial pain syndromes. Duloxetine hydrochloride is used anecdotally in the prophylactic management of migraine, but in the only efficacy analysis performed as a retrospective chart review, duloxetine demonstrated minimal effectiveness (67).

Antiepileptic Drugs (AEDs)

The AEDs are thought of as modulators or stabilizers of peripheral and central pain transmission and are commonly used for the management of neuropathic, headache, and face pain syndromes. There are no trials specific to CeH with AEDs. Only topiramate and gabapentin have been evaluated as prophylactic treatment of CDH in randomized, double-blind, placebo-controlled, or active comparator-controlled trials (68). Zonisamide, in an open-label study of 34 patients with refractory migraine, titrated to dosages of 400 mg per day was statistically significant for improvement (69), while in a chart review of 23 patients with CeH, subtype transformed migraine, zonisamide was ineffective at an average daily dose of 337.9 ± 146.3 mg for an average duration of treatment of 186.4 ± 174.0 days (70).

Antispasticity Agents

There are no studies of baclofen or tizanidine for CeH in the peer-reviewed literature. Baclofen, an agent that acts centrally via GABA(A) receptors, has only two open preventative trials conducted in migraine and cluster headache (71). Both of these studies support its use. Tizanidine, with both a possible peripheral and central effect, has been studied in several clinical trials. One well controlled trial, conducted as a follow-up to an open-label trial in the preventive treatment of chronic daily headache, reported tizanidine as having a statistically significant benefit over placebo (72).

Botulinum Neurotoxins

There are no controlled studies of botulinum neurotoxins for CeH in the peer-reviewed literature. In a double-blind, placebo-controlled single center trial of a refractory, unilateral, cervicothoracic, paraspinal, myofascial pain syndrome, no difference was found between placebo and 50 or 100 units of botulinum neurotoxin A (BoNTA) (73). These same authors in another paper concluded that a single dose treatment of BoNTA without physical therapy is not effective for chronic neck pain (74). Additionally, for the prophylactic treatment of tension-type headache and migraine, no sufficient positive evidence for a successful treatment can be obtained from the randomized, double-blind, and placebo-controlled trials performed so far (75). For the treatment of chronic daily headache (including medication-overuse headache), there is inconsistent positive evidence for subgroups (e.g., patients without other prophylactic treatment) (75,76). The most recent study to date performed in a single headache specialty center analyzed responders compared to nonresponders in two subtypes of CDH, chronic migraine (CM), and chronic tension-type headache (CTTH). A greater percentage of patients with CM responded to BoNTA than patients with CTTH. Predictors of response to BoNTA were headaches that were predominantly unilateral in location, and had scalp allodynia and pericranial muscle tenderness in CM, whereas in CTTH, pericranial muscle tenderness may be a predictor of response (77).

Other Options?
In an open-label pilot study of six patients, infliximab, a biological agent that acts as a cytokine monoclonal antibody against TNF-α, was administered (78). These subjects had severe CeH refractory to local repeated corticosteroid treatment. The protocol used 3 mg/kg and timed infusions at weeks 0, 2, 6, 14 and then every 8 weeks. Infliximab treatment was associated with rapid and sustained effects on CeH pain scores and self-administered analgesic consumption. (Date unpublished) (78). Specific data and longer term observation of this approach to CeH in a larger series of patients are mandatory to confirm the early results of this pilot study before widespread implementation (35).

Physical and Manual Modes of Therapy
To date the effectiveness of physical therapy or exercise in headache has hardly been analyzed (79). Physical and manual modes of therapy are important for the rehabilitation of CeH (80,81). A recent review about manual therapy in CeH found strong evidence that spinal manipulative therapy was effective for reducing headache intensity, duration, and medication intake in CeH, but insufficient to support or refute the efficacy for tension-type HA (79,82,83). A controlled trial of the effectiveness of therapeutic exercise and manipulative treatment for 200 subjects with CeH found no consistent pattern of predictors, although the absence of light-headedness indicated higher odds of success and efficacy was not substantially affected by age, gender, or moderate or severe intensity or headache chronicity suggesting that all patients with CeH could benefit from a trial of manual modes of therapy and physical conditioning (84). In a multicenter, randomized controlled trial of 200 CeH subjects with unblinded treatment for six weeks and blinded outcome assessment at 3, 6, and 12 months, Jull compared the effectiveness of manipulative therapy and a low-load exercise program when used alone and in combination with a control group for CeH (85). At the 12-month follow-up assessment, both manipulative therapy and specific exercise showed significantly reduced headache frequency and intensity, and the neck pain and effects were maintained for all active treatments. The combined therapies were not significantly superior to either therapy alone, but the effect sizes were at least moderate and clinically relevant with 10% more patients gaining relief with the combination (85). In this same study population, the concept of external locus of control, which refers to a high level of belief that results of treatment are influenced primarily by healthcare providers, was examined. Participants with relatively high external Headache-Specific Locus of Control scores were more likely to achieve a reduction in CeH frequency if they received the

combined manipulative therapy and exercise therapy, compared with the control group. The analysis of results reveals the pattern of findings suggesting that characteristics of the therapy were more pertinent than characteristics of the therapist (86). Physical treatment modalities are generally better tolerated when initiated with gentle muscle stretching and manual cervical traction. Therapy can be advanced slowly as tolerated to include strengthening and aerobic conditioning. Biondi, in a review, reported that the efficacy of physical treatment modalities for the long-term prevention and control of headaches appears greatest in patients who are involved in ongoing exercise and physical conditioning programs (81). Biondi also believes that using anesthetic blockade and neurolytic procedures for temporary pain relief can enhance the efficacy and advancement of physical modes of therapy (81).

Injections and Other Invasive Modes of Therapy
If diagnostic blockade of one or other appropriate structures abolishes the pain or, as some suggest, provides substantial pain relief, but temporary as anticipated, treatment can then proceed to consideration of one of a number of invasive procedures. GON and LON blockades are not, at present, considered a long-term treatment modality (35).

Cervical epidural injection with corticosteroids has no place in CeH therapy (35). Surgical procedures such as liberation of the occipital nerves, microvascular decompression of cervical roots and ganglion, neurolysis or neurectomy, and dorsal rhizotomy are not recommended without compelling radiologic evidence for a surgically correctable pathologic condition or a history of refractoriness to all reasonable treatment modalities (2). Surgical decompression via anterior disk surgery with segmental immobilization is increasingly championed (86). Radiofrequency thermal neurolysis is probably most frequently employed, but it is still a controversial therapy (87–89).

Injections

Greater and lesser occipital nerves
Similar relief from headache is achieved with local injections in patients with attacks of strictly unilateral primary headache, migraine, or cluster. This suggests that local injections block the cervico-trigeminal relay. In a subgroup of 41 subjects (VAS <40 mm) with CeH, Vincent reported a significant relief from headache during a seven-day period following infiltration of 0.5% bupivacaine 1 to 2 mL around the ipsilateral greater occipital nerve. The pain was significantly reduced both immediately and as long as seven days after the blockade, with improvement less marked during the first two days (90,91). Of 128 subjects suffering from CeH, injections of depot methylprednisolone into the region of the GON and LON produced complete relief from headache in 169 out of 180 patients for a period ranging from 10 to 77 days, with a mean duration of 23.5 days (92). A published report from Turkey suggested that repeated greater occipital nerve blockade provided efficacy similar to repeated blockade of the C2 and C3 nerves (42). In a different series, repeated nerve stimulator-guided occipital nerve blockade relieved 47 CeH subjects with no recurrence for at least six months in addition to alleviation of associated symptoms. 41/47 (87%) required more than one injection to achieve six month relief (93). The blockade involved

the use of three anesthetics, fentanyl, and clonidine in the mixture (93). These reports suggest that repeated greater occipital nerve blockade in the office setting or anesthesia department are a reasonable treatment option before considering referral for more invasive or more expensive interventions (2), especially with the patient actively participating in physical therapy and exercise modalities. Nevertheless, long-lasting headache relief has only been achieved using local injection therapy in isolated cases (35).

Cervical blocks
Pfaffenrath performed C2 nerve block five times at weekly intervals and the results were successful. In this study, 17 months' pain relief was observed (94). Inan et al. performed a C2/C3 diagnostic blockade with two follow-up therapeutic blocks in 14 CEH patients in comparison with 14 CeH patients with GON blockade with equal pain relief in each group (42).

Epidural therapy
Cervical epidural corticosteroids in nine patients with CeH were compared to a control group of six patients with tension-type headache (95,96). All received a cervical epidural injection with 40 mg methylprednisolone in 3 to 4 ML of saline. The one-month follow-up results revealed CeH subjects with significantly lower scores on the Numeric Pain Intensity Scale. Progressive clinical worsening occurred during a six-month follow-up in the CeH group.

Other Invasive Modes of Therapy

Liberation or neurolysis of the occipital nerve
Surgical liberation of the greater occipital nerve cannot be recommended (97). One hypothesis for such a procedure is that the GON is "entrapped" in the trapezius muscle or surrounding connective tissues. In 50 CeH subjects, surgical liberation, generally under local anesthetic, provided substantial one-week relief that was only temporary. Forty-six percent were pain free and 36% had some relief but with gradual return in 46 of 50 patients over 16 months of follow-up (96). Such a probable compression of the nerve could also be seen at autopsy of presumably headache-free individuals (98,99). Similarly, only temporary pain relief is observed after surgical transaction of the greater occipital nerve (97). Intensification of pain or anesthesia dolorosa is a potential adverse outcome that must be seriously considered when contemplating the use of surgical interventions (2).

Cryoanalgesia
There is no peer-reviewed literature on this technique. After local anesthesia, a cryosonde is brought close to the GON with temperature reduced to $-60°C$ to $-70°C$ for two to three minutes. Analgesia reportedly lasts three months, requiring repeat three to four times per year. Success is claimed in probable CeH to be approximately 60% (30).

Operative decompression of the C2 root and ganglion
Decompression of the C2 root and ganglion requires ligamentous and venous structure removal. Electrocautery of small vessels is essential. For this reason,

Stechison suggests that traumatization of C2 by electrocautery may explain improvements (100). Jansen reported 14/16 with "relieved" to "relative" improvement in a series of 16 subjects with recurrence in 4 (101). Pikus reported 79% improvement in a series of 31 CeH subjects who had, collectively, 35 procedures performed, 80% of whom had prior history of trauma involving the head or neck (102). Operative findings included venous compression of C2 in 86% of cases and a scarred and thickened dorsal atlanto-epistrophic ligament in 66% of cases with bilateral cases amounting to 88%. The two sides did not harbor exactly the same pathology in any case (102). Mean follow-up was 19 months; initial C2 root decompression was successful in achieving long-term, pain-free outcomes in 37% of patients. Another 51% of cases gained adequate relief. Recurrence occurred in 13%, with an average follow-up of 25 months (102). In 2000, Jansen reported on a series of 102 subjects with severe CeH unresponsive to treatment who underwent ganglionectomy or ventral and dorsal decompressive operations. About 80% were relieved of pain or improved during a long period of follow-up (103).

Cervical spine decompression/stabilization: the Smith–Robinson procedure
Nearly, all subjects reported having had spondylosis and osteochondrosis narrowing the spinal canal with radicular pain (cervicobrachialgia) (104). In a preliminary study of 32 patients, cervical levels C4-5, C5-6, C6-7 were singled out as the levels of affection by neurological examination, MRI, CT, anesthetic blockades (positive in all patients), and functional X-ray examinations for cervical decompression/stabilization. Blockades were principally carried out in two ways: (*i*) as localized, extradural, anesthetic procedures ($n = 28$, all positive), and/or (*ii*) as specific root blockades ($n = 8$). These 32 chronic, hard-to-treat, and partly suicidal (no other data) CeH subjects were studied prospectively with removal of one or two disks at one of these levels (5). Of 48 levels operated upon, 26 operations were carried out at the level of C5-6, 14 at C6-7, 8 at C4-5, and 2 at C3-4 (104). During a one- to three-month follow-up of collar wearing, patients generally reported being pain free. Pain recurrence occurred in 12 (not all follow-ups are known to the authors) with recurrence between 1 and 58 months. The mean time for recurrence was 14.8 months. Five patients were well at 3+ years. The authors concluded that this operation should be used in selected, chronic, severely afflicted, preferably elderly CeH patients (5). The authors extended this report to 60 patients: 32 unilateral and 28 bilateral, with 63% of unilateral cases and 64% of bilateral cases enjoying long-lasting pain freedom or >50% improvement. Secondary deterioration occurred in 37% of unilateral patients with mean follow-up of 19.8 months and 36% of bilateral patients with mean follow-up of 25.5 months (104).

Radiofrequency procedures (RF)
The RF procedure is widely used in parts of the world, including the Netherlands, Australia, and the United States, but remains controversial (30).

Under fluoroscopic guidance in RF procedures, the point of a special RF needle is attached to a radiofrequency generator and heated to approximately 80°C coagulating nerve fibers targeted most frequently at the facet joint or nerve innervations from C2-C3 down to C6-C7. The aim is to damage pain fibers thereby reducing the painful stimuli from the joint (30). RF, by its very nature, indicates thermal destruction unless otherwise qualified, as in pulsed RF, which uses very high density brief current pulses to allow for use of less heated probes (maximum 42°C) and no tissue destruction (105,106). According to Bogduk, significant differences exist between thermal and pulsed radiofrequency (106). These differences must be known by practitioners utilizing these techniques. To achieve a good result in the individual patient, nerve roots and disks are targets one needs to treat, in many instances, next to the facet joint (105). A placebo-controlled trial of 24 whiplash subjects showed that the effects of cervical medial branch RF neurotomy were genuine (104,107). Follow-up studies showed that in responders the median duration of complete relief from pain was over 400 days, and that if symptoms recurred, relief could be reinstated by repeat RF neurotomy (87,107). Outcome did not differ according to the operator, the type of electrode used, litigation status (108), or the type of diagnostic block used.

In a small, prospective, uncontrolled study of 15 patients meeting CeH criteria without diagnostic blocks, 12 (80%) significantly reduced headache severity, both at short term and long term (109). Controlled diagnostic blocks confirmed the clinical diagnosis of CeH in 49 patients subjected to RF neurotomy of the third occipital nerve (110). Forty-three (88%) successfully achieved freedom from pain (110). The criteria for successful outcome were complete relief from pain for at least 90 days associated with restoration of normal activities of daily living, and no use of drug treatment for the headache. In a smaller randomized, sham-controlled, patient- and evaluator-blinded study of only 12 patients who were diagnosed clinically and not based on diagnostic blocks, the 6 treated with RF neurotomy were somewhat improved at 3 months; but later, no marked difference between groups existed. These patients had diagnostic blocks performed but not used in allocation. None of the study's subjects responded completely to blocks, and therefore none should have been expected to obtain relief from RF and none did (111). Finally, in an RCT, a group of 15 patients received a sequence of radiofrequency treatments (cervical facet joint denervation, followed by cervical dorsal root ganglion lesions when necessary). Another group of 15 patients underwent local injections with steroid and anesthetic at the greater occipital nerve, followed by transcutaneous electrical nerve stimulation (TENS) when necessary. There were no statistically significant differences between the two treatment groups at any time point such that the RF procedural group was not better than GON infiltration followed by TENS (112). These most recent studies have fueled uncertainty and controversy about this approach in CeH.

Neurostimulation
Neurostimulation must be considered experimental at the time of this writing with patients deserving enrollment in RCTs. Occipital nerve stimulation by subcutaneous implant has been reported twice for intractable occipital neuralgia, but to date, no reports are available for CeH (113,115).

EVIDENCE-BASED MEDICINE
A few published, randomized, controlled trials exist analyzing the effectiveness of spinal manipulation and/or mobilization for TTH, migraine, or CeH in which methodological quality of the studies is low (114). For the prophylactic treatment of CeH, there is evidence that both neck exercise (low-endurance training)

and spinal manipulation are effective in the short and long term when compared to no treatment. There is also evidence that spinal manipulation is effective in the short term when compared to massage or placebo spinal manipulation, and weaker evidence when compared to spinal mobilization (115).

REFERENCES

1. Blau JN, MacGregor EA. Migraine and the neck. Headache 1994; 34:88–90.
2. Biondi DM. Cervicogenic headache: A review of diagnostic and treatment strategies. JAOA 2005; 105(4):16–22.
3. Sjaastad O, Saunte C, Hovdahl H, et al. "Cervicogenic" headache. A hypothesis. Cephalalgia 1983; 3:249–256.
4. Göbel H, Edmeads JG. Disorder of the skull and cervical spine. In: Olesen J, Goadsby PJ, Ramadan NM, et al., eds. The Headaches. 3rd ed. Philadelphia: Lippincott Williams & Wilkins, 2006:1003–1011.
5. Jansen J, Sjaastad O. Cervicogenic headache: Long-term prognosis after neck surgery. Acta Neurol Scand 2007; 115(3):185–191.
6. Sjaastad O, Fredriksen TA, Pfaffenrath V. Cervicogenic headache: Diagnostic criteria. Headache 1990; 30:725–726.
7. Laimi K, Erkintalo M, Metsähonkala L, et al. Adolescent disc degeneration—No headache association. Cephalalgia 2007; 27:14–21.
8. Bono G, Antonaci F, Ghimai S, et al. The clinical profile of cervicogenic headache as it emerges from a study based on the early diagnostic criteria. Funct Neurol 1998; 13:75–77.
9. Edmeads J. The cervical spine and headache. Neurology 1988; 38(12):1874–1878.
10. Sjaastad O, Bakketeig LS. Prevalence of cervicogenic headache. Vågå study of headache epidemiology. Acta Neurol Scand 2008; 117:173–180.
11. Haldeman S, Dagenais S. Cervicogenic headaches: A critical review. Spine J 2001; 1(1):31–46.
12. Fredriksen TA, Hovdal H, Sjaastad O. "Cervicogenic headache": Clinical manifestation. Cephalalgia 1987; 7:147–160.
13. Cervicogenic Headaches. In: Merskey H, Bogduk N, eds. Classification of Chronic Pain:Descriptions of Chronic Pain Syndromes and Definitions of Pain Terms. 2nd ed. Seattle: IASP Press, 1994.
14. Sjaastad O, Fredriksen TA, Pfaffenrath V. Cervicogenic headache: Diagnostic criteria. Headache 1998; 38:442–445.
15. van Suijlekom JA.Cervicogenic headache. Thesis. University of Maastricht. Maastricht; Formaris bv 2001; ISBN 90-9014845-0.
16. Headache Classification Subcommittee of the International Headache Society. The International Classification of Headache Disorders. 2nd ed. Cephalalgia 2004; 24(Suppl 1):1–151.
17. Leone M, D'Amico D, Frediani F, et al. Clinical considerations on side-locked unilaterality in long-lasting primary headaches. Headache 1993; 33:381–384.
18. D'Amico D, Leone M, Bussone G. Side-locked unilaterality and pain localization in long-lasting headaches: Migraine, tension-type headache, and cervicogenic headache. Headache 1994; 34:526–530.
19. Leone M, D'Amico D, Moschiano F, et al. Possible identification of cervicogenic headache among patients with migraine: An analysis of 374 headaches. Headache 1995; 35:461–464.
20. Zwart JA. Neck mobility in different headache disorders. Headache 1997; 37:6–11.
21. Sjaastad O, Bovim G. Cervicogenic headache: The differentiation from common migraine. An overview. Funct Neurol 1991; 6:93–100.
22. Sjaastad O, Fredriksen TA, Stolt-Nielsen A, et al. Cervicogenic headache: A clinical review with special emphasis on therapy. Funct Neurol 1997; 12:305–317.
23. Sjaastad O, Salvesen R, Jansen J, et al. Cervicogenic headache: A critical view on pathogenesis. Funct Neurol 1998; 13:71–74.

24. Sjaastad O. Reliability of cervicogenic headache diagnosis. Cephalalgia 1999; 19(9):767–768.
25. Tfelt-Hansen P, Lous I, Olesen J. Prevalence and significance of muscle tenderness during common migraine attacks. Headache 1981; 21(2):49–54.
26. Kaniecki RG. Migraine and tension-type headache: An assessment of challenges in diagnosis. Neurology 2002; 58(9 Suppl 16):S15–S20.
27. Diener HC, Kaminski M, Stappert G, et al. Lower cervical disc prolapse may cause cervicogenic headache: Prospective study in patients undergoing surgery. Cephalalgia 2007; 27:1050–1054.
28. Sjaastad O, Fredriksen TA, Petersen H, et al. Features indicative of cervical abnormality. A factor to be reckoned with in clinical headache work and research? Funct Neurol 2003; 18:195–203.
29. Frese A, Evers S. Biological markers of cervicogenic headache. Cephalalgia 2008; 28(Suppl 1):21–23.
30. Fredriksen TA. Cervicogenic headache: Invasive procedures. Cephalalgia 2008; 28(Suppl 1):39–40.
31. Pfaffenrath V, Dandekar R, Pöllmann W. Cervicogenic headache: The clinical picture, radiological findings and hypotheses on its pathophysiology. Headache 1987; 27: 495–499.
32. Fredriksen TA, Fougner R, Tangerud A, et al. Cervicogenic headache: Radiological investigations concerning head/neck. Cephalalgia 1989; 9:139–146.
33. Coskun O, Ucler S, Karakurum B, et al. Magnetic resonance imaging of patients with cervicogenic headache. Cephalalgia 2003; 23:842–845.
34. Pöllmann W, Keidel M, Pfaffenrath V. Headache and the cervical spine: A critical review. Cephalalgia 1997; 17:501–516.
35. Martelletti P, van Suijlekom H. Cervicogenic headache: Practical approaches to therapy. CNS Drugs 2004; 18:793–805.
36. Bovim G, Sand T. Cervicogenic headache, migraine without aura and tension-type headache. Diagnostic blockade of greater occipital and supra-orbital nerves. Pain 1992; 51:43–48.
37. Anthony M. Headache and the greater occipital nerve. Clin Neurol Neurosurg 1992; 94:297–301.
38. Gawel MJ, Rothbarth PJ. Occipital nerve block in the management of headache and cervical pain. Cephalalgia 1992; 12:9–13.
39. D'Amico D, Leone M, Bussone G. Side-locked unilaterality and pain localization in long-lasting headaches: Migraine, tension-type headache, and cervicogenic headache. Headache 1994; 34(9):526–530.
40. Caputi C, Firetto V. Therapeutic blockade of greater occipital and supraorbital nerves in migraine patients. Headache 1997; 37:174–179.
41. Bovim G, Berg R, Dale LG. Cervicogenic headache, anesthetic blockades of cervical nerves (C2-C5) and facet joint (C2/C3). Pain 1992; 49:315–320.
42. Inan N, Ceyhan A, Inan L, et al. C2/C3 nerve blocks and greater occipital nerve block in cervicogenic headache treatment. Funct Neurol 2001; 16:239–243.
43. Leone M, D'Amico D, Grazzi L, et al. Cervicogenic headache: A critical review of the current diagnostic criteria. Pain 1998; 78:1–5.
44. Bogduk N. The anatomical basis for cervicogenic headache. J Manipulative Physiol Ther 1992; 15:67–70.
45. Kerr FWL, Olafson RA. Trigeminal and cervical volleys. Arch Neurol 1961; 5: 171–178.
46. Kerr FWL. A mechanism to account for frontal headaches in cases of posterior fossa tumors. J Neurosurg 1961; 18:605–609.
47. Goadsby PJ, Bartsch T. On the functional neuroanatomy of neck pain. Cephalalgia 2008; 28(Suppl 1):1–7.
48. Frese A, Schilgen M, Edvinsson L, et al. Calcitonin gene-related peptide in cervicogenic headache.Cephalalgia 2005; 25:700–703.
49. Martelletti P, Stirparo G, Giacovazzo M. Proinflammatory cytokines in cervicogenic headache. Funct Neurol 1999; 14(3):159–162.

50. Martelletti P. Proinflammatory pathways in cervicogenic headache. Clin Exp Rheumatol 2000; 18(2 Suppl 19):S33–S38.
51. Zicari A, Giacovazzo M, Martelletti P. Nitric oxide: Emerging implications for headache mechanics. J Headache Pain 2001; 2:67–72.
52. Stovner LJ, Obelieniene D. Whiplash headache is transitory worsening of a pre-existing primary headache. Cephalalgia 2008; 28(Suppl 1):28–31.
53. Obilieniene D, Bovim G, Schrader H, et al. Headache after whiplash: A historical cohort study outside the medico-legal context. Cephalalgia 1998; 18: 559–564.
54. Vincent MB. Is a de novo whiplash-associated pain most commonly cervicogenic headache? Cephalalgia 2008; 28(Suppl 1):32–34.
55. Drottning M, Staff PH, Sjaastad O. Cervicogenic headache after whiplash injury. Cephalalgia 2002; 22:165–171.
56. Drottning M, Staff PH, Sjaastad O. Cervicogenic headache (CEH) six years after whiplash injury. Funct Neurol 2007; 22:145–149.
57. Drottning M. Cervicogenic headache after whiplash injury. Curr Pain Headache Rep 2003; 7:384–386.
58. Sjaastad O, Fredriksen TA. Cervicogenic headache: Lack of influence of pregnancy. Cephalalgia 2002; 22:667–671.
59. Grgić V. Cervicogenic headache: Etiopathogenesis, characteristics, diagnosis, differential diagnosis and therapy. Lijec Vjesn 2007; 129(6–7):230–236.
60. Bovim G, Sjaastad O. Cervicogenic headache: Responses to nitroglycerin, oxygen, ergotamine, and morphine. Headache 1993; 33:249–252.
61. Pascual J, Rivas MT, Leira R. Testing the combination beta-blocker plus topiramate in refractory migraine. Acta Neurol Scand 2007; 115(2):81–83.
62. Pascual J, El Berdei Y, Gómez-Sánchez JC. How many migraine patients need prolonged (>1 year) preventive treatment? Experience with topiramate. J Headache Pain 2007; 8(2):90–93.
63. Saarto T, Wiffen PJ. Antidepressants for neuropathic pain. Cochrane Database Syst Rev 2007; (4):CD005454.
64. Bendtsen L. Efficacy of antidepressants in headache prophylaxis. In: Olesen J, Silberstein S, Tfelt-Hansen P, eds. Preventive Pharmacotherapy of Headache Disorders. 12th ed. New York: Oxford University Press, 2004:103–111.
65. Feng FL, Schofferman J. Chronic neck pain and cervicogenic headaches. Curr Treat Options Neurol 2003; 5(6):493–498.
66. Ozyalcin SN, Talu GK, Kiziltan E, et al. The efficacy and safety of venlafaxine in the prophylaxis of migraine. Headache 2005; 45(2):144–152.
67. Taylor AP, Adelman JU, Freeman MC. Efficacy of duloxetine as a migraine preventive medication: Possible predictors of response in a retrospective chart review. Headache 2007; 47(8):1200–1203.
68. Mathew NT. The prophylactic treatment of chronic daily headache. Headache 2006; 46(10):1552–1564.
69. Drake ME Jr, Greathouse NI, Renner JB, et al. Open-label zonisamide for refractory migraine. Clin Neuropharmacol 2004; 27(6):278–280.
70. Ashkenazi A, Benlifer A, Korenblit J, et al. Zonisamide for migraine prophylaxis in refractory patients. Cephalalgia 2006; 26(10):1199–1202.
71. Freitag FG. Preventative treatment for migraine and tension-type headaches: Do drugs having effects on muscle spasm and tone have a role? CNS Drugs 2003; 17(6):373–381.
72. Saper JR, Lake AE 3rd, Cantrell DT, et al. Chronic daily headache prophylaxis with tizanidine: A double-blind, placebo-controlled, multicenter outcome study. Headache 2002; 42(6):470–482.
73. Wheeler AH, Goolkasian P, Gretz SS. A randomized, double-blind, prospective pilot study of botulinum toxin injection for refractory, unilateral, cervicothoracic, paraspinal, myofascial pain syndrome. Spine 1998; 23(15):1662–1666.
74. Wheeler AH, Goolkasian P, Gretz SS. Botulinum toxin A for the treatment of chronic neck pain. Pain 2001; 94(3):255–260.

75. Evers S. Status on the use of botulinum toxin for headache disorders [Review]. Curr Opin Neurol 2006; 3:310–315.
76. Dodick DW, Mauskop A, Elkind AH, et al. Botulinum toxin type a for the prophylaxis of chronic daily headache: Subgroup analysis of patients not receiving other prophylactic medications: A randomized double-blind, placebo-controlled study. Headache 2005; 45(4):315–324.
77. Mathew NT, Kailasam J, Meadors L. Predictors of response to botulinum toxin type A (BoNTA) in chronic daily headache. Headache 2008; 48(2):194–200.
78. Martelletti P. Inflammatory mechanisms in cervicogenic headache: An integrative view. Curr Pain Headache Rep 2002; 6:315–319.
79. Fernández-de-Las-Peñas C. Physical therapy and exercise in headache [Review]. Cephalalgia 2008; 28(Suppl 1):36–38.
80. Nilsson N, Christensen HW, Hartvigsen J. The effect of spinal manipulation in the treatment of cervicogenic headache. J Manipulative Physiol Ther 1997; 20:326–330.
81. Biondi D. Physical treatments for headache: A structured review. Headache 2005; 45:1–9.
82. Fernandez-de-las-Penas C, Alonso-Banco C, Cuadrado ML, et al. Spinal manipulative therapy in the management of cervicogenic headache. Headache 2005; 45:1260–1263.
83. Fernandez-de-las-Penas C, Alonso-Banco C, Cuadrado ML, et al. Are manual therapies effective in reducing pain from tension-type? A systematic review. Clin J Pain 2006; 22:278–285.
84. Jull GA, Stanton WR. Predictors of responsiveness to physiotherapy management of cervicogenic headache. Cephalalgia 2005; 25:101–108.
85. Jull G, Trott P, Potter H, et al. A randomized controlled trial of exercise and manipulative therapy for cervicogenic headache. Spine 2002; 27:1835–1843.
86. Stanton WR, Jull GA. Cervicogenic headache: Locus of control and success of treatment. Headache 2003; 43:956–961.
87. Lord SM, Barnsley L, Wallis BJ, et al. Percutaneous radio-frequency neurotomy for chronic cervical zygapophyseal-joint pain. N Engl J Med 1996; 335:1721–1726.
88. McDonald GJ, Lord SM, Bogduk N. Long-term follow-up of patients treated with cervical radiofrequency neurotomy for chronic neck pain. Neurosurgery 1999; 45: 61–67.
89. Blume HG. Cervicogenic headaches: Radiofrequency neurotomy and the cervical disc and fusion. Clin Exp Rheumatol 2000; 18(Suppl 19):S53–S58.
90. Vincent MB, Luna RA, Scandiuzzi D, et al. Greater occipital nerve blockade in cervicogenic headache. Arq Neuropsiquiatr 1998; 56(4):720–725.
91. Vincent M. Greater occipital nerve blockades in cervicogenic headache. Funct Neurol 1998; 13(1):78–79.
92. Anthony M. Cervicogenic headache: Prevalence and response to local steroid therapy. Clin Exp Rheumatol 2000; 18(2 Suppl 19):S59–S64.
93. Naja ZM, El-Rajab M, Al-Tannir MA, et al. Repetitive occipital nerve blockade for cervicogenic headache: Expanded case report of 47 adults. Pain Pract 2006; 6: 278–284.
94. Pfaffenrath V, Kaube H. Diagnostics of cervicogenic headache [Review]. Funct Neurol 1990; 5:159–164.
95. Martelletti P, Di Sabato F, Granata M, et al. Epidural corticosteroid blockade in cervicogenic headache. Eur Rev Med Pharmacol Sci 1998; 2:25–30.
96. Martelletti P, Di Sabato F, Granata M, et al. Failure of long-term epidural steroid injection in cervicogenic headache [letter]. Funct Neurol 1998; 13:148.
97. Bovim G, Fredriksen TA, Stolt-Nilsen A, et al. Neurolysis of the greater occipital nerve in cervicogenic headache. A follow-up study. Headache 1992; 32:175–179.
98. Bogduk N. The anatomy of occipital neuralgia. Clin Exp Neurol 1980; 17:167–184.
99. Bovim G, Bonamico L, Fredriksen T, et al. Topographic variations in the peripheral course of the greater occipital nerve. An autopsy study with clinical correlations. Spine 1991; 16:475–478.

100. Stechison M. Outcome of surgical decompression of the second cervical root for cervicogenic headache. Neurosurgery 1997; 40:1105–1106.
101. Jansen J, Markakis E, Rama B, et al. Hemicranial attacks or permanent hemicrania—A sequel of upper cervical root compression. Cephalalgia 1989; 9(2):123–130.
102. Pikus H, Phillips J. Characteristics of patients successfully treated for cervicogenic headache by surgical decompression of the second cervical root. Headache 1995; 35:621–629.
103. Jansen J. Surgical treatment of non-responsive cervicogenic headache. Clin Exp Rheumatol 2000; 18(2 Suppl 19):S67–S70.
104. Jansen J. Surgical treatment of cervicogenic headache. Cephalalgia 2008; 28(Suppl 1):41–44.
105. Sluijter M, Cosman E, Rittman I, et al. The effects of pulsed radiofrequency applied to the dorsal root ganglion—A preliminary report. Pain Clin 1998; 11:109–117.
106. Bogduk N. Position paper: Pulsed radiofrequency. Pain Med 2006; 7:396–497.
107. Lord SM, McDonald GJ, Bogduk N. Percutaneous radiofrequency neurotomy of the cervical medial branches: A validated treatment for cervical zygapophyseal joint pain. Neurosurg Q 1998; 8:288–308.
108. Sapir DA, Gorup JM. Radiofrequency medial branch neurotomy in litigant and non-litigant patients with cervical whiplash. Spine 2001; 26:E268–E273.
109. van Suijlekom HA, van Kleef M, Barendse GA. Radiofrequency cervical zygapophyseal joint neurotomy for cervicogenic headache: A prospective study of 15 patients. Funct Neurol 1998; 13:297–303.
110. Govind J, King W, Bailey B, et al. Radiofrequency neurotomy for the treatment of third occipital headache. J Neurol Neurosurg Psychiatry 2003; 74:88–93.
111. Bogduk N. Editorial. Cephalalgia 2004; 10:819–820.
112. Haspeslagh SRS, Van Suijlekom HA, Lamé IE, et al. Randomised controlled trial of cervical radiofrequency lesions as a treatment for cervicogenic headache. BMC Anesthesiol. 2006; 6:1–11.
113. Kapural L, Mekhail N, Hayek SM, et al. Occipital nerve electrical stimulation via the midline approach and subcutaneous surgical leads for treatment of severe occipital neuralgia: A pilot study. Anesth Analg 2005; 101:171–174.
114. Slavin KV, Nersesyan H, Wess C. Peripheral neurostimulation for treatment of intractable occipital neuralgia. Neurosurgery 2006; 58:112–119.
115. Fernandez-de-las-Penas C, Alonso-Banco C, San-Roman J, et al. Methodological quality of randomized controlled trials of spinal manipulation and mobilization in tension-type headache, migraine, and cervicogenic headache. J Orthop Sports Phy Ther 2006; 36(3):160–196.
116. Bronfort G, Nilsson N, Haas M, et al. Non-invasive physical treatments for chronic/recurrent headache. Cochrane Database Syst Rev 2004; 3:CDOO1878.

Frederick G. Freitag

Diamond Headache Clinic, Chicago, Illinois, U.S.A.

Perhaps the first description of cluster headache is from Gerhard Van Swieten in 1745. He wrote "Viro sano, robusto, mediae aetatis, quotidie eadem hora oriebatur molesti doloris sensus in eodem loco supraorbitam oculi sinistri." This translates to "A healthy robust man of middle age was suffering from troublesome pain, which came on every day at the same hour at the same spot above the orbit of the left eye." Later Wilfred Harris (1) described a clinical syndrome that he termed "migrainous neuralgia." The term cluster headache originated with an article by Kunkel (2). However, Horton (3) did the first accurate description of this disorder. The astuteness of his observations continues to have recognition into the present (4). The literature is replete with terms that appear to be synonymous for cluster headache. These include "red migraine," erythromyelgia," "Sluder's syndrome," "sphenopalatine neuralgia," "histaminic cephalgia," and "Horton's headache."

THE DISORDER

Clinical Features of Cluster Headache

Epidemiology

Cluster headache is rare compared to migraine headache. Population studies estimate the incidence from 0.1% (5) to as high as 0.9% (6) of population. This variability is not related to ethnicity or geography. Rather it appears related to sampling methodology. There is a strong male predominance of the disorder estimated as high as 85% of cases. This, however, is changing along with other lifestyle factors linked to cluster headache. The gender prevalence was 6.2 to 1 male *versus* female in the pre-1960 era. By the 1990s, the ratio shifted to 1.7 to 1. During this time, increased employment of women and increased use of tobacco among women occurred (7). The causal relationship with the change in sexual preponderance of these lifestyle changes is dubious, whereas improved disease recognition of cluster headache is not.

The first attack of cluster headache is uncommon in childhood or adolescence. It becomes more common in the 20s where the peak incidence of the disorder also occurs for both males and females with episodic cluster headache and for men with chronic cluster headache (8). Like migraine headache, the prevalence of the disorder begins to decline past age 50 with the headache only rarely seen in elderly individuals past age 70.

Clinical Description

Clinicians such as John Graham painted a physical and emotional picture of cluster headaches that is dubious in its relation to the headache disorder itself. Some describe patients with cluster headaches as having distinguishing facial characteristics such as peau d'orange skin, deep vertical facial creases, a ruddy complexion, and frequent facial telangiectasia (9). They are heavy smokers, characteristically and historically (10). These features were commonly seen during the age of common use of tobacco products, even as medicinal treatments. The heavy use of tobacco products, by themselves, without having cluster headache produces these facial characteristics. Therefore, attributing these characteristics to either cluster headache or cigarette smoking may both be correct. Table 1 lists the clinical features of cluster headache. Perhaps the heavy use of tobacco resulted from patients' use of it to treat the individual attack of cluster headache. Rapid smoking of a cigarette rarely helps in aborting an acute attack of cluster. Other characteristic attributes that have been associated with cluster headache include a propensity to be the tallest individuals in their family as well as having hazel colored eyes.

Graham characterized cluster patients as having a leonine appearance (9). This attribute relates to their coarse facial characteristics and having full heads of hair. He described a unique personality to cluster patients. The typical cluster patient he saw as being a tall, rugged male with an anticipated personality to match (11). However, these same patients typically came to their office visit with a diminutive wife who, rather than her husband, would have the domineering personality, frequently answering the questions for the patient, herself.

The use of alcoholic beverages may serve a trigger for cluster headaches when a patient is in cycle. It is rare to find a patient with cluster headache who will not have an acute attack of headache that is precipitated within minutes of ingestion of even minimal amounts of alcohol. This sensitivity only occurs when the patient is in the active cycle of headache. The use of alcohol is more common in patients than in the population (10) and may play a contributory role in the disorder.

TABLE 1 Clinical Features of Cluster Headache

Males more commonly than females
Peak occurrence in 20 seconds
Tobacco and alcohol use common
Distinct facial characteristics
Cycles begin near summer and winter solstices
Individual attacks occur same time of day in given patient
Attacks commonly occur during sleep
Pain lasts 15 minutes to 2 hours
Strictly unilateral
Eye and temple region
"Hot poker" pain description
Rhinorrhea
Lacrimation
Partial Horner's syndrome

Circadian and Circannual Features

The term, cluster headache, seems appropriate since the attacks occur in a group of headaches with a frequency from once to multiple times per day over a period of several weeks to many months; a pain-free period occurs spontaneously only to have the cluster headache recur at a later time. A typical cycle of cluster headache lasts two weeks to about three months. Rarely is the cycle shorter, but it can be longer and can recur persistently for a year without respite. There are variants on this, which I discuss later. During a cycle of cluster headache, a patient will have one or multiple attacks per day. Both circadian and circannual elements are often present in patients with cluster headache. The attacks of cluster headache often occur at night and occur near the end of a sleep cycle. Patients awaken 1.5 to 2 hours after retiring to bed. Commonly, patients can predict the time of onset of their cluster headache attacks to within several minutes producing bizarre habits aimed at attempting to avoid the attacks. A circannual pattern is also common for patients. The series of headaches may occur multiple times a year or there may be remissions of up to 20 years. The onset of a cycle typically begins within several weeks of the summer or winter solstices (12). Others have their attacks occur in the spring or fall (13). Each patient with cluster headache tends to have his or her own unique pattern of both circadian and circannual patterns (14,15).

Individual Attack Features

An individual attack of cluster headache is brief compared to other headaches lasting 15 minutes to 2 hours. The key question in the diagnosis of cluster headache is whether there are individual attacks of cluster headache lasting over 4 hours. Though brief, the pain of cluster headache is extremely severe. The intensity of pain is such that it is called "suicide headache" by some patients. The pain is strictly unilateral and typically in the temporal and periorbital region. Unlike migraine, it does not become bilateral or switch sides in a given attack or even a cycle of cluster headache. Occasionally, the attacks may occur on the opposite side in some cluster headache cycles. The pain description is of a boring intense pain compared to the sore throbbing pain of migraine. A patient may use the description of a "hot poker being pushed into the eye." While the Migraineurs retire to the dark, quiet of their bed, the patients with cluster headache sit and rock, or pace about the room clutching their head. Patients may also experience a less intense deep ache in the upper ipsilateral cervical paraspinal region during their attack and may have residual soreness in the temporal region between the individual attacks of cluster headache.

Only rarely do patients with cluster headache have associated symptoms similar to migraine with aura (16), nausea, vomiting, and photophobia. More commonly, patients demonstrate evidence of autonomic dysfunction with injection of the conjunctiva, tearing, nasal congestion, and rhinorrhea. These are ipsilateral to the pain. Patients may also have other autonomic symptoms such as flushing, sweating, and bradycardia.

Chronic Cluster

Roughly 10% of patients with cluster headache experience, at some time in their lives, a nonremitting stage of the disorder termed chronic cluster headache. This variation characteristically exhibits a failure of a remission of the cluster headaches to occur over a one-year period. The most common form of chronic cluster occurs when the patient with episodic cluster headache fails to experience the expected remission. This makes up about 90% of all patients with chronic cluster headache. Predisposing factors for this transformation are the onset of cluster later in life, a high frequency of cluster periods with brief remissions (17), heavy use of tobacco products or alcohol intake and head trauma (18).

The remaining 10% of chronic cluster have primary chronic cluster. These patients have never experienced a remission period from the inception of their cluster headache history.

More than the loss of a remission of the headaches characterizes chronic cluster headache. In chronic cluster patients, the attack frequency is greater. The circadian pattern of the individual attacks typical of episodic cluster headache is lost. Lastly, the response to treatment is less reliable and prone to tachyphylaxis and eventual loss of response.

DIAGNOSIS

The diagnosis of cluster headache rests upon satisfying the ICHD-II criteria established in 2004 (19). In general, diagnosis of cluster headaches requires that the patient have at least four attacks that meet the criteria described as individual attacks of severe and strictly unilateral pain. The location of pain is orbital, supraorbital, temporal or as a combination of these locations. Individual attacks of pain will last from 15 to 180 minutes. The attacks occur as seldom as once every other day to as often as eight times a day. One or more symptoms are associated with the attacks and all are ipsilateral to the headache. These symptoms are conjunctival injection, lacrimation, nasal congestion, rhinorrhea, forehead and facial sweating, miosis, ptosis, and eyelid edema. Additionally, most patients describe being restless or agitated during an attack. Episodic cluster headache is characterized by attacks occurring in periods lasting seven days to one year separated by pain-free periods lasting 1 month or longer. Chronic cluster, on the other hand, has no remission in at least a year, or if there are remissions, they are brief and last less than one month.

PATHOPHYSIOLOGY

Like migraine headache, our understanding of cluster headache mechanism has evolved from a hypothesis that rested on its being, primarily, a vascular disorder with secondary neurologic sequella to one in which the neurobiology of the disorder is the focal point and the involvement of other biologic and biochemical changes occur as secondary effects.

In cluster headache, a specific active locus in the posterior hypothalamus serves as the focal point (20). Along with this, there are changes in calcitonin gene-related peptide (CGRP) release and vasoactive intestinal peptide (VIP), which appear to be involved in a trigeminal-vascular mechanism like migraine along with facial involvement. Clues to the role of the hypothalamic involvement arose from clinical and laboratory observations of circadian biological changes and neuroendocrine disturbances (21). Beyond these effects related to hypothalamic function, there are a host of other effects that may occur related to the hypothalamus that also relate to cluster headache such as effects on cardiorespiratory interactions and efferent sympathetic functions (22). Studies of the posterior hypothalamus through implantation of a deep brain implanted stimulator show that there are also effects on a variety of other structures. Besides the ipsilateral hypothalamic gray matter, there is also activation of the ipsilateral thalamus, somatosensory cortex and praecuneus, the anterior cingulate cortex, and the ipsilateral trigeminal nucleus and ganglion. Pain modulation in cluster headache occurs through the trigeminal nucleus and, directly, from the posterior hypothalamic gray matter (23). The effect on cardiovascular effects related to hypothalamic function may be important in cluster headache. Alteration in sympathetic activity (24) may contribute to the clinical symptoms through inhibition of sympathetic activity. Kudrow has further suggested that their may be dysregulation of autoregulatory chemoreceptors for oxygen in the carotid circulation that may contribute to the vascular changes associated with cluster headache (25,26).

Autonomic system involvement in cluster headache is strongly suggested by its clinical features (27). Parasympathetic activation is suggested by the symptoms of lacrimation, conjunctival injection and rhinorrhea; sympathetic impairment by miosis and ptosis; and additional parasympathetic mediated effects in the form of nasal congestion, eyelid edema and forehead sweating. The autonomic system is also active in the cluster headache variant, chronic paroxysmal hemicrania (28). Similar changes in CGRP and VIP occur in these patients and normalize with adequate treatment with response to indomethacin. Inhibition of the sympathetic system occurs both in the periphery and in the CNS and cerebrospinal fluid (29). Decreased plasma norepinephrine levels occur in patients with cluster headache compared with the control group. These changes also correlate with the duration, intensity, and frequency of the cluster headaches. Furthermore, there are changes in cerebrospinal fluid levels of norepinephrine and its metabolites that are consistent with central changes in the nervous system underlying cluster headache.

Examination of parasympathetic system activity demonstrated alteration in clinical parameters of its function that extended to the interval between cluster headache cycles suggesting a chronic alteration in this part of the autonomic system (30).

The occurrence of autonomic symptoms is typical of cluster headache. There are patients, however, who lack the associated cranial autonomic symptoms occurring as part of their cluster headaches (31). These patients compared to other cluster headache patients are more likely to have milder headache attacks or be a female cluster headache patient or to have chronic cluster headache.

While many studies support a central basis for cluster headache, others have suggested that cluster headache may have a substantial basis involving peripheral neural changes. A trigeminal-cervical reflex may be present in cluster headache patients suggested by a shortened latency of response for sternocleidomastoid muscle stimulation of the trigeminal nerve during a cluster series (32), and alteration of occipital nerve reflexes such as the blink reflex (33). Although the use of occipital nerve blocks, which may influence the reflex response, suggests that the mechanism of pain relief from these is through central inhibitory effects on the trigeminal-vascular basis of cluster headache, not peripheral analgesic effects.

Drummond has made a strong argument for a combined central and peripheral autonomic disturbance occurring in cluster headache (34). Lacrimation and nasal secretion during attacks of cluster headache appear to be due to massive trigeminal-parasympathetic discharge. In addition, the presence of ocular-sympathetic deficit and loss of thermoregulatory sweating and flushing on the symptomatic side of the forehead indicate that the cervical sympathetic pathway to the face is injured in a subgroup of cluster headache patients. In this review, the argument is that a peripheral rather than a central lesion produces signs of cervical sympathetic inhibition, resulting from compression of the sympathetic fibers traversing the internal carotid artery arising from the cervical sympathetic chain, although trigeminally mediated discharge of the parasympathetic system appears to be the main trigger for vasodilation during attacks. This may also account for the increased sensitivity seen to the neurotransmitter, vasoactive intestinal polypeptide. Although neither trigeminally mediated parasympathetic discharge nor cervical sympathetic deficit appears to be the primary trigger for attacks of cluster headache, these autonomic disturbances could contribute to the rapid escalation of pain once the attack begins. He hypothesizes that a pericarotid inflammatory process stimulates trigeminal nociceptors. Activation of these nociceptors initiates a neurogenic inflammation and trigeminally mediated parasympathetic vasodilation. These processes may culminate with provocation of the release of mast cell products, further aggravating the inflammation and intensifying trigeminal discharge.

Increased plasma levels of plasma cortisol and ACTH that occur in patients with CH, especially in the morning and in the evening, suggest an alteration of the feedback circuit involving the hypothalamus, the pituitary, and the adrenal gland suggesting an alteration of the circadian rhythm (35). These significant relationships between biochemical parameters and the clinical patterns suggest a complex interplay between the hypothalamus, neuroendocrinological parameters, activity of the autonomic nervous system, and the pain of CH.

Further evidence for central hypothalamic dysfunction on the genesis of cluster headache suggests that the effects may be via modulation of other hormonal factors and, specifically, testosterone (36). For years, the male cluster patient's description was one with very strong masculine features. In addition to the impacts on corticotrophin level, other work suggests that gonatropins are also involved, and these along with sleep factors lead to involvement of pineal gland levels of melatonin. Testosterone levels were consistently low in the study by Stillman, which involved chronic cluster headache, primarily, and males, for the most part. Melatonin's effects may be far ranging beyond its putative role in sleep (37). Among the mechanisms that are influenced by melatonin that have implications for cluster headache include its anti-inflammatory effect, its role as a toxic free radical scavenger, and its ability to reduce proinflammatory cytokine production. Other effects that are of interest in cluster headache include the impact on nitric oxide synthase activity and inhibitory effects on dopaminergic neurons. Melatonin also modulates analgesia via positive effects on GABA-mediated pain mechanisms as well as on opioid induced analgesia.

Melatonin modulates glutamate and serotonin levels. It has neuroprotective effects as well. Involvement of the opioid-mediated pain process in cluster headache has been shown by our group (38) to demonstrate marked decline in enkephalin levels during a cluster cycle coupled with a marked alteration in the metabolism of this system. PET scanning also demonstrates decreases in pineal gland binding of opioids and declines in these receptors in both the hypothalamus and cingulated cortex with long-standing cluster headache (39).

Nitric oxide pathways may play a role in the genesis of cluster headache. In my experience, it may be involved in the mast cell regulation of the inflammatory response that may modulate refractoriness of cluster headache. Genetic studies have failed to find a relationship of cluster headache with either nitric oxide synthase (40) or histamine metabolism (41); however, several genes associated with inflammatory modulation upregulate in a cycle of cluster headache (42) compared to interictal periods or from population controls.

The pathogenesis of cluster headache appears to be a central disorder involving an alteration of the hypothalamus characterized by its increased activity and subsequent increase in parasympathetic activity and changes in hypothalamically mediated hormonal activity and opioid-related analgesia. The linkage to the pineal gland neurologically and endocrinolgically modulates the circadian components of the disorder. However, a central basis for the disorder is important, and the excessive parasympathetic activity that may be needed to produce the disorder of the sympathetic system in the periphery is also involved through an inhibitory process. Modulation of the pain, itself, occurs via the trigeminal vascular system, which may account for peripheral cervical spinal nerves in the clinical presentation.

TREATMENT

Treatment of cluster headache, as other primary headaches, may be directed at both the acute relief of a single episode (Table 2) and preventative treatment (Table 3) aimed at alleviating a cycle of cluster headache. The brief nature of cluster headache attacks, their severity, and underlying physiology coupled with their frequency of occurrence both within a day and during a cluster period lead to increased reliance on the preventative therapy as being the mainstay of treatment. There is little that makes an impact on the nature of cluster headache from a nonpharmacologic methodology; however, lifestyle adjustments in a given series of attacks may have benefit. Invasive procedures have been utilized in patients whose headaches are refractive to medical intervention with variable results.

Abortive Treatments

Oxygen

The mainstay of acute treatment for cluster headache is the inhalation of oxygen. 100% oxygen given via a facemask at rates of 8–10 L/min is effective and well

TABLE 2   Acute Treatment of Cluster Headache

Drug	Dose
Oxygen	100% at 8–10 L/min for up to 15 minutes
Lidocaine	4% aqueous drops instilled into ipsilateral nostril
Olanzapine	2.5–10 mg PO at onset
Dihydroergotamine	1 mg IV, IM or SC at onset. Repeat q 1 hour up to 3 mg per day and 5 mg per week
	or
	1–mg NS at onset. Repeat in 1 hour if needed. Limit 6 mg per week
Sumatriptan	6 mg SC at onset. Repeat in 1 hour if needed. Limit 2 doses per day and 6 doses per week
	or
	20 mg NS repeat in 1 hour if needed. Limit 2 sprays per day. Limit to 6 sprays per week
Zolmitriptan	2.5–10 mg (PO or NS) at onset. Limit to 10 mg per day. Limit to 30 mg per week

TABLE 3 Preventive Therapy

Drug	Dose
Prednisone	40 mg per day to start for 3 to 5 days. Taper by 5 mg decrements over no more than 3 weeks
Dihydroergotamine	1 mg IV q 8 hours for 9 doses. Requires inpatient admission and observation
Ergotamine tartrate	2 mg qhs
Sumatriptan	100 mg TID for up to 7 days at a treatment
Naratriptan	2.5 mg BID for up to 7 days at a treatment
Lithium	300 mg BID to QID. Titrate dose on tolerability and efficacy. Monitor blood levels
Verapamil	80 mg BID to 240 mg TID
Divalproex sodium	250–1000 mg BID or up to 1000 mg qhs
Topiramate	25–200 mg BID or up to 200 mg qhs

tolerated in the majority of patients. The mechanism by which oxygen alleviates the acute of attack of cluster headache is not fully understood. The increased concentrations of arterial oxygen may reverse the noted decline associated with the attack. It may also reverse the vasodilatation and increased cranial blood flow during attacks of cluster headache by direct vasoconstrictive mechanisms.

In addition to several clinical reports of its efficacy, there are two controlled trials of oxygen therapy for cluster headache. The first, by Kudrow, demonstrated that 70% of attacks aborted within 15 minutes in 75% of patients studied (43). Subsequently a blinded trial comparing inhalation of 100% oxygen compared to inhaling compressed air found that 80% of attacks were relieved promptly in the majority of patients using oxygen but only 7% of those breathing air had comparable results (44). There are few contraindications or adverse effects associated with oxygen inhalation, with proper use, for treating cluster headache. Patients with severe obstructive pulmonary disease need to use oxygen with caution, and patients should not fall asleep with the oxygen mask in place where it might allow the cornea to be exposed to the high oxygen flow rate for a prolonged period. While safe and highly effective and reliable, oxygen is not a terribly practical tool for acute treatment of cluster headache if the patient has attacks of cluster headache occurring other than at home. For these situations, other therapies need consideration.

Local Anesthetics and Dopaminergics

Kittrele (45) noted the historical use of cocaine for the treatment of acute headache but felt it to be impractical. He suggested the alternative use of lidocaine applied intranasal reporting benefit in a small number of patients. Cocaine possesses a modest vasoconstrictive effect in addition to its local anesthetic effect, which might make it superior to other local anesthetics. It is addictive and requires compounding as a solution, which is unstable. The application of lidocaine requires installation into the nostril on the side of the headache (46,47). Ideally, it is applied by using a long nasal pledgett placed down the nares to the posterior pharyngeal wall then withdrawn about one inch. This would place in proximity to the underlying sphenopalatine ganglia. Application of lidocaine into this region would be expected to provide an anesthetizing effect in the region of the pain of cluster headache. This is not a practical technique for the patient to use who must rather instill drops into the nasal passage while lying recumbent, the head extended and turned toward the side of the pain.

A small open trial of olanzapine (48) at doses between 2.5 and 10 mg was conducted in patients with cluster headache. The majority of the five patients using the medication experienced a reduction or elimination of their acute attacks within 20 minutes.

5HT Agonists

More effective and with greater ease of use are the $5HT_{1B/1D}$ agonist agents. This includes dihydroergotamine mesylate, sumatriptan, and zolmitriptan. The use of dihydroergotamine mesylate (DHE) in cluster headache has been a first-line therapy since it became available in the 1945. Horton describes its use as an intramuscular preparation (49). Administration is via intravenous, intramuscular, and subcutaneous routes by injection or as a nasal spray. The intravenous administration is well suited for use in the office, emergency department, and inpatient treatment situations. Repetitive dosing of DHE has been recommended as a means of interrupting a cycle of cluster headache (50). The intramuscular and subcutaneous routes, which have essentially identical pharmacokinetic properties, are suited for self-administration by the patient in addition to the health care professional administration. The usual dose is 1 mg IV, IM, or SC with repeated doses 1 hour apart up to 3 mg per day and 5 mg per week. The nasal spray formulation may also be effective as an acute therapy for cluster headaches with its lack of traumatic administration and rapid onset of activity similar to the injectable routes. Since it is incompletely absorbed, doses of 2–3 mg may be required to treat an attack. A single trial of it using only 1 mg as the treating dose reduced the intensity of cluster attacks significantly compared to placebo (51). Its establishment as a therapeutic agent in cluster headache, while not supported by significant clinical trials, is as an important therapy based on its widespread use by headache specialists treating cluster headache over nearly six decades.

DHE is as active at the $5HT_{1B/1D}$ receptor sites as are the newer therapies in the class of drugs known as the triptans. Studies exist for several of the triptans in the acute cluster headache treatment. Sumatriptan has the greatest amount of research and clinical experience of these agents as a therapy for cluster headache. Sumatriptan has been examined as the injectable and intranasal formulations in cluster headache. Multiple large clinical trials using doses up to 12 mg subcutaneously for the acute attack of cluster headache (52–55) demonstrated that it is rapidly effective and highly reliable. It appears to be without evidence of tachyphylaxis despite repetitive treatments in use of up to one year. Some patients have been studied using doses far in excess of product labeling recommendations without significant occurrence of adverse events (56,57). Several small trials have reported at least modest results with the 20 mg nasal spray formulation of sumatriptan (58,59). The lower results seen for nasal spray compared to the subcutaneous formulation in these trials occur because of the relatively small comparative dose of the drug.

Zolmitriptan (60) administered as an oral tablet at doses of up to 10 mg was effective for the treatment of acute attacks of episodic cluster headache compared to placebo. Unfortunately, it had no benefit in patients with chronic cluster headache. In general, it was well tolerated. By comparison, however, the intranasal formulation has proven rapidly effective in placebo-controlled trials with doses as low as 5 mg being superior to placebo for headache relief and pain freedom within 30 minutes and showing efficacy by 10 minutes. Adverse events were comparable to other clinical trials even at the 10 mg intranasal dose (61).

Preventative Treatment
Wide varieties of therapies exist for the preventative treatment of cluster headache. Unfortunately, rigorous placebo-controlled trials exist for only a few of them. Despite the lack of well-controlled trials, the uniformity of response with many of these treatments has led to their acceptance as standards of care.

Brief Therapies
Corticosteroids are a treatment of first choice for cluster headache. The mechanism is likely to be unrelated to their anti-inflammatory effects. Onset of activity occurs within 24 hours of initiating treatment. Activity at the level of the hypothalamus may be nominative circadian alterations and parasympathetic outflow.

Horton (62) was the first to describe the use of corticosteroids as a treatment for cluster headache. Reports by Kudrow (63) and by Couch and Ziegler (64) both found that doses of approximately 40 mg per day of prednisone produced a favorable response in approximately 80% of patients. Short-term treatment at this dose is well tolerated and, after a period of three to five days, may allow for a rapid taper of up to three weeks with good interim control of the cluster headaches. The rapid onset of activity and good tolerability in the short course of the corticosteroid allows for starting other preventative medications and giving them the opportunity to exert their effect on control of the cluster cycle by the time tapering begins with the corticosteroids. A recurrence of the cluster headaches occurs in the majority of patients once the dose of prednisone reaches the physiologic daily production equivalent of 20 mg of prednisone when used by itself. Longer term use of the corticosteroids may be associated with an increased risk of adverse effects. These include glucose intolerance, altered lipid metabolism, weight gain, fluid retention, moon facies, and even aseptic necrosis of the hip.

Interrupting the cycle of cluster headache abruptly occurs with the intravenous administration of dihydroergotamine mesylate (50) in a series of doses over three days. While highly effective, repetitive IV DHE requires hospitalization. Recurrence of the cluster headaches is likely without instituting other preventative treatments.

Once commonly used, now rarely used as a treatment, is ergotamine. Typically, if the attacks are strictly nocturnal, ergotamine given once daily at bedtime is effective (65). The usual dose is 2 mg orally. There is substantial literature on methysergide prevention for cluster headache. This serotonergic agent, related to ergotamine, is no longer distributed in the United States.

Sumatriptan has been studied at doses of up to 100 mg three times a day as a preventive therapy for cluster headache. Patients' treatment lasted for up to seven days. The study failed to find significant benefits of treatment with sumatriptan in this manner (66). Encouraging results with naratriptan given as a preventive agent occur in cluster headache (67).

Long-Term Therapy
Lithium has been one of the commonly used preventive medications (68) since the late seventies. The mechanism of action has not been determined. Theories

suggest that it may influence several neurotransmitters (69). It is more commonly used for the treatment of chronic cluster than episodic cluster. Both adverse events and time to onset of activity influence this decision. Monitor blood levels of the drug periodically (70); baseline and follow-up thyroid testing should be obtained as the drug may induce hypothyroidism with long-term use. In comparison to their use in mood disorders, the blood levels that are effective for treatment tend to be lower. The typical dosage is 300 mg twice to four times a day. Side effects are often dose related but can include decreased coordination, tremor, and nausea. It is important to avoid restriction of salt intake, which may increase the risk of toxicity. Avoidance of thiazide diuretics occurs for this reason.

The advent of the calcium channel blockers in the early 80s found them to be effective in migraine and cluster headache. As is the case with lithium, the mechanism of action of the calcium channel blockers is unknown. Possible mechanisms include the direct effect on calcium channels in vascular smooth muscle as well-mediating effects on serotonin. A variety of calcium channel blockers have been shown to be effective in management (71). Verapamil (72,73) has remained the one most consistently used. Onset of activity occurs in less than a week in patients at dose of 240 mg/day. Some patients, especially those with chronic cluster headache where up to 720 mg/day has been used, may require higher doses. Perform vital sign monitoring along with monitoring of the electrocardiogram if doses of greater than 360 mg day are prescribed. Hypotension, bradycardia, and development of heart block may occur at higher doses. Calcium channel blockers may interact with beta-blockers to produce cardiovascular complications. Verapamil also interacts with digitalis, albeit a rare concern in the typical cluster headaches patient. More important may be the interactions with lithium, which can be both advantageous and problematic. A controlled trial (74) demonstrated that verapamil was as effective as lithium but had better tolerability and quicker onset of action. The only common side effect seen with verapamil at normal therapeutic doses is constipation.

Several anti-epileptic drugs have shown activity in cluster headache. There is demonstration of effectiveness with divalproex sodium. The mechanism of action is unknown. Central inhibition of serotonergic pathways is suggested by studies as a mechanism. Kuritsky (75) demonstrated efficacy in an open trial with doses of up to 2 g per day. Roughly 75% of patients responded in this open trial as well as in another open trial (76) of divalproex. Subsequently, we demonstrated similar results with a relatively smaller dose. We found the average dose to be 750 mg per day. There does not appear to be much difference in the dose for episodic *versus* chronic cluster headache. Recently, a double-blind, placebo-controlled trial (77) failed to find evidence of effectiveness of divalproex sodium. The trial was hampered rendering conclusions difficult because of a high placebo response rate of 62% compared to a 50% response rate for the active group. The most likely explanation for the high placebo response rate relates to spontaneous remission of the cluster headaches. Adverse effects include fatigue, gastrointestinal upset, transient hair loss with prolonged used, and weight gain, which may occur and is more significant in men compared to women. Avoid the drug in women of childbearing potential without adequate contraception because of the risk of neural tube defects.

Topiramate has been shown to be effective as well. Several small open trials (78,79) have found that approximately 75% of patients treated with dose averaging 87.5 mg but ranging up to 200 mg had a substantial reduction in the frequency of their cluster headaches attacks.

Gabapentin (80) was studied in a small group of patients with chronic cluster headache as an add-on treatment with favorable results lasting up to 18 months.

Miscellaneous Therapies

The circadian and circannual characteristics of cluster headache have lead to investigation of melatonin as a treatment for cluster headache. This hormone, secreted by the pineal gland and intimately involved in these processes, has been studied as a preventive for cluster headache. After several case reports (81) suggested that melatonin might be useful for treatment, a larger study was conducted (21). This failed to demonstrate positive results in patients with episodic or chronic cluster headache as an adjunctive therapy to their usual medications.

Solomon has reported (82) on the use of capsaicin applied topically intranasal as a treatment for cluster headache. The results were suggestive of efficacy. Adverse effects, however, have proven limiting with this hot pepper extract. Working along similar lines, a derivative of capsaicin, civamide, was studied in a placebo-controlled trial again demonstrating modest reductions in cluster headaches but with improved tolerability (83).

Botulinum toxin type A has been used in a small group of patients with a 50-unit administration per patient (84). It was ineffective in episodic cluster headache and produced partial results as an add-on treatment in one-third of those with chronic cluster headache.

A number of other therapeutic agents have had limited exposure in cluster headache but may have effectiveness in some patients. These include methylphenidate (85), baclofen (86), hallucinogens (87), clonidine (88), and ACE inhibitors, which may act via blocking endorphin and enkephalin metabolism (89).

Other injection techniques such as greater occipital nerve blocks have been studied with mixed results. One study of 15 patients found little if any response (90). Another study though found 13 of 22 patients responded robustly for up to 3 weeks following a single injection, in part, predicted by tenderness over the GON prior to injection (91). As a transition therapy while awaiting effects of more standard preventative treatment, there may be a limited role based on a study by Silberstein and colleagues (92) where a modest reduction was seen in the first week after injection.

Though the responses to greater occipital nerve blocks to date have been marginal, it may have provided the impetus to investigation of other surgical approaches such as the greater occipital nerve stimulator.

Patients with episodic cluster headache will typically respond to the same successful regimen with each bout of the attacks. Once the clusters have remitted for two weeks, it may be possible to taper the patient off their regimen without recurrence of the cluster attacks in that cycle. Alternatively, patients may be continued through the period that their cluster cycle usually lasts and then taper off their treatment more rapidly. A staged approach to managing the cluster headaches is often very successful and well tolerated (Table 4).

Patients with chronic cluster headache are often more difficult to treat. The expected response to typical therapies for cluster headache may not occur. They may also require higher doses of the preventive medications and may

TABLE 4 An Approach to Cluster Headache Management

Acute	Preventive
Oxygen	Prednisone 40 mg daily (not for first-line use in diabetic patients) for 5 days then taper by 5 mg daily and stop
If cluster attacks away from home	Begin at same time verapamil 80 mg TID or divalproex sodium 250 mg qhs titrating up to 750 mg qhs over 6 days or as tolerated or
Add sumatriptan SC or lidocaine IN	Topiramate 25 mg qhs titrating up to 100 mg qhs over 9 days
If failed response to oxygen	If fail one of above give trial of another
Use sumatriptan SC or NS or zolmitriptan PO or NS or dihydroergotamine mesylate NS	Alternatively may start lithium 300 mg BID and titrate
AVOID opioid analgesics	If patient fails single drug regimen refer

need dosing increases over time to maintain control. They may also become spontaneously refractive to an agent that had been successfully controlling the cluster headaches. Co-pharmaceutical approaches may become mandatory for treatment in some of these patients. In those patients who become refractive to standard therapies, other alternative treatments may need to be used.

Intractable Cluster Headache Treatment

Surgery

Advances in technology have permitted neuromodulation to be explored as potential therapy in medically refractive conditions. Deep brain implants to modulate the poster hypothalamus have been studied (93) in 18 patients with some positive results but also potentially significant complications. Mixed results were seen in a report from Germany of six patients, half of whom lost the effects within the course of months (94).

A less invasive approach to neuromodulation makes use of an implanted occipital nerve stimulator (95). The authors reported on eight patients implanted for about 20 months. Only two of eight patients over the course of months of use achieved near complete remission of their cluster headaches; and another four experienced reductions that they found of sufficient benefit to continue using the stimulator, despite only a 20% reduction in the attacks. The effects of occipital nerve stimulation were lost almost at once when the device was disconnected.

Surgical approaches to cluster headache date back over several decades. Their success is predicated upon the response seen in trigeminal neuralgia. A hopeful approach since it is noninvasive was a radiosurgical approach. While nearly half of patients initially responded well to the treatment over the course of weeks to years the effect was lost. The remainder of the patients experienced little if any benefit (96). Complications to the treatment can include a variety of trigeminal abnormalities of trigeminal sensation.

Invasive procedures have been advocated as treatment for refractive cluster headache. The most complicated of the procedures that have been used is microvascular decompression of the trigeminal nerve (Janetta procedure). It has been reported to be effective in nearly 75% of patients with a 50% or greater reduction in the frequency of cluster attacks. Patients were followed up for up to 5.3 years in this trial (97). Over time, the procedure became ineffective in about a third of the patients who initially responded. Repeat surgery had no benefit in the majority of cases. A less invasive procedure that has been effective is the percutaneous retrogasserian injunction (98) with glycerol to perform rhizolysis of the second division of the trigeminal nerve. Avoiding the first division of the nerve reduced the risk of developing corneal anesthesia. As with the Janetta procedure, over three-fourths of patients improved with good long-term results of over five years in about 50% of patients. Radiofrequency rhizotomy of the sphenopalatine ganglion has been performed in patients who have failed medical management (99). About 60% of patients with episodic cluster headache have had pain-free responses of up to two years. In chronic cluster, the results are not as positive, with a response rate of about 30%. Recently, gamma knife disruption of the trigeminal root outlet has been suggested as a procedure (100). Five of six patients treated with this technique improved. While various authors have reported successful outcomes with these procedures, there may be significant risks associated with them including corneal anesthesia, anesthesia dolorosa, and recurrence of the cluster headaches.

Histamine Desensitization

At the Diamond Headache Clinic, we have had outstanding success with the use of intravenous histamine desensitization in aiding the treatment of patients with chronic cluster that has become refractive to treatment. The use of IV histamine desensitization in the treatment of cluster headache has been used since the 1930s when Bayard Horton, M.D. at Mayo Clinic (3) developed it. Review of his case reports and description of cluster headache has been noted (4) to be of such clarity as to have allowed inclusion of patients with other than cluster headache unlikely. Over his years at Mayo between 1936 and 1940, Horton treated approximately 184 patients with histamine (101). Of these, 63 patients met the majority of clinical features for what he was then calling "histaminic cephalgia." However, 12 of the 63 cases had some atypical features in their presentation. Of the 51 cases meeting all the criteria, 48 demonstrated relief from chronic cluster headaches with IV Histamine desensitization for variable periods, the majority of which developed a prolonged remission from their attacks. Other (102–104) headache experts including Blumenthal (102) and Ryan (104), who were fellows under Horton, had high success rates with IV Histamine desensitization therapy in the treatment of chronic cluster headache. Kunkle et al. (2) reported on 30 patients; 11 had received histamine treatments elsewhere without success, though he never utilized the treatment for his own patients. Subsequently, Friedman and Mikropouolos (105) reported only 15% of 35 patients as benefiting from histamine desensitization. Like Kunkle, the treatment with histamine was performed elsewhere; apparently, they are not utilizing it. These later anecdotal reports led to histamine desensitization falling into disrepute in the following years by the neurology community. We have reported previous studies (106,107) of IV Histamine desensitization as part of the treatment of intractable cluster headache that failed to respond to traditional medical therapies for cluster headache. Both of these initials reports showed marked clinical improvement in patients with chronic cluster headache that had become refractive to standard medical therapy. Most recently, we have been able to demonstrate a superior response of intravenous histamine compared to intravenous repetitive doses of dihydroergotamine (Fred Freitag, DO, Chicago, Illinois, unpublished data, January 2001). We were also able to show aspects of the chronic cluster headache patient and previous treatment, which would be helpful in determining who might require only more standard medical therapy *versus* who would benefit from intravenous histamine desensitization.

The mechanism by which IV histamine desensitization may act in cluster headache treatment has not been determined. Exposure of neural origin cells, however, to increasing concentrations of histamine has been shown to inhibit the production of cyclic guanosine $3'$, $5'$ monophosphate (cGMP) (108). They also demonstrated that this was not a calcium-dependent phenomenon suggesting that it was not related to the formation of cGMP. Increased cGMP activity correlates with increased formation of nitric oxide (NO) via nitric oxide synthetase (NOS) (109). Though not studied in cluster headache, this system of cellular mediation has been linked to chronic daily headache and migraine (110–113). Cluster headache patients have been found to have higher levels of plasma nitrites than controls (114) suggesting that this system may be activated even between acts thus predisposing patients to their cluster headache attacks. These studies suggest that histamine desensitization may be an active agent in the prevention of cluster headache by downregulating the cGMP-NO-*l*-arginine pathway by the persisting high levels of histamine present during the treatment process.

EVIDENCE-BASED MEDICINE

There is little evidence-based medicine available for the treatment of cluster headache. Most therapeutic approaches have been used in open-label paradigms. There are only single controlled trials *versus* placebo for Oxygen and DHE injections as being safe and effective. In multiple, placebo-controlled trials sumatriptan injections 6 mg and zolmitriptan nasal spray 5 and 10 mg doses demonstrate efficacy and safety consistently. There is minimal evidence for sumatriptan nasal spray at a 20 mg dose because of the numbers enrolled, though the results were favorable. There is only a single comparative trial for evidence of verapamil being effective and safe compared to lithium, which was also effective but had more adverse events. There is evidence not to use divalproex based on a single controlled trial, though the results had a high placebo response. There is positive evidence for civamide based on a single controlled trial.

There is positive evidence for IV histamine being more effective than IV DHE based on a comparative trial. There is only open-label and case study information available for the remainder of the treatments that are discussed above in cluster headache. Based on even these open-label studies, there is no evidence for melatonin, cyproheptadine or other antihistamines, deep brain stimulation of the hypothalamus, occipital nerve stimulators, botulinum toxin type A, or radiosurgical procedures. For the remainder of the approaches, the open-label evidence while favorable is insufficient to make a recommendation for utilization.

CONCLUSION

Cluster headache is a relatively rare condition, especially in family practice. Recognition of this disorder is important to provide optimal therapy. The treatment of cluster headache focuses on preventive therapies because of the high frequency of attacks that patients may experience. Acute therapies such as oxygen are highly reliable and safe. One can stage preventive therapies to provide early response such as may occur with corticosteroids and longer term, better-tolerated treatments of a variety of types. Patients with chronic cluster headache tend to become refractive to medical therapies and may require specialized medical therapies or surgery for intractable cases.

REFERENCES

1. Boes CJ, Capobianco DJ, Matharu MS, et al. Wilfred Harris' early description of cluster headache. Cephalalgia 2002; 22:320–326.
2. Kunkle EC, Pfeiffer JB, Wilhout WM, et al. Recurrent brief headaches in "cluster" pattern. Trans Am Neurol Assoc 1952; 77:240–243.
3. Horton BT, Maclean AR, Craig WMcK. A new syndrome of vascular headache: results of treatment with Histamine: Preliminary Report. Proc Staff Meet Mayo Clin 1939; 14:257–260.
4. Sjaastad O. Cluster headache syndrome. Maj Prob Neurol 1992; 23:16–17.
5. Moskowitz MA. Basic mechanisms in vascular headache. Neurol Clin 1990; 8:802–816.
6. Kudrow L. Cluster Headache: Mechanisms and Management. New York: Oxford University Press, 1980.
7. Manzoni GC. Gender ratio of cluster headache over the years: a possible role of changes in lifestyle. Cephalalgia 1988; 18:138–142.
8. Ekbom K, Svensson DA, Traff H, et al. Age at onset and sex ratio in cluster headache: observations over three decades. Cephalalgia 2002; 22:94–100.
9. Graham JR. Cluster headache. Headache 1972; 11:175–185.
10. Manzoni GC. Cluster headache and lifestyle: remarks on a population of 374 male patients. Cephalalgia 1999; 19:88–94.
11. Rogardo AZ, Harrison RH, Graham JR. Personality profiles in cluster headache, migraine and normal controls. Arch Neurol (Madr) 1974; 37:227–241.
12. Kudrow L. The cyclic relationship of natural illumination to cluster period frequency. Cephalalgia 1987; 7(Suppl 7):76–78.
13. Graham J. Cluster headache. The relation to arousal, relaxation and autonomic tone. Headache 1990; 30:145–151.
14. Pringsheim T. Cluster headache: evidence for a disorder of circadian rhythm and hypothalamic function. Can J Neurol Sci 2002; 29:33–40.
15. Costa A, Leston JA, Cavallini A, et al. Cluster headache and periodic affective illness: common chronobiologic features. Funct Neurol 1998; 13:263–272.
16. Silberstein SD, Niknam R, Rozen TD, et al. Cluster headache with aura. Neurology 2000; 54:219–221.
17. Torelli P, Manzoni GC. What predicts evolution from episodic to chronic cluster headache? Curr Pain Headache Rep 2002; 6:65–70.
18. Torelli P, Cologno D, Cadmartiri C, et al. Possible predictive factors in the evolution of episodic to chronic cluster headache. Headache 2000; 40:798–808.
19. Headache Classification Subcommittee of the International Headache Society. International Classification of Headache Disorders. Cephalalgia 2004; 24(Suppl 1): 44–48.
20. Edvinsson L, Uddman R. Neurobiology in primary headaches. Brain Res Rev 2005; 48:438–456.
21. Goadsby PJ. Pathophysiology of cluster headache: a trigeminal autonomic cephalgia. Lancet Neurol 2002; 1:251–257.
22. Leone M, Proietti Cecchini A, Franzini A, et al. Lessons from 8 years' experience of hypothalamic stimulation in cluster headache. Cephalalgia 2008; 28:787–797.
23. May A, Leone M, Boecker H, et al. Hypothalamic deep brain stimulation in positron emission tomography. J Neurosci 2006; 26:3589–3593.

24. Cortelli P, Guaraldi P, Leone M, et al. Effect of deep brain stimulation of the posterior hypothalamic area on the cardiovascular system in chronic cluster headache patients. Eur J Neurol 2007; 14:1008–1015.
25. Kudrow L. The pathogenesis of cluster headache. Curr Opin Neurol 1994; 7: 278–282.
26. Kudrow L, Kudrow DB. The role of chemoreceptor activity and oxyhemoglobin desaturation in cluster headache. Headache 1993; 33:483–484.
27. Gouveia RG, Parreira E, Pavão Martins I. Autonomic features in cluster headache. Exploratory factor analysis. J Headache Pain 2005; 6:20–23.
28. Goadsby PJ, Edvinsson L. Neuropeptide changes in a case of chronic paroxysmal hemicrania—evidence for trigemino-parasympathetic activation. Cephalalgia 1996; 16:448–450.
29. Strittmatter M, Hamann GF, Grauer M, et al. Altered activity of the sympathetic nervous system and changes in the balance of hypophyseal, pituitary, and adrenal hormones in patients with cluster headache. Neuroreport 1996; 7:1229–1234.
30. Meineri P, Pellegrino G, Rosso MG, et al. Systemic autonomic involvement in episodic cluster headache: a comparison between active and remission periods. J Headache Pain 2005; 6:240–243.
31. Martins IP, Gouveia RG, Parreira E. Cluster headache without autonomic symptoms: why is it different? Headache 2005; 45:190–195.
32. Nardone R, Ausserer H, Bratti A, et al. Trigemino-cervical reflex abnormalities in patients with migraine and cluster headache. Headache 2008; 48:578–585.
33. Busch V, Jakob W, Juergens T, et al. Occipital nerve blockade in chronic cluster headache patients and functional connectivity between trigeminal and occipital nerves. Cephalalgia 2007; 27:1206–1214.
34. Drummond PD. Mechanisms of autonomic disturbance in the face during and between attacks of cluster headache. Cephalalgia 2006; 26:633–641.
35. Strittmatter M, Hamann GF, Grauer M, et al. Altered activity of the sympathetic nervous system and changes in the balance of hypophyseal, pituitary and adrenal hormones in patients with cluster headache. Neuroreport 1996; 7:1229–1234.
36. Stillman MJ. Testosterone replacement therapy for treatment refractory cluster headache. Headache 2006; 46:925–933.
37. Peres MF. Melatonin, the pineal gland and their implications for headache disorders. Cephalalgia 2005; 25:403–411.
38. Mosnaim AD, Wolf ME, Lee G, et al. Plasma degradation of methionine–enkephalin by cluster headache patients (in vitro studies). Headache Q 1990; 1:79–83.
39. Sprenger T, Willoch F, Miederer M, et al. Opioidergic changes in the pineal gland and hypothalamus in cluster headache: a ligand PET study. Neurology 2006; 66: 1108–1110.
40. Sjöstrand C, Modin H, Masterman T, et al. Analysis of nitric oxide synthase genes in cluster headache. Cephalalgia 2002; 22:758–764.
41. Platform presentation by Frederick G. Freitag, at the National Headache Foundation Research Summit. Genetics of Headache: Do the Genetics of Histamine Metabolism Predict Response to Treatment with Histamine in Cluster Headache? Palm Springs, California, February 10, 2004.
42. Sjöstrand C, Duvefelt K, Steinberg A, et al. Gene expression profiling in cluster headache: a pilot microarray study. Headache 2006; 46:1518–1534.
43. Kudrow L. Response of cluster headache attacks to oxygen inhalation. Headache 1981; 21:1–4.
44. Fogan L. Treatment of cluster headache: a double blind comparison of oxygen versus air inhalation. Arch Neurol 1985; 4:362–363.
45. Kittrelle JP, Grouse DS, Seybold ME. Cluster headache local anesthetic abortive agents. Arch Neurol 1985; 42:496–498.
46. Kudrow L, Kudrow DB. Intranasal lidocaine. Headache 1995; 35:565–566.
47. Kudrow L, Kudrow DB, Sandweiss JH. Rapid and sustained relief of migraine attacks with intranasal lidocaine: preliminary findings. Headache 1995; 35:79–82.

48. Rozen TD. Olanzapine as an abortive agent for cluster headache. Headache 2001; 41:813–816.
49. Horton BT, Peters GA, Blumenthal LS. A new product in the treatment of migraine: a preliminary report. Proc Staff Meet Mayo Clin 1945; 20:241–248.
50. Mather PJ, Silberstein SD, Shulman EA, et al. The treatment of cluster headache with repetitive intravenous dihydroergotamine. Headache 1991; 31:525–532.
51. Andersson PG, Jespersen LT. Dihydroergotamine nasal spray in the treatment of attacks of cluster headache. A double blind trial versus placebo. Cephalalgia 1986; 6:51–54.
52. The Sumatriptan Cluster Headache Study Group. Treatment of acute cluster headache with sumatriptan. N Engl J Med 1991; 325:322–326.
53. Ekbom K, Krabbe A, Miceli G, et al. Cluster headache attacks treated for up to three months with subcutaneous sumatriptan (6 mg). Cephalalgia 1995; 15:230–236.
54. The Sumatriptan Cluster Headache Study Group. Subcutaneous sumatriptan in the acute treatment of cluster headache: a dose comparison study. Acta Neurol Scand 1993; 88:63–69.
55. Gobel H, Lindner V, Heinze A, et al. Acute therapy for cluster headache with sumatriptan: findings of a one year long term study. Neurology 1998; 51:908–911.
56. Centonze V, Bassi A, Causarano V, et al. Sumatriptan overuse in episodic cluster headache: lack of adverse events, rebound syndromes, drug dependence and tachyphylaxis. Funct Neurol 2000; 15:167–170.
57. Centonze V, Polito BM, Attolini E, et al. Use of high sumatriptan dosages during episodic cluster headache: three clinical cases. Headache 1996; 36:389–391.
58. Schuh-Hofer S, Reuter U, Kinze S, et al. Treatment of acute cluster headache with sumatriptan 20 mg nasal spray—an open pilot study. J Neurol 2002; 249:94–99.
59. Hardebo JE, Dahlof C. Sumatriptan nasal spray (20 mg/dose) in the acute treatment of cluster headache. Cephalalgia 1998; 18:487–489.
60. Bahra A, Gawel MJ, Hardebo JE, et al. Oral zolmitriptan is effective in the acute treatment of cluster headache. Neurology 2000; 54:1832–1839.
61. Rapoport AM, Mathew NT, Silberstein SD, et al. Zolmitriptan nasal spray in the acute treatment of cluster headache: a double-blind study. Neurology 2007; 69:821–826.
62. Horton B. Histaminic cephalgia. Lancet 1952; 2:92–98.
63. Kudrow L. Comparative results of prednisone, methysergide, and lithium therapy in cluster headache. In: Greene R, ed. Current Concepts in Migraine Research. New York: Raven Press, 1978:159–163.
64. Couch JR, Ziegler DK. Prednisone therapy for cluster headache. Headache 1978; 18:219–221.
65. Kudrow L. Diagnosis and treatment of cluster headache. Med Clin North Am 191; 75:579–593.
66. Monstad I, Krabbe A, Miceli G, et al. Preemptive oral treatment with sumatriptan during a cluster period. Headache 1995; 35:607–613.
67. Loder E. Naratriptan in the prophylaxis of cluster headache. Headache 2002; 42:56–57
68. Ekbom K. Lithium for cluster headache: review of the literature and preliminary result of long term treatment. Headache 1981; 21:132–139.
69. Treiser SL, Cascio CS, O'Donohue TL, et al. Lithium increases serotonin release and decreases serotonin receptors in the hippocampus. Science 1981; 213:1529–1531.
70. Okusa MD, Lux Jovita TC. Clinical manifestations and management of acute lithium intoxication. Am J Med 1994; 97:383–389.
71. Meyer JS, Hardenberg J. Clinical effectiveness of calcium entry blockers in prophylactic treatment of migraine and cluster headache. Headache 1983; 23:266–277.
72. Gabai IJ, Spierings ELH. Prophylactic treatment of cluster headache with verapamil. Headache 1989; 29:167–168.
73. Leone M, d'Amico D, Frediani F, et al. Verapamil in the prophylaxis of episodic cluster headache: a double-blind study versus placebo. Neurology 2000; 54:1382–1385.

74. Bussone G, Leone M, Peccarisi C, et al. Double blind comparison of lithium and verapamil in cluster headache prophylaxis. Headache 1990; 30:411–417.
75. Hering R, Kuritsky A. Sodium valproate in the treatment of cluster headache: an open clinical trial. Cephalalgia 1989; 9:195–198.
76. Gallagher RM, Mueller LL, Freitag FG. Divalproex sodium in the treatment of migraine and cluster headaches. J Am Osteopath Assoc 2002; 102:92–94.
77. El Amrani M, Massiou H, Bousser MG. A negative trial of sodium valproate in cluster headache: methodological issues. Cephalalgia 2002; 22:205–208.
78. Wheeler SD, Carrazana EJ. Topiramate-treated cluster headache. Neurology 1999; 53:234–236.
79. Mathew NT, Kailasam J, Meadors L. Prophylaxis of migraine, transformed migraine, and cluster headache with topiramate. Headache 2002; 42(8):796–803.
80. Schuh-Hofer S, Israel H, Neeb L, et al. The use of gabapentin in chronic cluster headache patients refractory to first-line therapy. Eur J Neurol 2007; 14:694–696.
81. Peres Mf, Rozen TD. Melatonin in the preventive treatment of chronic cluster headache. Cephalalgia 2001; 21:993–995.
82. Solomon GD, Kunkel RS, Frame Jr. Intranasal capsaicin cream in cluster headache. In: Rose FC, ed. New Advances in Headache Research 3. London: Smith-Gordon, 1993.
83. Saper JR, Klapper J, Mathew NT, et al. Intranasal civamide for the treatment of episodic cluster headaches. Arch Neurol 2002; 59:990–994.
84. Sostak P, Krause P, Förderreuther S, et al. Botulinum toxin type-A therapy in cluster headache: an open study. J Headache Pain 2007; 8:236–241.
85. Mellick GA, Mellick LB. Cluster headache management with methylphenidate (Ritalin). Headache 1998; 38:710–712.
86. Hering-Hanit R, Gadoth N. The use of baclofen in cluster headache. Curr Pain Headache Rep 2001; 5:79–82.
87. Sewell RA, Halpern JH, Pope HG Jr. Response of cluster headache to psilocybin and LSD. Neurology 2006; 66:1920–1922.
88. D'Andrea G, Perini F, Granella F, et al. Efficacy of transdermal clonidine in short-term treatment of cluster headache: a pilot study. Cephalalgia 1995; 15:430–433.
89. Sicuteri F. Enkephalinase inhibition relieves pain syndromes of central dysnociception (migraine and related headache). Cephalalgia 1981; 1:229–232.
90. Busch V, Jakob W, Juergens T, et al. Occipital nerve blockade in chronic cluster headache patients and functional connectivity between trigeminal and occipital nerves. Cephalalgia 2007; 27:1206–1214.
91. Afridi SK, Shields KG, Bhola R, et al. Greater occipital nerve injection in primary headache syndromes—prolonged effects from a single injection. Pain 2006; 122:126–129.
92. Peres MF, Stiles MA, Siow HC, et al. Greater occipital nerve blockade for cluster headache. Cephalalgia 2004; 24:239.
93. Proietti Cecchini A, Mea E, Tullo V, et al. Long-term experience of neuromodulation in TACs. Neurol Sci 2008; 29(Suppl 1):S62–S64.
94. Bartsch T, Pinsker MO, Rasche D, et al. Hypothalamic deep brain stimulation for cluster headache: experience from a new multicase series. Cephalalgia 2008; 28:285–295.
95. Burns B, Watkins L, Goadsby PJ. Treatment of medically intractable cluster headache by occipital nerve stimulation: long-term follow-up of eight patients. Lancet 2007; 369:1099–1106.
96. McClelland S 3rd, Tendulkar RD, Barnett GH, et al. Long-term results of radiosurgery for refractory cluster headache. Neurosurgery 2006; 59:1258–1262.
97. Lovely TJ, Kotsiakis X, Jannetta PJ. The surgical management of chronic cluster headache. Headache 1998; 38:590–594.
98. Pieper DR, Dickerson J, Hassenbusch SJ. Percutaneous retrogasserian glycerol rhizolysis for the treatment of chronic intractable cluster headaches: long term results. Neurosurgery 2000; 46:363–368.

99. Sanders M, Zuurmond WW. Efficacy of sphenopalatine ganglion blockade in 66 patients suffering from cluster headache: a 12 to 70 month follow-up evaluation. J Neurosurg 1997; 87:876–880.
100. Ford RG, Ford KT, Swaid S, et al. Gamma knife treatment of refractory cluster headache. Headache 1998; 38:3–9.
101. Horton BT. The use of histamine in the treatment of specific types of headache. JAMA 1941; 116:377–383.
102. Blumenthal LS. Current histamine therapy. Mod Med 1950; 18:51–53.
103. Stern FH. Histamine cephalalgia—an often overlooked cause of headache. Psychosomatics 1969; 10:53–56.
104. Ryan RE Sr, Ryan RE Jr. Cluster headache. Otolaryngol Clin North Am 1989; 22:1131–1144.
105. Friedman AP, Mikropouolos HE. Cluster headache. Neurology 1958; 8:653–663.
106. Diamond S, Freitag FG, Prager J, et al. Treatment of intractable cluster. Headache 1986; 26:42–46.
107. Diamond S, Freitag FG, Diamond ML, et al. IV histamine desensitization therapy in intractable cluster headache. Headache Q 1998; 9:55–59.
108. Taylor JE, Richelson E. Desensitization of histamine H_1 receptor-mediated cyclic GMP formation in mouse neuroblastoma cells. Mol Pharmacol 1979; 15:462–471.
109. Akerman S, Williamson DJ, Kaube H, et al. Nitric oxide synthetase inhibitors can antagonize neurogenic and calcitonin gene-related peptide induced dilation of dural meningeal vessels. Br J Pharmacol 2002; 137:62–68.
110. Sarchielli P, Alberti A, Floridi A, et al. L-Arginine/nitric oxide pathway in chronic tension type headache: relation with serotonin content and secretion and glutamate content. J Neurol Sci 2002; 198:9–15.
111. Sarchielli P, Alberti A, Codini M, et al. Nitric oxide metabolites, prostaglandins and trigeminal vasoactive peptides in internal jugular vein blood during spontaneous migraine attacks. Cephalalgia 2000; 20:907–918.
112. Thomsen LL. Investigation into the role of nitric oxide and the large intracranial arteries in migraine headache. Cephalalgia 1997; 17:873–985.
113. Olesen J, Thomsen LL, Lassen LH, et al. The nitric oxide hypothesis of migraine and other vascular headaches. Cephalalgia 1995; 15:94–100.
114. D'Amico D, Ferraris A, Leone M, et al. Increased plasma nitrites in migraine and cluster headache patients in the interictal period: basal hyperactivity of L-arginine-NO-pathway? Cephalalgia 2002; 22:33–36.

6   Trigeminal Autonomic Cephalalgias

Gary D. Klasser

Department of Oral Medicine and Diagnostic Sciences, University of Illinois at Chicago, College of Dentistry, Chicago, Illinois, U.S.A.

Trigeminal autonomic cephalalgias (TACs) are a collective term for headache disorders that are characterized by unilateral head and/or face pain with accompanying autonomic features (1,2). The International Classification of Headache Disorders II (ICHD-II) classifies TACs as (*i*) episodic or chronic cluster headache (CH); (*ii*) episodic or chronic paroxysmal hemicrania (PH); and (*iii*) short-lasting unilateral neuralgiform headache attacks with conjunctival injection and tearing (SUNCT) (2). This chapter is aimed at increasing awareness and providing information regarding PH and SUNCT (information regarding CH is presented in Chap. 5) as patients often consult with health care providers for symptoms and management of these types of headaches (3–7). For purposes of clarity, TACs will refer to CH, PH and SUNCT in this chapter.

PAROXYSMAL HEMICRANIA

The Disorder

Sjaastad and Dale (8) were the first to recognize and describe PH as a "new and treatable headache entity." They later named the headache "chronic PH" to better describe and identify the headache (9). The early cases of PH seemed to involve only patients who complained of daily and unremitting headaches and it was assumed that there was only a chronic form of PH. However, it is now reported that there exists an episodic form whereby the headache bouts are separated by periods of complete remission (10–13). Hence, the term "episodic PH" is currently used to better describe the remitting variant of PH (10). These two various forms of PH have been classified in the ICHD-II (Table 1).

    Unfortunately, data regarding prevalence for PH are lacking in the literature. However, it is thought to represent a small proportion of headaches (1–3%) in comparison to CH (14). Prevalence of PH is described as equivalent to 1 case per 50,000 persons in the general population with the chronic form (80%) of PH being more prevalent than the episodic form (20%) (15). The episodic form is rare with fewer than 30 cases reported in the literature (1,16,17). PH has a female preponderance with a female-to-male ratio ranging between 1.6 and 2.36 to 1 (14,18). However, this prevailing view of PH as being a female-dominated condition may arise from males being incorrectly diagnosed with CH instead of PH because CH is the more common disorder with a male preponderance. PH lacks any geographic boundaries (19–21) or racial tendencies (21). The typical age of onset for PH is between 20 and 30 years (14,22) with a mean age of 34 years (23). However, PH can occur at any age (range between 6 and 81 years) (23) with

TABLE 1   The International Classification of Headache Disorders II for Paroxysmal
Hemicrania (2)

Diagnostic criteria
A. At least 20 attacks fulfilling criteria B–D
B. Attacks of severe unilateral orbital, supraorbital or temporal pain lasting 2–30 minutes
C. Headache is accompanied by at least one of the following:
    1. Ipsilateral conjunctival injection and/or lacrimation
    2. Ipsilateral nasal congestion and/or rhinorrhea
    3. Ipsilateral eyelid edema
    4. Ipsilateral forehead and facial sweating
    5. Ipsilateral miosis and/or ptosis
D. Attacks have a frequency above 5 per day for more than half of the time, although
   periods with lower frequency may occur
E. Attacks are prevented completely by therapeutic doses of indomethacin[a]
F. Not attributed to another disorder[b]
Episodic
Diagnostic criteria
A. Attacks fulfilling criteria A–F for paroxysmal hemicrania (see above)
B. At least two attacks lasting 7–365 days and separated by pain-free remission periods
   ≥ 1 month
Chronic
Diagnostic criteria:
A. Attacks fulfilling criteria A–F for paroxysmal hemicrania (see above)
B. Attacks recur over > 1 year without remission periods or with remission period lasting
   < 1 month

[a]In order to rule out incomplete response, indomethacin should be used in a dose of ≥ 150 mg daily orally or
rectally, or ≥ 100 mg by injection, but for maintenance smaller doses are often sufficient.
[b]History and physical and neurological examination do not suggest any of the disorders listed in groups 5–
12, or history and/or physical and/or neurological examinations do suggest such disorder but it is ruled out
by appropriate investigations, or such disorder is present but attacks do not occur for the first time in close
temporal relationship to the disorder.

reports of occurrence in children as young as the age of 3 years (24–26). Interestingly, there has only been one report of PH with a familial link which involved a
mother and daughter (27).

PH is characterized by severe, almost always unilateral pain (without side
shift) attacks localized to orbital, supraorbital, temporal, or combinations of
these sites accompanied by one or more ipsilateral autonomic features. However,
there have been reports of side shifts in PH attacks, albeit, only a few (28,29) and
one report of bilateral PH attacks (30). PH pain is also reported to be present
in and around the maxilla and frontal regions (2,15) and may also involve
the neck and occiput (15,22). It is not uncommon for the pain to involve the
orofacial structures thereby confusing the health care provider as to the true
source of the pain. This misinterpretation often results in a referral to a dentist
where, unfortunately, the delivery of inappropriate dental procedures may be
undertaken (4–7,31–34).

The intensity of PH pain is excruciating and extreme with the quality typically described as aching or throbbing initially and elevating to boring or stabbing at peak intensity (1,35). Most patients suffer from the chronic form of PH,
which is, essentially, unremitting. However, 20% of PH patients have the episodic
form which involves bouts of PH ranging from 2 weeks to 4.5 months with a
mean duration of 13.3 ± 12.2 years accompanied by periods of remission lasting

between 1 and 36 months (14,36). Typically, episodic PH progresses into chronic PH (35) but may also transform into another form of headache termed hemicrania continua (37). Although less likely, chronic PH can evolve to the episodic form (35). The individual PH attack usually begins abruptly with duration of 2 to 30 minutes and can persist up to 2 hours (2,14,15).

PH attacks are characterized by an abrupt onset and cessation accompanied by mild pain and tenderness between attacks (1). The frequency of PH attacks is between 1 and 40 attacks per day (14) with a mean of 6 to 14 attacks per day (18,38). PH attacks occur regularly at all hours of the day. There is no preponderance for nocturnal attacks (as present with CH); however, nocturnal attacks, in association with rapid eye movement sleep phase, have been reported (39). One-third of PH patients report pain or discomfort between PH attacks (14).

Almost all PH attacks exhibit ipsilateral cranial and facial autonomic features (2,15) with lacrimation, conjunctival injection, nasal congestion and rhinorrhea being the most frequently observed (14). Less frequent autonomic features such as eyelid edema, ptosis, miosis and facial sweating may also occur with PH attacks (2,15). Interestingly, there have been reports of bilateral autonomic features in PH (14) as well as PH attacks without autonomic features (40) and autonomic features during PH attacks without pain (29).

Approximately 50% of PH sufferers report sitting still or resting in bed during attacks and 50% prefer pacing (14,41). In a recent prospective study of 31 PH cases (42), it was found that the majority of patients (80%) were agitated or restless or both with the pain and 26% were aggressive. Migraine-like features such as photophobia (21%) and nausea (14%) are familiar complaints during PH attacks (14) with occasional vomiting and phonophobia reported (14,15).

The majority of PH attacks are spontaneous; however, individuals report that certain triggers initiate attacks. Alcoholic drinks (7%) (14) and mechanical rotation or bending of the head with external pressure against certain points (10%) (43) have been reported to be such triggers. Additionally, the application of external pressure to the transverse process of C4–5, C2 root or greater occipital nerve can also precipitate a PH attack (43,44).

Diagnosis
The key feature to PH diagnosis is based on the history from previous attacks. These include the classical presentations of rapid onset, location, quality, and duration of the pain, temporal pattern of episodes, trigger factors, and associated autonomic features (2). A differential diagnosis is necessary prior to establishing a working diagnosis for PH as many other conditions can mimic PH (Table 2). A potential difficulty with the differential diagnosis of PH is the considerable overlap with CH. They may be differentiated, as PH has a purported female preponderance, shorter duration and more frequent headache attacks (2,45). There are also a few case reports of PH coexisting with other primary headaches and orofacial pains including trigeminal neuralgia (PH-tic syndrome) (46), CH (47), migraine (48), primary cough headache (49), and red ear syndrome (50). It is important to differentiate PH from other coexisting conditions as they require different treatments.

Another differentiating and almost pathognomonic feature between PH and other disorders is the responsiveness to oral indomethacin, 25 mg three times a day. If there is a lack of response after 10 days, oral indomethacin may be

TABLE 2 Differential Diagnosis for Paroxysmal Hemicrania (1,2,4,7)

Symptomatic paroxysmal hemicrania
- Vascular causes
- Tumors

TACs including
- Hemicrania continua
- Short-lasting unilateral neuralgiform headache attacks with cranial Autonomic symptoms (SUNA)

Other primary headaches
- Primary stabbing headache
- Primary cough headache
- Primary exertional headache
- Primary headache associated with sexual activity
- Hypnic headache

Trigeminal neuralgia
  Temporomandibular disorders
  Dental pain

increased gradually to a maximum of 75 mg three times a day if PH is strongly suspected in the differential diagnosis. An absolute resolution of the headache should be apparent within two days of an effective dose of oral indomethacin (45). Another available diagnostic test is the "Indotest," which involves the use of intramuscular injections of indomethacin (between 50 and 100 mg) resulting in sustained pain relief (between 493 and 668 minutes) (51). The advantage of the Indotest is that it allows for immediate diagnosis of PH, but further validation of this test is needed (45,51). In patients who do not respond to indomethacin, the working diagnosis of PH should be reconsidered (45). However, patients with classical presentation of PH have been reported to be unresponsive to indomethacin (18,52). Although the diagnosis of PH may be obvious, underlying pathology (symptomatic PH) is common and must be considered (18). Therefore, a neurological examination and an MRI should be performed routinely regardless of the clinical presentation (45). Symptomatic PH may involve vascular pathology including middle cerebral artery infarct (53); collagen vascular disease (54); and parietal arteriovenous malformation (53); and tumors such as a Pancoast tumor (55), pituitary microadenoma (56), and macroprolactinoma (57). Therefore, if necessary, additional tests to rule out these diseases, such as complete blood count (58), vasculitis screen (54), lumbar puncture (59), chest radiograph (58), and electrocardiography (60), may be necessary.

Since PH is a phenomenon that has been described relatively recently, there is a paucity of literature on its longitudinal natural history and long-term prognosis.

Pathophysiology

The pathophysiology of PH is unknown, yet it appears that TACs share somewhat of a common pathophysiology. Functional neuroimaging studies in PH provide evidence for hypothalamic involvement (61). It appears that there is persistent activation of certain regions of the brain, termed the pain neuromatrix, during acute PH attacks and interictal pain-free states off indomethacin that is deactivated by the administration of indomethacin. Furthermore, during the untreated PH state, there is significant activation of the contralateral posterior hypothalamus and contralateral ventral midbrain, which extends over the red nucleus and substantia nigra. The conclusion is that these activated subcortical structures, particularly the hypothalamus, are pivotal in the pathophysiology of this disorder.

There are two interesting features regarding the pathophysiology of PH with one being rather unique to this headache disorder. It appears that the involvement of the trigeminal–autonomic reflex pathway is a shared feature among TACs. The unique feature only found with PH seems to be absolute responsiveness of this disorder to indomethacin.

Trigeminal–Autonomic Reflex Pathway

Two key aspects characterizing the pathophysiology of PH and other TACs are the source and trigeminal distribution of pain, and the ipsilateral cranial and facial autonomic features. The trigeminal–autonomic reflex involves the trigeminal afferents and the brain stem connections between nucleus caudalis and superior salivary nucleus. Activation of the superior salivary nucleus is responsible for the cranial and facial parasympathetic outflow via the facial nerve. Given the anatomical connections, trigeminal efferent activation also results in pain in the distribution of the trigeminal and upper cervical nerves in addition to stimulating the facial nerve parasympathetic outflow (1,35,62). Due to the anatomical extension of the nucleus caudalis to upper cervical nerves (1), PH pain may also involve the neck and occiput (22). It has also been reported that neurotransmitters such as calcitonin gene-related peptide (CGRP) and vasoactive intestinal polypeptide (VIP) released by sensitized trigeminal neurons are elevated during PH attacks and return to normal after treatment (1) implicating involvement of trigeminal afferents. This is supported by experimental studies whereby stimulation of the trigeminal ganglion results in local release of CGRP, substance P, and VIP from parasympathetic nerves mimicking the occurrence during PH attacks (63).

Absolute Responsiveness to Indomethacin

The rationale for the absolute effectiveness of indomethacin in the treatment of PH is unknown. It appears that indomethacin is effective in a mechanism other than that of prostaglandin synthesis inhibition as other nonsteroidal anti-inflammatory drugs (NSAIDs) have been found to be ineffective in PH treatment (64). Possible explanations for the efficacy of indomethacin may be related to its unique ability to decrease intracranial pressure (64), its inhibitory effects on the central nociceptive system (65), and its ability to reduce cerebral blood flow (66,67). However, the most current theory for the efficacy of indomethacin is related to its ability to inhibit the production of nitric oxide by endothelial and inducible nitric oxide synthase (64,68,69). The rationale for this is that glycerol trinitrate (a nitric oxide donor), a known trigger of CH and migraine (59), colocalizes nitric oxide with VIP in parasympathetic nerves in addition to activating the release of CGRP from trigeminal fibers (64,70). Therefore, indomethacin may be effective by antagonizing one or more steps in the nitric oxide pathway, hence, returning the elevated levels of CGRP and VIP to a state of normalcy (64). Further studies are required to better elucidate the relationship between indomethacin responsiveness and PH pathophysiology.

Treatment

The management for PH is prophylactic use of indomethacin. The recommended dose is 75 mg per day for three days, followed, if necessary, by 150 mg per day for another three days (71). The usual therapeutic doses range between 50 and 125 mg per day; however, higher doses of 200–250 mg per day may be necessary to abort pain during an exacerbation (72). Patients who are nonresponsive at these higher doses are unlikely to benefit from this medication. For responsive patients, the pain usually disappears within 24 hours with a range of a few hours to 5 days (14). When indomethacin is discontinued, symptoms often reappear within 12 hours to several days (73); therefore, continuous use of indomethacin for an undetermined period of time is the preferred management strategy (74). Unfortunately, it has been reported that the therapeutic effectiveness of indomethacin may decrease with time (14,73) for reasons unrelated to drug tolerance (75). However, there have also been reports where discontinuation of indomethacin has not resulted in the reoccurrence of PH symptoms, allowing the patients to be symptom-free for lengthy periods of time (7,76). Health care providers should be alerted to situations in which persistently high doses of indomethacin are utilized, if patients suddenly become refractory to their therapeutic dose or require escalating doses, as this may be indicative of an underlying pathologic condition (15,72,77). This should immediately prompt reevaluation of the diagnosis of PH (45). Unfortunately, there are several common side effects associated with the use of indomethacin such as dyspepsia, anorexia, nausea, and abdominal discomfort. In order to prevent these gastrointestinal complications, prostaglandin analogues (misoprostol), gastroprotective antacids, histamine-2 receptor antagonists, or proton pump inhibitors can be prescribed (1,7) and should always be considered for long-term treatment. The contraindications for indomethacin use include those patients who have asthma, anemia, impaired hepatic, and/or renal functions.

Intolerable side effects, contraindications, or nonresponsiveness to indomethacin necessitates trials with other medications. Other NSAIDs such as aspirin, naproxen, diclofenac, and ketoprofen have been used (14,78,79). The COX-2 inhibitor, celecoxib, has also been reported to be effective in PH management (16,80). Calcium channel blockers such as verapamil have also been used in PH management (79,81,82). Acetazolamide, a diuretic with anticonvulsant properties that is also known to reduce intraocular pressure, may be used for PH with some positive results reported (52). Sumatriptan, which shows effectiveness in migraine and CH, was reported to benefit a patient with bilateral PH (59) and a unilateral case (83), although its effectiveness in other cases is questionable (84,85). Topiramate, an anticonvulsant used in the treatment of other primary headache disorders and pain syndromes, was effective in treating a patient who experienced epigastric symptoms with indomethacin (86). Steroids, due to anti-inflammatory effects, have been employed in the treatment of PH (78). Anesthetic blockades of pericranial nerves have been reported to be ineffective (87). Contrary to this, responses to greater occipital nerve blockade have shown positive results (88). It appears that other than indomethacin, all other medications or procedures are rather inconsistent and have only been used in isolated refractory or nonresponsive cases and in very small clinical trials.

SHORT-LASTING UNILATERAL NEURALGIFORM HEADACHE WITH CONJUNCTIVAL INJECTION AND TEARING

The Disorder

SUNCT was first described by Sjaastad and colleagues in 1978 (89). Awareness and recognition for SUNCT was enhanced by subsequent papers that characterized this disorder, which, in turn, led to a diagnostic criteria proposal to validate SUNCT as a headache entity (1,90–92). Consequently, the committee for the ICHD-II developed and implemented classification criteria for SUNCT as one of the TACs (Table 3) (2).

SUNCT is an extremely rare disorder with fewer than 100 cases reported in the literature. Due to its rarity, the prevalence and incidence of SUNCT have not been well categorized. Williams and Broadley (93) estimated the incidence of SUNCT and/or a variant of SUNCT to be 1.2 per 100,000 and the prevalence to be approximately 6.6 per 100,000. However, SUNCT may be more common than the literature suggests due to the commonalities and possible misdiagnosis with trigeminal neuralgia, primary stabbing headache, CH and PH (94). In fact, recent studies suggest that SUNCT may be at least as common as PH (95,96). Less than a decade ago, SUNCT was reported to have a male preponderance with a male-to-female ratio of 3.75 to 1 in a sample based on 19 patients (97). Following this, Matharu et al. (98) reported a male-to-female ratio of 1.3 to 1 based on 50 patients suggesting only a modest male preponderance. The typical age of onset for SUNCT is between 35 and 65 years with a mean age of 50 years (98). However, SUNCT can occur at any age (15) with reports of occurrence in individuals as young (99) as 5 and as old (100) as 88 years. Additionally, there does not appear to be any geographic propensity with SUNCT (100–103). Whether or not SUNCT has a familial link is yet to be determined as there has only been one report of SUNCT in a family (104).

The headache attacks in SUNCT are characteristically unilateral without side shift in most patients (88%) and present more frequently on the right side (60%) compared to the left side (36%) (97,98). However, there are reports of side shifts between attacks (105,106) as well as bilateral SUNCT attacks (97,107).

TABLE 3 International Classification of Headache Disorders II for Short-Lasting Unilateral Neuralgiform Headache Attacks with Conjunctival Injection and Tearing (SUNCT) (2)

Diagnostic criteria
B. At least 20 attacks fulfilling criteria B–D
C. Attacks of unilateral orbital, supraorbital or temporal stabbing or pulsating pain lasting 5–240 seconds
D. Pain is accompanied by ipsilateral conjunctival injection and lacrimation
E. Attacks occur with a frequency from 3 to 200 per day
F. Not attributed to any other disorder[a]

[a]History and physical and neurological examination do not suggest any of the disorders listed in groups 5–12, or history and/or physical and/or neurological examinations do suggest such disorder, but it is ruled out by appropriate investigations, or such disorder is present, but attacks do not occur for the first time in close temporal relationship to the disorder.

The pain is localized and most intense in the periorbital, temporal, and frontal region and, occasionally, involves the neck, occiput, side, and top of the head, ear, nose, cheek, palate, and throat (2,97,98,105,108,109). Interestingly, 33% and 21% of SUNCT patients report pain localized to the maxillary branch of the trigeminal nerve and teeth, respectively (95).

The intensity of SUNCT pain can be excruciating and extreme. In a recent study, 84% of SUNCT patients reported pain as 10/10 (most severe pain imaginable) on a verbal rating scale (95). The pain quality of SUNCT is typically neuralgic-like (97) with 70% of patients describing the pain as stabbing, sharp, burning, pricking, piercing, shooting, lancinating, or electric-shock like. Other descriptions of pain quality include pulsatile, throbbing, steady, spasmodic, and staccato-like (98).

Most patients suffer from episodic periods of symptoms with alternating periods of remission without any pattern. Typically, the symptomatic period persists for several days to months with one to two bouts a year. Remission of SUNCT episodes have been reported to last for a few months, although it has also been reported to be as little as 1 week and prolonged for up to 8.5 years (110). Also, remission periods tend to decrease with time (97). There are numerous cases that report a chronic form of SUNCT exists with symptomatic periods lasting between 1 and 17 years. The longest reported duration of a symptomatic period is 48 years (97). Also, SUNCT attacks may have a chronic pattern from onset, evolve from an initially episodic form to a chronic form, or even alternate between the episodic form and chronic form (98). Interestingly, a distinction between the chronic form and episodic form was not incorporated into the ICHD-II criteria for SUNCT as has been with the other TACs (2).

The individual SUNCT attack usually begins abruptly with maximum intensity within 2 to 3 seconds and may persist between 2 and 600 seconds (97,105,111,112). Although rare, prolonged attacks lasting up to two hours have been described in a patient with otherwise classical SUNCT. SUNCT attacks usually have an abrupt onset and rapid cessation with pain-free periods between attacks (97,98). However, not all periods between attacks are pain-free, as previously stated; rather, there are reports of dull interictal discomfort in the site of pain between attacks that may be intermittent or continuous (113). In addition to the classic "plateau-like pattern," other temporal patterns exist for individual SUNCT attacks, including a "repetitive pattern of spike-like paroxysms" (short lasting attacks in rapid succession), "saw-tooth pattern" (consecutive spike-like paroxysms without reaching pain-free baseline), and a "plateau-like pattern plus exacerbation" (one- to two-second jabs superimposed over the classic plateau-like pattern) (94,114).

The frequency of SUNCT attacks varies both intraindividually and interindividually (98). The attack frequency varies from less than once a day to more than 60 attacks per hour (112). Pareja et al. (92), in a study involving objective assessment of the attack frequency in four SUNCT patients, reported a mean of 16 attacks per day with a range between 1 and 86 attacks daily. Also status-like pattern lasting one to three days has been reported in SUNCT (115) as well as frequent, repetitive attacks that last for hours or days (112,116,117). SUNCT attacks occur predominantly during the day; typically, with bimodal distribution in the morning and afternoon or evening. Only 1.2% of SUNCT attacks are nocturnal and usually occur during severe periods (92). A recent study reported that 7%

of SUNCT patients experience attacks in their sleep (95). Similarly, others have argued that although SUNCT attacks predominately occur during the day, it is overstated, claiming that nocturnal attacks are more frequent than reported in the literature (98).

Almost all SUNCT attacks exhibit ipsilateral cranial and facial autonomic features, namely conjunctival injection and tearing (2,15). Matharu et al. (98), in a review of 50 SUNCT patients, reported ipsilateral conjunctival injection and tearing to occur in 100% and 94%, respectively. Other less frequent cranial and facial autonomic features include rhinorrhea (54%), nasal congestion (48%), eyelid edema (26%), ptosis (12%), miosis (4%), facial sweating (8%), or redness (2%) (98). The autonomic features essentially occur in tandem, one to two seconds after the attacks, and abort within a few seconds of the pain ceasing (97). In addition, generalized systemic autonomic accompaniments may be observed during SUNCT attacks, such as increased systemic blood pressure, decreased heart rate, and hyperventilation (118,119). Unlike CH sufferers and some PH sufferers, reports have suggested that SUNCT patients do not typically report restlessness during attacks (97). Contrary to early reports, Cohen et al. (95) stated that 62% of SUNCT patients reported being agitated during an attack. Studies also suggested that migraine-like features including nausea, vomiting, photophobia, phonophobia, and osmophobia, are not associated with SUNCT (95,98). However, it was reported that 49% of SUNCT patients reported a history of migraine or having a first-degree relative with migraine (95).

The majority of SUNCT attacks occur spontaneously with an innocuous triggering mechanism. There are only a few reports of purely spontaneous attacks but no reports of patients having only attacks by a triggered event (98). Others have argued that spontaneous attacks may be subclinically triggered and merely unnoticed by the observer (94). Typically, attacks may be triggered almost immediately by touching certain trigger zones within the trigeminal nerve distribution and, rarely, an extratrigeminal area (94,97). Common cutaneous triggers include touching or washing the face or scalp, shaving, eating, brushing teeth, talking, and coughing (97). Additionally, neck movement may trigger an attack, and in some patients, continuous rotation of the neck may lessen or abort the attacks (90,97). In spite of almost neuralgia-like triggers in SUNCT, there are no refractory periods as seen in trigeminal neuralgia (97). There have only ever been two cases of SUNCT with absolute refractory periods (95,120). Whether a lack of refractory period is truly the case with SUNCT or the result of poor awareness and under-reporting remains unanswered (98).

There are reports of SUNCT being preceded by trigeminal neuralgia involving the ophthalmic branch of the trigeminal nerve. This suggests that SUNCT may merely represent a variant of trigeminal neuralgia (121–123). Further research is needed to ascertain information on the relationship between SUNCT and trigeminal neuralgia.

A variant of SUNCT is the headache disorder termed short-lasting unilateral neuralgiform headache attacks with cranial autonomic features (SUNA) that is classified in the appendix section of the International Headache Society's ICDH-II. The rationale behind including SUNA in the ICDH-II classification was to recognize a broader category of headache entities that present similarly to SUNCT. Unlike SUNCT, SUNA may be diagnosed with only one of the cranial or facial autonomic features regardless of the presence of rhinorrhea or tearing.

In addition, pain in SUNA may be longer in duration (less than 10 minutes) compared to SUNCT (2). Further research is required to validate SUNA as a distinct headache entity (94).

Diagnosis

Once again, the key to SUNCT diagnosis is based on the history from previous attacks. These include the rapid onset, location, intensity, quality and duration of pain, temporal patterns of episodes, triggering factors, and associated autonomic features (2). The physical examination in SUNCT is usually normal with a few reports of mild cutaneous allodynia, hypoesthesia or hyperesthesia over the trigeminal nerve distribution as well as corneal hyperesthesia (97,103,108). A differential diagnosis is necessary prior to establishing a definitive diagnosis for SUNCT as other conditions such as trigeminal neuralgia, primary stabbing headaches, hypnic headache, CH, and PH can mimic SUNCT (Table 4).

Health care providers should be alerted to the fact that underlying central nervous system pathology (symptomatic SUNCT) commonly presents like primary SUNCT and must be ruled out (77). Therefore, it is prudent that a neurological examination and an MRI be performed routinely regardless of the clinical presentation (98). Most cases of symptomatic SUNCT involve posterior fossa abnormalities such as ipsilateral cerebellopontine angle arteriovenous malformation (124), brainstem cavernous hemangioma (125), and ischemic brainstem infraction (126). Also, patients with prolactinomas (pituitary adenomas) with resultant pituitary-related symptoms such as hormonal imbalance may present with symptomatic SUNCT (98,127). Therefore, blood studies to evaluate imbalances in basal hormone levels should be utilized. The hormones to be investigated should include prolactin, thyroid stimulating hormone, free thyroxine, cortisol, adrenocorticotrophic hormone, luteinizing hormone, follicle-stimulating hormone, estrogen, testosterone, and growth hormone (98).

Health care providers need to be cognizant of both the similarities between SUNCT and trigeminal neuralgia and the need to differentiate SUNCT from other orofacial pains including dental pain. There are many similarities between SUNCT and trigeminal neuralgia. Some of the common characteristics are unilaterality, not side alternating, the high frequency of attacks, the triggerability of the attacks, and the periodic appearance and localization of symptoms (117). A possible differentiating factor between these two conditions is that autonomic signs are not usually associated with neuralgias (1); however, cranial autonomic features have been reported in trigeminal neuralgia affecting the ophthalmic branch (128). Also, there are reports of the coexistence of trigeminal neuralgia and SUNCT (121,129). There are also case reports in which SUNCT patients, in addition to facial pain, complain of pain radiating to adjacent teeth. This has prompted referral to dentists resulting in the delivery of definitive interventions such as tooth extraction, occlusal splints, and incorrect pharmacology (130–132). Unfortunately, the commonality of these two conditions may result in misdiagnosis with the delivery of unnecessary and inappropriate treatments.

Pathophysiology

The pathophysiology of SUNCT is unknown but thought to be similar to other TACs (1). Although there are differences in their clinical presentation, SUNCT shares commonalities with respect to the source and trigeminal distribution of

TABLE 4 Differentiating Features of Short-Lasting Headaches and Other Facial Pains[a]

Feature	Cluster headache	Paroxysmal hemicrania	SUNCT	Trigeminal neuralgia	Primary stabbing headache	Hypnic headache
Sex (male:female)	5:1	1:2	2:1	1.6:1	5:1	5:3
Age (years)	20–40	30	40–70	50	30–40	60
Pain						
Type	Boring	Boring	Electric-like	Electric-like	Stabbing	Dull
Severity	Very severe	Very severe	Severe	Very severe	Severe	Moderate
Location	Orbital	Orbital	Orbital	V2/V3>V1	V1	Generalized
Duration	15–180 minutes	2–30 minutes	15–240 seconds	<1–30 seconds	<30 seconds	15–180 minutes
Frequency	1–8/day	2–40/day	3–200/day	Variable	Variable	1–3/night
Autonomic	Yes	Yes	Yes	No	No	No
Trigger	Alcohol, nitrates	Alcohol, mechanical	Cutaneous	Mucocutaneous	No	Sleep

[a]This table provides a general overview and is a broad diagnostic guide without specific rules for the presentations of the various short lasting headaches and other facial pains.

pain and ipsilateral cranial and facial autonomic features of the other TACs. The same trigeminal–autonomic reflex processes involved in the pathophysiology of PH also occur with SUNCT. Similarly to PH, the hypothalamus may also be a trigger for trigeminal activation and cranial autonomic activation in SUNCT. In fact, functional magnetic resonance imaging studies revealed hypothalamic activation during SUNCT attacks (133,134) that may cause central disinhibition of the trigeminal–autonomic reflex (135). Therefore, an abnormality in the hypothalamus results in the central disinhibition of the trigeminal–autonomic reflex, which, in turn, causes trigeminovascular activation (pain) as well as cranial and facial autonomic activation (autonomic features) (98). However, knowledge about SUNCT is in its infancy; and further studies are required to better elucidate its pathophysiology.

Treatment
SUNCT is considered to be relatively resistant to treatment (136). Nevertheless, different approaches for the management of this headache have been attempted. These approaches involve pharmacological treatments as well as several surgical approaches. The surgical approaches can be subdivided into three main groups: local anesthetic blockades, invasive procedures involving the trigeminal nerve, and neurosurgical procedures.

Pharmacological Treatments
Several classes of medications used in other headache disorders and pain syndromes have been tried for the treatment of SUNCT but have been found to be either minimally or not at all effective. These include nonsteroidal anti-inflammatory drugs and cyclooxygenase 2 inhibitors (indomethacin and nimesulide), analgesics (acetaminophen and opiates), 5-hydroxytryptamine agonists (triptans, ergotamine, and dihydroergotamine), beta-blockers (propranolol and timolol), alpha adrenoreceptor agonists (clonidine), histamine desensitization and antagonists, tricyclic antidepressants (amitriptyline, nortriptyline, and desipramine), calcium channel blockers (nifedipine, flunarizine, and diltiazem), lithium, phenytoin, valproic acid, clonazepam, and baclofen (90,105,107,111,117, 121,125,129,136–138). In fact, certain medications such as the calcium channel blockers, verapamil, and amlodipine, when utilized to treat SUNCT, have not only been ineffective but have worsened the symptoms (1,97,110). Inhalation of 100% oxygen (7–10 L/min) has been attempted to abort an attack in one patient with SUNCT without a positive outcome (125).

Currently, based on case reports, the anticonvulsant drug, lamotrigine, has been reported to be highly effective in a number of patients with SUNCT (105,139–143). The dosing in these studies ranged between 100 and 300 mg per day resulting in either complete remission or an 80% improvement. The dosing was initiated gradually with titration to a therapeutic dose over several weeks. However, there were other case reports that reported a lack of effectiveness with lamotrigine (111,134,144).

The mechanism of action by which lamotrigine exerts its effect is thought to be its ability to stabilize neuronal sodium channels with consequent inhibition of glutamate and aspartate release (145). It is by way of this effect that lamotrigine is also used in the treatment of neuropathic pains; most notably, trigeminal neuralgia (129,146,147). If lamotrigine is utilized, the prescriber must be aware of the significant risk of Stevens–Johnson syndrome (0.3% incidence in adults) or toxic epidermal necrolysis during the initial phase of lamotrigine therapy (148). Even though lamotrigine is empirically considered first-line treatment for SUNCT, the ultimate confirmation of the usefulness of this medication must be based on randomized, double-blind, placebo-controlled clinical trials (98,149).

Two other anticonvulsant medications can be considered as second-line treatments for SUNCT (98,149). Gabapentin has been trialed in nine patients with SUNCT. It was highly effective in three patients by completely suppressing the attacks at dosages between 800 and 2700 mg daily (108,137,150) and ineffective in six patients (111,112,117,120,151). Topiramate has been reported to be effective in a small number of patients with doses ranging between 50 and 300 mg per day (120,129,152,153) but has also been reported to be ineffective in two patients (111).

Patients have occasionally claimed that corticosteroids were of some benefit. A total of 19 reported patients were treated with medications within this class of drugs. Prednisone (12 patients), prednisolone (2 patients), and methylprednisolone (5 patients) have been employed (108,112,116,123,136,144,151,152, 154,155). Of the 12 patients on prednisone, 5 had a positive response with 1 patient having complete relief. A total of three patients on the other two corticosteroids received treatment in combination with carbamazepine and reported a favorable response. The use of corticosteroids may be considered as a treatment option but caution must be exercised due to the potential serious side effects associated with prolonged use (98).

Lidocaine, both intravenously and intranasally, has been used for the treatment of SUNCT. Lidocaine by intravenous infusion was reported to be highly effective at completely suppressing the attacks in four patients with recurrence after cessation of treatments (144). In contrast, a bolus infusion of lidocaine was reported to be ineffective when administered to two patients (136). These approaches are not clinically practical and can only occur in an inpatient setting with continuous monitoring of cardiac function, control of nausea and awareness of psychiatric manifestations. It has been suggested that this approach should be reserved in patients exhibiting "SUNCT status" (156). Intranasal lidocaine has been reported to be ineffective in a small trial of patients (120,136). Intranasal local anesthetic (exact agent was not stated) was stated to be ineffective in one case (157). Interestingly, lidocaine mouthwash has been reported to produce a slight improvement in two of five patients (136).

Carbamazepine, in doses between 600 and 1200 mg per day, has been tried in 43 patients. As a single agent, carbamazepine had no effect in 27 patients, partial or transitory responses in 13 patients and produced a complete or near complete relief in three patients (103,106,107,111,112,120,123,134,136,139,142,144,152, 157–161). Carbamazepine has also been used in combination with various other medications with mixed results in terms of reliability over time (98). The use of carbamazepine may be as an adjunctive agent when other agents are ineffective (98). The lack of an absolute response to carbamazepine in SUNCT supports the view that trigeminal neuralgia and SUNCT are distinctive entities (160).

Oxcarbazepine was reported to be effective at a dose of 600 mg per day in a solitary case report. A spontaneous remission was ruled out because when the drug was stopped a recurrence of the attacks ensued with reinstitution of the drug resulting in the relief of the attacks (162).

The common mechanism of action of lamotrigine, topiramate, lidocaine, carbamazepine, and oxcarbazepine is the blockage of sodium channels. Therefore, the possibility exists that the therapeutic effect of these drugs on SUNCT is mediated by this mechanism. However, valproic acid, and phenytoin, which also share a similar mechanism of action, do not appear to have beneficial effects for SUNCT patients. Advances in understanding the pathophysiology of SUNCT and further characterization of the mechanism of actions of pharmacologic agents will likely result in more efficacious treatment for this disorder.

Local Anesthetic Blockades
SUNCT patients have been trialed with local anesthetic blockades of various anatomical structures including peripheral branches of the trigeminal nerve including the supraorbital, infraorbital, and lacrimal nerves, the greater occipital nerve, orbicularis oculi muscle, stellate, sphenopalatine and superior cervical ganglions, and the retrobulbar region The basis for the efficacy of these blocks is to interrupt pain impulses being conveyed by these peripheral nerve fibers and/or to interrupt the afferent and efferent pathways of abnormal reflex mechanisms (163). The various local anesthetic agents tried include lidocaine, bupivacaine, alcohol or phenol, and opioids (107,117,125,136). Generally, the blockades are ineffective in suppressing spontaneous attacks, although in a few cases, it was more difficult to precipitate attacks by touching the anesthetized trigger areas.

Invasive Procedures
There are only a few case reports involving surgical procedures directed at the trigeminal nerve. A few patients who have undergone these procedures, such as percutaneous trigeminal ganglion compression (151), microvascular decompression of the trigeminal nerve root (134,164,165), retrogasserian glycerol rhizolysis (117), and balloon compression of the trigeminal nerve root (117,166), have obtained an improvement in their symptoms. However, negative results and postoperative complications (anesthesia dolorosa, unilateral deafness, chronic vertigo, and disequilibrium) of several surgical procedures such as glycerol rhizotomy, gamma knife radiosurgery, trigeminal radiofrequency thermocoagulation, and microvascular decompression of the trigeminal nerve have also been reported (111,117,144). Due to the uncertainty of the outcomes from these invasive surgical procedures and the potential for serious complications, surgery should only be considered as a last resort after pharmacologic options have been exhausted.

Neurosurgical Approaches
There is one case report of a patient with drug resistant SUNCT who received deep brain stimulation by implantation of an electrode in the posterior inferior hypothalamus (167). This site was chosen based on functional MRI findings that this area is activated during times of crisis (133) as well as the evidence that stimulation of this area produces pain relief in CH (168–171). Prolonged stimulation of the posterior inferior hypothalamus resulted in long-lasting pain relief without side effects. Interestingly, when the electrode stimulation was discontinued without the knowledge of the patient, the pain reappeared but gradually

disappeared when the device was turned back on. These observations, in addition to the lasting pain relief, appear to exclude a placebo effect (167). Neurosurgical procedures involving hypothalamic stimulation may be a treatment alternative for patients with intractable SUNCT.

REFERENCES

1. Goadsby PJ, Lipton RB. A review of paroxysmal hemicranias, SUNCT syndrome and other short-lasting headaches with autonomic feature, including new cases. Brain 1997; 120(Pt 1):193–209.
2. The International Classification of Headache Disorders: 2nd edition. Cephalalgia 2004; 24(Suppl 1):9–160.
3. van Vliet JA, Eekers PJ, Haan J, et al. Features involved in the diagnostic delay of cluster headache. J Neurol Neurosurg Psychiatry 2003; 74:1123–1125.
4. Sarlani E, Schwartz AH, Greenspan JD, et al. Chronic paroxysmal hemicrania: a case report and review of the literature. J Orofac Pain 2003; 17:74–78.
5. Delcanho RE, Graff-Radford SB. Chronic paroxysmal hemicrania presenting as toothache. J Orofac Pain 1993; 7:300–306.
6. Moncada E, Graff-Radford SB. Benign indomethacin-responsive headaches presenting in the orofacial region: eight case reports. J Orofac Pain 1995; 9: 276–284.
7. Benoliel R, Sharav Y. Paroxysmal hemicrania. Case studies and review of the literature. Oral Surg Oral Med Oral Pathol Oral Radiol Endod 1998; 85:285–292.
8. Sjaastad O, Dale I. Evidence for a new (?), treatable headache entity. Headache 1974; 14:105–108.
9. Sjaastad O, Dale I. A new (?) Clinical headache entity "chronic paroxysmal hemicrania" 2. Acta Neurol Scand 1976; 54:140–159.
10. Kudrow L, Esperanca P, Vijayan N. Episodic paroxysmal hemicrania? Cephalalgia 1987; 7:197–201.
11. Blau JN, Engel H. Episodic paroxysmal hemicrania: a further case and review of the literature. J Neurol Neurosurg Psychiatry 1990; 53:343–344.
12. Newman LC, Gordon ML, Lipton RB, et al. Episodic paroxysmal hemicrania: two new cases and a literature review. Neurology 1992; 42:964–966.
13. Newman LC, Lipton RB, Solomon S. Episodic paroxysmal hemicrania: 3 new cases and a review of the literature. Headache 1993; 33:195–197.
14. Antonaci F, Sjaastad O. Chronic paroxysmal hemicrania (CPH): a review of the clinical manifestations. Headache 1989; 29:648–656.
15. Lance JW, Goadsby P. Mechanism and Management of Headache. Philadelphia: Elsevier, 2005.
16. Siow HC. Seasonal episodic paroxysmal hemicrania responding to cyclooxygenase-2 inhibitors. Cephalalgia 2004; 24:414–415.
17. Rossi P, Di Lorenzo G, Faroni J, et al. Seasonal, extratrigeminal, episodic paroxysmal hemicrania successfully treated with single suboccipital steroid injections. Eur J Neurol 2005; 12:903–906.
18. Boes CJ, Dodick DW. Refining the clinical spectrum of chronic paroxysmal hemicrania: a review of 74 patients. Headache 2002; 42:699–708.
19. Petty RG, Rose FC. Chronic paroxysmal hemicrania: first reported British case. Br Med J (Clin Res Ed) 1983; 286(6363):438.
20. Tehindrazanarivelo AD, Visy JM, Bousser MG. Ipsilateral cluster headache and chronic paroxysmal hemicrania: two case reports. Cephalalgia 1992; 12:318–320.
21. Joubert J, Powell D, Djikowski J. Chronic paroxysmal hemicrania in a South African black. A case report. Cephalalgia 1987; 7:193–196.
22. Sjaastad O. Chronic paroxysmal hemicrania (CPH). In: Vinken PJ, Bruyn GK, Klawans HL, Rose FC, eds. Handbook of Clinical Neurology. Amsterdam: Elsevier Science, 1986:257–266.

23. Newman LC, Goadsby P. The paroxysmal hemicranias, SUNCT syndrome, and hypnic headache. In: Silberstein SD, Lipton RB, Dalessio DJ, eds. Wolff's Headache and other Head Pain. Oxford: Oxford University Press, 2001:310–324.
24. Talvik I, Koch K, Kolk A, et al. Chronic paroxysmal hemicrania in a 3-year, 10-month-old female. Pediatr Neurol 2006; 34:225–227.
25. de Almeida DB, Cunali PA, Santos HL, et al. Chronic paroxysmal hemicrania in early childhood: case report. Cephalalgia 2004; 24:608–609.
26. Broeske D, Lenn NJ, Cantos E. Chronic paroxysmal hemicrania in a young child: possible relation to ipsilateral occipital infarction. J Child Neurol 1993; 8:235–236.
27. Cohen AS, Matharu MS, Goadsby PJ. Paroxysmal hemicrania in a family. Cephalalgia 2006; 26:486–488.
28. Pelz M, Merskey H. A case of pre-chronic paroxysmal hemicrania. Cephalalgia 1982; 2:47–50.
29. Pareja JA. Chronic paroxysmal hemicrania: dissociation of the pain and autonomic features. Headache 1995; 35:111–113.
30. Pollmann W, Pfaffenrath V. Chronic paroxysmal hemicrania: the first possible bilateral case. Cephalalgia 1986; 6:55–57.
31. Benoliel R, Elishoov H, Sharav Y. Orofacial pain with vascular-type features. Oral Surg Oral Med Oral Pathol Oral Radiol Endod 1997; 84:506–512.
32. Graff-Radford SB. Paroxysmal hemicrania. Oral Surg Oral Med Oral Pathol Oral Radiol Endod 1998; 86:138.
33. Alonso AA, Nixdorf DR. Case series of four different headache types presenting as tooth pain. J Endod 2006; 32:1110–1113.
34. Graff-Radford SB. Headache problems that can present as toothache. Dent Clin North Am 1991; 35:155–170.
35. Boes CJ, Swanson JW. Paroxysmal hemicrania, SUNCT, and hemicrania continua. Semin Neurol 2006; 26:260–270.
36. Newman LC, Lipton RB. Paroxysmal hemicranias. In: Goadsby P, Silberstein SD, eds. Headache. Boston: Butterworth-Heinemann, 1997:243–250.
37. Castellanos-Pinedo F, Zurdo M, Martinez-Acebes E. Hemicrania continua evolving from episodic paroxysmal hemicrania. Cephalalgia 2006; 26:1143–1145.
38. Russell D. Chronic paroxysmal hemicrania: severity, duration and time of occurrence of attacks. Cephalalgia 1984; 4:53–56.
39. Kayed K, Godtlibsen OB, Sjaastad O. Chronic paroxysmal hemicrania IV: "REM sleep locked" nocturnal headache attacks. Sleep 1978; 1(1):91–95.
40. Bogucki A, Szymanska R, Braciak W. Chronic paroxysmal hemicrania: lack of pre-chronic stage. Cephalalgia 1984; 4:187–189.
41. Stein HJ, Rogado AZ. Headache rounds. Chronic paroxysmal hemicrania: two new patients. Headache 1980; 20:72–76.
42. Cittadini E, Matharu MS, Goadsby PJ. Paroxysmal hemicrania: a prospective clinical study of 31 cases. Brain 2008; 131:1142–1155.
43. Sjaastad O, Russell D, Saunte C, et al. Chronic paroxysmal hemicrania: VI. Precipitation of attacks. Further studies on the precipitation mechanism. Cephalalgia 1982; 2:211–214.
44. Sjaastad O, Saunte C, Graham JR. Chronic paroxysmal hemicrania. VII. Mechanical precipitation of attacks: new cases and localization of trigger points. Cephalalgia 1984; 4:113–118.
45. Matharu MS, Boes CJ, Goadsby PJ. Management of trigeminal autonomic cephalgias and hemicrania continua. Drugs 2003; 63:1637–1677.
46. Boes CJ, Matharu MS, Goadsby PJ. The paroxysmal hemicrania-tic syndrome. Cephalalgia 2003; 23:24–28.
47. Centonze V, Bassi A, Causarano V, et al. Simultaneous occurrence of ipsilateral cluster headache and chronic paroxysmal hemicrania: a case report. Headache 2000; 40:54–56.
48. Pareja J. Chronic paroxysmal hemicrania coexisting with migraine. Differential response to pharmacological treatment. Headache 1992; 32:77–78.

49. Mateo I, Pascual J. Coexistence of chronic paroxysmal hemicrania and benign cough headache. Headache 1999; 39:437–438.
50. Boes CJ, Swanson JW, Dodick DW. Chronic paroxysmal hemicrania presenting as otalgia with a sensation of external acoustic meatus obstruction: two cases and a pathophysiologic hypothesis. Headache 1998; 38:787–791.
51. Antonaci F, Pareja JA, Caminero AB, et al. Chronic paroxysmal hemicrania and hemicrania continua. Parenteral indomethacin: the "indotest". Headache 1998; 38:122–128.
52. Warner JS, Wamil AW, McLean MJ. Acetazolamide for the treatment of chronic paroxysmal hemicrania. Headache 1994; 34:597–599.
53. Newman LC, Herskovitz S, Lipton RB, et al. Chronic paroxysmal headache: two cases with cerebrovascular disease. Headache 1992; 32:75–76.
54. Medina JL. Organic headaches mimicking chronic paroxysmal hemicrania. Headache 1992; 32:73–74.
55. Delreux V, Kevers L, Callewaert A. Paroxysmal hemicrania preceding Pancoast's syndrome. Rev Neurol (Paris) 1989; 145:151–152.
56. Gatzonis S, Mitsikostas DD, Ilias A, et al. Two more secondary headaches mimicking chronic paroxysmal hemicrania. Is this the exception or the rule? Headache 1996; 36:511–513.
57. Sarov M, Valade D, Jublanc C, et al. Chronic paroxysmal hemicrania in a patient with a macroprolactinoma. Cephalalgia 2006; 26:738–741.
58. MacMillan JC, Nukada H. Chronic paroxysmal hemicrania. N Z Med J 1989; 102:251–252.
59. Hannerz J, Jogestrand T. Intracranial hypertension and sumatriptan efficacy in a case of chronic paroxysmal hemicrania which became bilateral (the mechanism of indomethacin in CPH). Headache 1993; 33:320–323.
60. Russell D, Storstein L. Chronic paroxysmal hemicrania: heart rate changes and ECG rhythm disturbances. A computerized analysis of 24 h ambulatory ECG recordings. Cephalalgia 1984; 4:135–144.
61. Matharu MS, Cohen AS, Frackowiak RS, et al. Posterior hypothalamic activation in paroxysmal hemicrania. Ann Neurol 2006; 59:535–545.
62. May A, Goadsby PJ. The trigeminovascular system in humans: pathophysiologic implications for primary headache syndromes of the neural influences on the cerebral circulation. J Cereb Blood Flow Metab 1999; 19:115–127.
63. Goadsby PJ, Edvinsson L. Neuropeptide changes in a case of chronic paroxysmal hemicrania—evidence for trigemino-parasympathetic activation. Cephalalgia 1996; 16:448–450.
64. Dodick D. Indomethacin-responsive headache syndromes. In: Noseworthy JH, ed. Neurological Therapeutics: Principles and Practice. London: Martin Dunitz, 2003: 142–150.
65. Burke A, Smyth E, FitzGerald G. Analgesic-antipyretic and antiinflammatory agents: pharmacotherapy of gout. In: Brunton LL, ed. Goodman and Gilman's the Pharmacological Basis of Therapeutics. New York: McGraw-Hill, 2006.
66. Imberti R, Fuardo M, Bellinzona G, et al. The use of indomethacin in the treatment of plateau waves: effects on cerebral perfusion and oxygenation. J Neurosurg 2005; 102:455–459.
67. Rasmussen M. Treatment of elevated intracranial pressure with indomethacin: friend or foe? Acta Anaesthesiol Scand 2005; 49:341–350.
68. Beasley TC, Bari F, Thore C, et al. Cerebral ischemia/reperfusion increases endothelial nitric oxide synthase levels by an indomethacin-sensitive mechanism. J Cereb Blood Flow Metab 1998; 18:88–96.
69. Hrabak A, Vercruysse V, Kahan IL, et al. Indomethacin prevents the induction of inducible nitric oxide synthase in murine peritoneal macrophages and decreases their nitric oxide production. Life Sci 2001; 68:1923–1930.
70. Akerman S, Williamson DJ, Kaube H, et al. Nitric oxide synthase inhibitors can antagonize neurogenic and calcitonin gene-related peptide induced dilation of dural meningeal vessels. Br J Pharmacol 2002; 137:62–68.

71. Pareja J, Sjaastad O. Chronic paroxysmal hemicrania and hemicrania continua. Interval between indomethacin administration and response. Headache 1996; 36:20–23.
72. Sjaastad O, Stovner LJ, Stolt-Nielsen A, et al. CPH and hemicrania continua: requirements of high indomethacin dosages—an ominous sign? Headache 1995; 35: 363–367.
73. Sjaastad O, Apfelbaum R, Caskey W, et al. Chronic paroxysmal hemicrania (CPH): the clinical manifestations. A review. Ups J Med Sci Suppl 1980; 31:27–33.
74. Pareja JA, Caminero AB, Franco E, et al. Dose, efficacy and tolerability of long-term indomethacin treatment of chronic paroxysmal hemicrania and hemicrania continua. Cephalalgia 2001; 21:906–910.
75. Sjaastad O, Antonaci F. Chronic paroxysmal hemicrania: a case report. Long-lasting remission in the chronic stage. Cephalalgia 1987; 7:203–205.
76. Jensen NB, Joensen P, Jensen J. Chronic paroxysmal hemicrania: continued remission of symptoms after discontinuation of indomethacin. Cephalalgia 1982; 2:163–164.
77. Trucco M, Mainardi F, Maggioni F, et al. Chronic paroxysmal hemicrania, hemicrania continua and SUNCT syndrome in association with other pathologies: a review. Cephalalgia 2004; 24:173–184.
78. Hannerz J, Ericson K, Bergstrand G. Chronic paroxysmal hemicrania: orbital phlebography and steroid treatment. A case report. Cephalalgia 1987; 7:189–192.
79. Evers S, Husstedt IW. Alternatives in drug treatment of chronic paroxysmal hemicrania. Headache 1996; 36:429–432.
80. Mathew NT, Kailasam J, Fischer A. Responsiveness to celecoxib in chronic paroxysmal hemicrania. Neurology 2000; 55:316.
81. Coria F, Claveria LE, Jimenez-Jimenez FJ, et al. Episodic paroxysmal hemicrania responsive to calcium channel blockers. J Neurol Neurosurg Psychiatry 1992; 55:166.
82. Shabbir N, McAbee G. Adolescent chronic paroxysmal hemicrania responsive to verapamil monotherapy. Headache 1994; 34:209–210.
83. Pascual J, Quijano J. A case of chronic paroxysmal hemicrania responding to subcutaneous sumatriptan. J Neurol Neurosurg Psychiatry 1998; 65:407.
84. Dahlof C. Subcutaneous sumatriptan does not abort attacks of chronic paroxysmal hemicrania (CPH). Headache 1993; 33:201–202.
85. Antonaci F, Pareja JA, Caminero AB, et al. Chronic paroxysmal hemicrania and hemicrania continua: lack of efficacy of sumatriptan. Headache 1998; 38:197–200.
86. Cohen AS, Goadsby PJ. Paroxysmal hemicrania responding to topiramate. J Neurol Neurosurg Psychiatry 2007; 78:96–97.
87. Antonaci F, Pareja JA, Caminero AB, et al. Chronic paroxysmal hemicrania and hemicrania continua: anaesthetic blockades of pericranial nerves. Funct Neurol 1997; 12:11–15.
88. Afridi SK, Shields KG, Bhola R, et al. Greater occipital nerve injection in primary headache syndromes—prolonged effects from a single injection. Pain 2006; 122:126–129.
89. Sjaastad O, Russell D, Horven I, et al. Multiple neuralgiform unilateral headache attacks associated with conjunctival injection and appearing in clusters: a nosological problem. In: Proceedings of the Annual Meeting, Scandinavian Migraine Society, Aarhus, 1978.
90. Sjaastad O, Saunte C, Salvesen R, et al. Short-lasting unilateral neuralgiform headache attacks with conjunctival injection, tearing, sweating, and rhinorrhea. Cephalalgia 1989; 9:147–156.
91. Sjaastad O, Zhao JM, Kruszewski P, et al. Short-lasting unilateral neuralgiform headache attacks with conjunctival injection, tearing, etc. (SUNCT): III. Another Norwegian case. Headache 1991; 31:175–177.
92. Pareja JA, Shen JM, Kruszewski P, et al. SUNCT syndrome: duration, frequency, and temporal distribution of attacks. Headache 1996; 36:161–165.
93. Williams MH, Broadley SA. SUNCT and SUNA: clinical features and medical treatment. J Clin Neurosci 2008; 15:526–534.
94. Pareja JA, Cuadrado ML. SUNCT syndrome: an update. Expert Opin Pharmacother 2005; 6:591–599.

95. Cohen AS, Matharu MS, Goadsby PJ. Short-lasting unilateral neuralgiform headache attacks with conjunctival injection and tearing (SUNCT) or cranial autonomic features (SUNA)—a prospective clinical study of SUNCT and SUNA. Brain 2006; 129:2746–2760.

96. Sjaastad O, Bakketeig LS. The rare, unilateral headaches. Vaga study of headache epidemiology. J Headache Pain 2007; 8:19–27.

97. Pareja JA, Sjaastad O. SUNCT syndrome. A clinical review. Headache 1997; 37:195–202.

98. Matharu MS, Cohen AS, Boes CJ, et al. Short-lasting unilateral neuralgiform headache with conjunctival injection and tearing syndrome: a review. Curr Pain Headache Rep 2003; 7:308–318.

99. Sekhara T, Pelc K, Mewasingh LD, et al. Pediatric SUNCT syndrome. Pediatr Neurol 2005; 33:206–207.

100. Vikelis M, Xifaras M, Mitsikostas DD. SUNCT syndrome in the elderly. Cephalalgia 2005; 25:1091–1092.

101. Schwaag S, Frese A, Husstedt IW, et al. SUNCT syndrome: the first German case series. Cephalalgia 2003; 23:398–400.

102. Chakravarty A, Mukherjee A, Roy D. Trigeminal autonomic cephalgias and variants: clinical profile in Indian patients. Cephalalgia 2004; 24:859–866.

103. Raimondi E, Gardella L. SUNCT syndrome. Two cases in Argentina. Headache 1998; 38:369–371.

104. Gantenbein AR, Goadsby PJ. Familial SUNCT. Cephalalgia 2005; 25:457–459.

105. D'Andrea G, Granella F, Ghiotto N, et al. Lamotrigine in the treatment of SUNCT syndrome. Neurology 2001; 57:1723–1725.

106. D'Andrea G, Granella F. SUNCT syndrome: the first case in childhood. Short-lasting unilateral neuralgiform headache attacks with conjunctival injection and tearing. Cephalalgia 2001; 21:701–702.

107. Sabatowski R, Huber M, Meuser T, et al. SUNCT syndrome: a treatment option with local opioid blockade of the superior cervical ganglion? A case report. Cephalalgia 2001; 21:154–156.

108. Graff-Radford SB. SUNCT syndrome responsive to gabapentin (Neurontin). Cephalalgia 2000; 20:515–517.

109. Wingerchuk DM, Nyquist PA, Rodriguez M, et al. Extratrigeminal short-lasting unilateral neuralgiform headache with conjunctival injection and tearing (SUNCT): new pathophysiologic entity or variation on a theme? Cephalalgia 2000; 20: 127–129.

110. Jimenez-Huete A, Franch O, Pareja JA. SUNCT syndrome: priming of symptomatic periods and worsening of symptoms by treatment with calcium channel blockers. Cephalalgia 2002; 22:812–814.

111. Black DF, Dodick DW. Two cases of medically and surgically intractable SUNCT: a reason for caution and an argument for a central mechanism. Cephalalgia 2002; 22:201–204.

112. Montes E, Alberca R, Lozano P, et al. Statuslike SUNCT in two young women. Headache 2001; 41:826–829.

113. Pareja JA, Joubert J, Sjaastad O. SUNCT syndrome. Atypical temporal patterns. Headache 1996; 36:108–110.

114. Pareja JA, Sjaastad O. SUNCT syndrome in the female. Headache 1994; 34:217–220.

115. Pareja JA, Caballero V, Sjaastad O. SUNCT syndrome. Status-like pattern. Headache 1996; 36:622–624.

116. Pareja JA, Pareja J, Palomo T, et al. SUNCT syndrome: repetitive and overlapping attacks. Headache 1994; 34:114–116.

117. Hannerz J, Linderoth B. Neurosurgical treatment of short-lasting, unilateral, neuralgiform hemicrania with conjunctival injection and tearing. Br J Neurosurg 2002; 16:55–58.

118. Kruszewski P, Fasano ML, Brubakk AO, et al. Shortlasting, unilateral, neuralgiform headache attacks with conjunctival injection, tearing, and subclinical forehead

sweating ("Sunct" syndrome): II. Changes in heart rate and arterial blood pressure during pain paroxysms. Headache 1991; 31:399–405.

119. Kruszewski P, White LR, Shen JM, et al. Respiratory studies in SUNCT syndrome. Headache 1995; 35:344–348.

120. Matharu MS, Boes CJ, Goadsby PJ. SUNCT syndrome: prolonged attacks, refractoriness and response to topiramate. Neurology 2002; 58:1307.

121. Bouhassira D, Attal N, Esteve M, et al. "SUNCT" syndrome. A case of transformation from trigeminal neuralgia? Cephalalgia 1994; 14:168–170.

122. Benoliel R, Sharav Y. Trigeminal neuralgia with lacrimation or SUNCT syndrome? Cephalalgia 1998; 18:85–90.

123. Calvo JF, Bruera OC, de Lourdes Figuerola M, et al. SUNCT syndrome: clinical and 12-year follow-up case report. Cephalalgia 2004; 24:900–902.

124. Morales F, Mostacero E, Marta J, et al. Vascular malformation of the cerebellopontine angle associated with "SUNCT" syndrome. Cephalalgia 1994; 14:301–302.

125. De Benedittis G. SUNCT syndrome associated with cavernous angioma of the brain stem. Cephalalgia 1996; 16:503–506.

126. Penart A, Firth M, Bowen JR. Short-lasting unilateral neuralgiform headache with conjunctival injection and tearing (SUNCT) following presumed dorsolateral brainstem infarction. Cephalalgia 2001; 21:236–239.

127. Massiou H, Launay JM, Levy C, et al. SUNCT syndrome in two patients with prolactinomas and bromocriptine-induced attacks. Neurology 2002; 58:1698–1699.

128. Pareja JA, Baron M, Gili P, et al. Objective assessment of autonomic signs during triggered first division trigeminal neuralgia. Cephalalgia 2002; 22:251–255.

129. Sesso RM. SUNCT syndrome or trigeminal neuralgia with lacrimation and conjunctival injection? Cephalalgia 2001; 21:151–153.

130. Benoliel R, Sharav Y. SUNCT syndrome: case report and literature review. Oral Surg Oral Med Oral Pathol Oral Radiol Endod 1998; 85:158–161.

131. Leone M, Mea E, Genco S, et al. Coexistence of TACS and trigeminal neuralgia: pathophysiological conjectures. Headache 2006; 46:1565–1570.

132. de Siqueira SR, Nobrega JC, Teixeira MJ, et al. SUNCT syndrome associated with temporomandibular disorders: a case report. Cranio 2006; 24:300–302.

133. May A, Bahra A, Buchel C, et al. Functional magnetic resonance imaging in spontaneous attacks of SUNCT: short-lasting neuralgiform headache with conjunctival injection and tearing. Ann Neurol 1999; 46:791–794.

134. Sprenger T, Valet M, Platzer S, et al. SUNCT: bilateral hypothalamic activation during headache attacks and resolving of symptoms after trigeminal decompression. Pain 2005; 113:422–426.

135. Bartsch T, Levy MJ, Knight YE, et al. Differential modulation of nociceptive dural input to [hypocretin] orexin A and B receptor activation in the posterior hypothalamic area. Pain 2004; 109:367–378.

136. Pareja JA, Kruszewski P, Sjaastad O. SUNCT syndrome: trials of drugs and anesthetic blockades. Headache 1995; 35:138–142.

137. Hunt CH, Dodick DW, Bosch EP. SUNCT responsive to gabapentin. Headache 2002; 42:525–526.

138. Hannerz J, Greitz D, Hansson P, et al. SUNCT may be another manifestation of orbital venous vasculitis. Headache 1992; 32:384–389.

139. D'Andrea G, Granella F, Cadaldini M. Possible usefulness of lamotrigine in the treatment of SUNCT syndrome. Neurology 1999; 53:1609.

140. Leone M, Rigamonti A, Usai S, et al. Two new SUNCT cases responsive to lamotrigine. Cephalalgia 2000; 20:845–847.

141. Gutierrez-Garcia JM. SUNCT syndrome responsive to lamotrigine. Headache 2002; 42:823–825.

142. Malik K, Rizvi S, Vaillancourt PD. The SUNCT syndrome: successfully treated with lamotrigine. Pain Med 2002; 3:167–168.

143. Chakravarty A, Mukherjee A. SUNCT syndrome responsive to lamotrigine: documentation of the first Indian case. Cephalalgia 2003; 23:474–475.

144. Matharu MS, Cohen AS, Goadsby PJ. SUNCT syndrome responsive to intravenous lidocaine. Cephalalgia 2004; 24:985–992.
145. Eisenberg E, Shifrin A, Krivoy N. Lamotrigine for neuropathic pain. Expert Rev Neurother 2005; 5:729–735.
146. Zakrzewska JM, Chaudhry Z, Nurmikko TJ, et al. Lamotrigine (lamictal) in refractory trigeminal neuralgia: results from a double-blind placebo controlled crossover trial. Pain 1997; 73:223–230.
147. Tremont-Lukats IW, Megeff C, Backonja MM. Anticonvulsants for neuropathic pain syndromes: mechanisms of action and place in therapy. Drugs 2000; 60:1029–1052.
148. Mockenhaupt M, Messenheimer J, Tennis P, et al. Risk of Stevens–Johnson syndrome and toxic epidermal necrolysis in new users of antiepileptics. Neurology 2005; 64:1134–1138.
149. May A. Update on the diagnosis and management of trigemino-autonomic headaches. J Neurol 2006; 253:1525–1532.
150. Porta-Etessam J, Benito-Leon J, Martinez-Salio A, et al. Gabapentin in the treatment of SUNCT syndrome. Headache 2002; 42:523–524.
151. Morales-Asin F, Espada F, Lopez-Obarrio LA, et al. A SUNCT case with response to surgical treatment. Cephalalgia 2000; 20:67–68.
152. Rossi P, Cesarino F, Faroni J, et al. SUNCT syndrome successfully treated with topiramate: case reports. Cephalalgia 2003; 23:998–1000.
153. Kuhn J, Vosskaemper M, Bewermeyer H. SUNCT syndrome: a possible bilateral case responding to topiramate. Neurology 2005; 64:2159.
154. Lain AH, Caminero AB, Pareja JA. SUNCT syndrome; absence of refractory periods and modulation of attack duration by lengthening of the trigger stimuli. Cephalalgia 2000; 20:671–673.
155. Pareja JA, Cuadrado ML, Caminero AB, et al. Duration of attacks of first division trigeminal neuralgia. Cephalalgia 2005; 25:305–308.
156. Alore PL, Jay WM, Macken MP. SUNCT syndrome: short-lasting unilateral neuralgiform headache with conjunctival injection and tearing. Semin Ophthalmol 2006; 21:9–13.
157. Becser N, Berky M. SUNCT syndrome: a Hungarian case. Headache 1995; 35:158–160.
158. van Vliet JA, Ferrari MD, Haan J. SUNCT syndrome resolving after contralateral hemispheric ischaemic stroke. Cephalalgia 2003; 23:235–237.
159. Prakash KM, Lo YL. SUNCT syndrome in association with persistent Horner syndrome in a Chinese patient. Headache 2004; 44:256–258.
160. Sjaastad O, Kruszewski P. Trigeminal neuralgia and "SUNCT" syndrome: similarities and differences in the clinical pictures. An overview. Funct Neurol 1992; 7:103–107.
161. Cohen AS, Matharu MS, Goadsby PJ. SUNCT syndrome in the elderly. Cephalalgia 2004; 24:508–509.
162. Dora B. SUNCT syndrome with dramatic response to oxcarbazepine. Cephalalgia 2006; 26:1171–1173.
163. Pareja JA, Caminero AB, Sjaastad O. SUNCT syndrome: diagnosis and treatment. CNS Drugs 2002; 16:373–383.
164. Gardella L, Viruega A, Rojas H, et al. A case of a patient with SUNCT syndrome treated with Jannetta procedure. Cephalalgia 2001; 21:996–999.
165. Lenarest M, Diederich N, Phuoe D. A patient with SUNCT cured by the Janetta procedure [letter]. Cephalalgia 1997; 17:460.
166. Ertsey C, Bozsik G, Afra J. A case of SUNCT syndrome with neurovascular compression [abstract]. Cephalalgia 2000; 20:325.
167. Leone M, Franzini A, D'Andrea G, et al. Deep brain stimulation to relieve drug-resistant SUNCT. Ann Neurol 2005; 57:924–927.
168. Leone M, Franzini A, Bussone G. Stereotactic stimulation of posterior hypothalamic gray matter in a patient with intractable cluster headache. N Engl J Med 2001; 345:1428–1429.

169. Franzini A, Ferroli P, Leone M, et al. Stimulation of the posterior hypothalamus for treatment of chronic intractable cluster headaches: first reported series. Neurosurgery 2003; 52:1095–1099.
170. Leone M, Franzini A, Broggi G, et al. Long-term follow-up of bilateral hypothalamic stimulation for intractable cluster headache. Brain 2004; 127:2259–2264.
171. Schoenen J,Di Clemente L, Vandenheede M, et al. Hypothalamic stimulation in chronic cluster headache: a pilot study of efficacy and mode of action. Brain 2005; 128:940–947.

7 Trigeminal Neuralgia

Gary. W. Jay

Clinical Disease Area Expert-Pain, Pfizer, Inc., New London, Connecticut, U.S.A.

Trigeminal neuralgia (TN), also known as tic douloureux, is possibly the best known and most prevalent facial neuralgia. It is typically disabling.

THE DISORDER

Osler (1) described TN in 1912. He noted that a patient's pain is paroxysmal and can be initiated by benign forms of external stimuli including a breeze, speaking, and inducing movement of facial muscles and/or the tongue, even swallowing. The disorder is not self-limited—it may become ferociously painful making life unbearable, with suicide a sometime occurrence. The morbidity can become overwhelming.

TN is described as a severe, lancinating, electrical-like pain in the territory of one or more branches of the trigeminal nerve. It is associated with electrical-like, facial pain associated with intra- and extraoral triggers. Not uncommonly, patients may be seen with only one side of their face shaved, or make up on only one side of their face, as they will not want to do anything to arouse a trigger to their pain.

DIAGNOSIS

The International Headache Society (2) (IHS) diagnostic criteria note two forms of TN: classical and symptomatic. The criteria for classical TN are as follows:

A. Paroxysmal attacks of pain lasting anywhere from a fraction of a second to two minutes, affecting one or more divisions of the trigeminal nerve and fulfilling criteria B and C.
B. Pain has at least one of the following characteristics:
    ○ Intense, sharp, superficial, or stabbing.
    ○ Precipitated from trigger areas or by trigger factors.
C. The attacks are stereotyped in the individual patient.
D. There is no clinically evident neurological deficit.

While the classical form of TN typically starts in the second or third divisions, the first (ophthalmic) division is affected in <5% of patients. The pain is side-locked—it doesn't change sides, but it may be bilateral (at which time a central cause such as multiple sclerosis should be considered).

Patients may experience a dull background pain in some long-standing cases. Typically, there is a refractory period after a painful paroxysm, during which the pain can not be triggered. In rare cases, the pain can be triggered not from a trigger point in the trigeminal area, but by somatosensory stimulation outside of the trigeminal region, such as a limb or secondary to other sensory stimulation such as bright lights and noises, and strong tastes (3). The patient may experience facial muscle spasm on the affected side, coinciding with the pain.

The main difference between classical and symptomatic TN is that the latter has a causative lesion other than vascular compression. Also neurological examination may determine a sensory impairment in the painful trigeminal division. Finally, there are no refractory periods after the paroxysmal pain, unlike that in classical TN (2).

Women are affected two to three times more frequently than men. Most cases develop in patients >50 years of age. There have been some pediatric cases (4) too. The prevalence of TN is 0.1 to 0.2 per thousand, with an incidence ranging from about 4–5/1000,000/year up to 20/100,000/year (5).

Differential diagnosis can include cluster headache, benign paroxysmal hemicrania, "atypical facial pain," Raeder's syndrome, and glossopharyngeal neuralgia.

There is another entity called "pretrigeminal neuralgia," which may be easily misdiagnosed. It has a "toothache"-like presentation. The pain is longer lasting and is often dull or aching in quality. Pretrigeminal neuralgia must be differentiated from small tumors inducing pain, atypical odontalgia or atypical facial pain, facial or "lower half" migraine, toothache of pulpal origin, sinusitis, and TMJ dysfunction. It is important to differentiate trigeminal neuralgia from pretrigeminal neuralgia from dental pain to avoid unnecessary tooth extraction (6,7).

It is worth mentioning a rare variant of TN, the cluster-tic syndrome, which consists of cluster headache and concurrent TN in a V2 distribution. This entity is very difficult to treat conservatively; surgical intervention may be needed.

PATHOPHYSIOLOGY

The age of onset may give information regarding the etiology of the disorder. People with onset in their twenties to thirties may have associated demyelinating disease (multiple sclerosis), compression of the trigeminal nerve root by myeloma, aneurysm or tumor, including schwannoma, Meckel's cave meningioma, epidermoid cyst, trigeminal neuroma, acoustic neuroma or chordoma, as well as pontine infarction (8,9).

In the elderly, vascular compression of the trigeminal nerve by abnormal arterial loops is found in 80% to 90% of patients when (and if) they are treated surgically (10).

The pathophysiology of TN is subject to a number of interpretations and conclusions, in that some authors feel that the disorder is centrally *versus* peripherally induced. While microvascular compression of the sensory root of cranial nerve V may be thought of as the cause of TN, other causes such as

It has been postulated that the origin of TN was vascular compression of the trigeminal nerve at the root entry zone. However, it appears to be more complex. One group notes that the disorder may be secondary to an abnormal discharge within the peripheral nervous system (11).

Still, the proponents of the "neurovascular conflict" note an artery, most often a loop of the superior or anteroinferior cerebellar artery compresses part of the trigeminal nerve root. This, in turn, triggers localized demyelination and ectopic triggering of neuronal discharges (12). This would explain the fact that anticonvulsant medications do relieve the condition.

After looking at experimental nerve injury preparations, one group proposed a hypothesis that indicated that trigger stimuli set off bursts of neuronal activity in a small cluster of trigeminal ganglion neurons that have become hyperexcitable as a result of trigeminal ganglion or trigeminal root damage. This trigeminal ganglion "ignition focus" of activity spreads the neuronal excitability to more widespread parts of the ganglion. After a short period of autonomous firing (seconds to minutes), the activity ends and a refractory period is begun by intrinsic suppressive (hyperpolarizing) processes which engage as a result of the rapid neuronal firing. Therefore, the primary abnormality is found in the trigeminal ganglion or root, and not the skin or other areas of the CNS. This would also explain the essentially normal neurological examination found between periods of ectopic paroxysmal trigeminal ganglionic discharge (13).

Members of this group later published on the "ignition hypothesis" of trigeminal neuralgia. It postulates that TN results from specific abnormalities of trigeminal afferent neurons in the trigeminal ganglion or root. Such injury creates a hyperexcitable state in the injured axons and axotomized somata. These hyperexcitable afferents then give rise to paroxysms of pain as a result of synchronized after-discharge activity. This would account for the major positive and negative symptoms and signs of TN, as well as its pathogenesis and treatment (14).

It was also noted that, in 12 patient biopsy specimens of trigeminal root (postmicrovascular decompression) there were pathophysiological changes including axonopathy and axonal loss, demyelination, a less severe myelin range of abnormalities (dysmyelination), residual myelin debris and the presence of excess collagen, including collagen masses in two cases. Also, within demyelinated zones, groups of axons were often closely opposed without intervening glial processes. It was thought that these findings were consistent with the ignition hypothesis of TN, and could, via axonopathy-induced changes in the electrical excitability of afferent axons in the trigeminal root and localized neuronal somata in the trigeminal ganglion induce ignition. The key pathological changes included ectopic impulse discharge, spontaneous and triggered after-discharge, and cross excitation found among closely placed afferent fibers (15).

Other groups also noted the demyelination found under the region of vascular compression (16,17).

Pathological review of a rhizotomy specimen from a patient with TN and multiple sclerosis demonstrated demyelination with intervening astrocyte processes, perivascular lymphocytes and lipid-laden macrophages, supporting the hypothesis that ephaptic transmission may also play a role in the pathogenesis of TN related to vascular compression (18).

TREATMENT

Medical

Carbamazepine has the only FDA approval for treating this indication. It is considered the "gold-standard." It has good initial efficacy, about 80% initially. It can be used as a diagnostic test for TN. It appears to work by depressing synaptic transmission in the spinal trigeminal nucleus. The drug can be used successfully at subantiepileptic dosages (100 mg bid–tid). The dose can then be escalated if pain continues and/or worsens. The maintenance dosage can range from 300 to 800 mg/day. Unfortunately, tachyphylaxis is common, this, too, causing the clinician to increase the dosage being used. Long-term efficacy with carbamazepine decreases to about 50% (19–21).

Initial side effects can include drowsiness, nausea, diplopia, dizziness, or ataxia. These symptoms are typically self-limited, and can resolve quickly by slowing the dose titration. Most typically, blood is checked QW or BIW for a month to evaluate for hepatotoxicity as well as aplastic anemia. The blood evaluation should occur then monthly for three months and then every six months or so. Lymphadenopathy, systemic lupus erythematosus and Stevens–Johnson syndrome may also occur, uncommonly, with the drug. Also, not all patients tolerate carbamazepine, up to 19% (19–21).

Carbamazepine should be used with caution in patients with cardiac conduction disturbances, Asian patients (who most commonly have a HLA-B*1502 allele, placing them with a higher risk of fatal dermatologic reactions, including toxic-epidermal necrolysis and Stevens–Johnson syndrome), as well as in patients with depression or a history of depression, particularly suicidal ideation. The drug may also impair the effectiveness/reliability of oral contraceptives. There are also other drug interactions that should be avoided, including erythromycin and prophoxphene (19–21).

Oxcarbazepine, a keto derivative of carbamazepine, has a less concerning side effect profile. It can be used at doses of 900 to 2400 mg/day with the typical maintenance dose being in the range of 300 to 600 mg BID. It is effective in about two-thirds of carbamazepine refractory patients (20). There are fewer drug reactions. Side effects include hyponatremia, part of the syndrome of inappropriate secretion of antidiuretic hormone (SIADH) (19–21).

Per Chesire, Solaro, et al. and Khan (22–24), gabapentin, while less useful than carbamazepine in TN, has better patient tolerance and fewer severe side effects. It works at the alpha-2-delta calcium channel. Its safety profile is better, possibly making it safer to use in the elderly patient. Dosages have varied in different studies, between 100 and 2400 mg/day. Main side effects may include dizziness or ankle edema (19,22). The drug may also be used as monotherapy or adjunctive therapy in the more difficult to treat multiple sclerosis patients with TN (23,24).

Baclofen, a gaba-aminobutyric acid (GABA) analog, depresses excitatory transmission and facilitates segmental inhibition in the trigeminal nucleus. It can be used adjunctively with carbamazepine or phenytoin. It has shown itself to be useful, while, like gabapentin, not FDA approved for this use (19,20,25,26).

A host of other anticonvulsant and other drugs have been evaluated for treatment of TN. These include, per Oberman, et al. (27), pregabalin, another "gabapentenoid" (150–600 mg/day in divided doses) (27); clonazepam (28); sumatriptan, a migraine abortive drug which is a $5\text{-}HT_{1A/1B/1D}$ receptor agonist, has been successfully used via subcutaneous injection followed by oral administration (29,30); intranasal lidocaine, 8% spray for second division trigeminal neuralgia (31); botulinum toxin (32); and cannabinoids (33).

Surgical

When medication therapy becomes unable to help, there are a number of different neurosurgical procedures that have been used in the treatment of TN. In one paper, they are grouped as follows (8):

1. Glycerol injection, 85% effective, minor procedure, easily repeatable; has slight facial sensory loss and highest recurrence rate;
2. Radiofrequency rhizotomy, 90% effective, minor procedure, associated with possible sensory loss, masseter weakness, corneal reflex loss, recurrence rate approximately 25%;
3. Microvascular decompression, >90% effective, is a major surgical procedure with possible serious side effects;

The most well-known procedure is the Janetta procedure (microvascular decompression) which involves an occipital craniotomy. Any vascular contacts with the fifth cranial nerve (trigeminal roots) are decompressed, with long-term benefit found in 80% to 100% of patients. Recurrence rates vary from 1% to 6%. Surgical mortality can be 1% and serious morbidity is seen in 7% (hemorrhage, hearing loss, or hematoma, CSF leak, infection). The procedure appears to be more effective when treating "typical" *versus* atypical trigeminal neuralgia (34–40).

In patients who have failed microvascular decompression, posterior fossa reexploration was found to be effective and safe for the treatment of recurrent TN (41).

The use of radiofrequency rhizotomy percutaneously works by thermally damaging C- and A-delta fibers. Recurrence rate is 9% to 28%. Complications, as noted above, include loss of corneal reflex in 70%, paresthesias in 10%, and anesthesia dolorosa in up to 4%, but the latter happened before the procedure was better refined (8,42–46).

Percutaneous glycerol injections, during which glycerol is injected percutaneously into the retrogasserian CSF cistern in Meckel's cavity (cave), is one of three percutaneous stereotactic procedures used to treat the pain of TN. The glycerol reportedly destroys already damaged myelinated axons which are involved in the central aspects of TN. The procedure is least likely to cause postoperative sensory loss but has a higher recurrence rate (10–43% at two years). The procedure is good for patients who are poor candidates for posterior fossa exploration/surgery (8,47–49).

Balloon compression and radiofrequency thermocoagulation are the other two common procedures used to relieve the pain of TN (8). Like the glycerol retrogasserian ganglion injection, they work to block the pain of TN by inducing a partial injury to the trigeminal ganglion. Both procedures may have recurrence rates of up to 25%. Anesthesia dolorosa can be found in between 1% and 10% of patients (50).

Gamma knife radiosurgery is being used more frequently secondary to its minimal invasiveness. A very focused beam of radiation is delivered to a small (4 mm) target area, which encompasses the retrogasserian cisternal aspect of the trigeminal nerve. Pain relief, initially, is found in 81% to 92% (51–54).

Evidence-Based Medicine

The RCTs demonstrating Carbamazepine's usefulness in the treatment of TN enabled the drug to attain FDA approval for this indication. There were four placebo-controlled studies of carbamazepine in TN (55–58). The number needed to treat (NNT) for effectiveness was 2.6 (CI 2.0–3.4) (59).

Another Cochrane Review looked at nine RCTs of different nonepileptic drugs involving 223 people. These drugs included Baclofen, L-baclofen, racemic Baclofen, tizanidine, tocainide, proparacaine hydrochloride 0.5%, pimozide, and clomipramine. Insufficient evidence was found to demonstrate significant benefit from these nonanticonvulsant medications in treating TN (60).

REFERENCES

1. Osler W. The Principles and Practice of Medicine. 8th ed. New York: D. Appleton and company, 1912:191–202.
2. Headache Classification Subcommittee of the International Headache Society. The international classification of headache disorders, 2nd ed. Cephalalgia 2004; 24(Suppl 1):1–151.
3. Terrence CF, Jensen TS. Trigeminal neuralgia and other facial neuralgias. In: Olesen J, Tfelt-Hansen P, Welch KMA, eds. The Headaches. 2nd ed. Philadelphia: Lippincott Williams & Wilkins, 2000:929–938.
4. Solth A, Veelken N, Gottschalk J, et al. Successful vascular decompression in an 11-year-old patient with trigeminal neuralgia. Childs Nerv Syst 2008; 24(6):763–766.
5. Manzoni GC, Torelli P. Epidemiology of typical and atypical craniofacial neuralgias. Neurol Sci 2005; 26(Suppl 2):S65–S67.
6. Jay GW. The Headache Handbook: Diagnosis and Treatment. New York: CRC Press, 1999:101–107.
7. Mitchell RG. Pre-trigeminal neuralgia. Br Dengt J 1980; 149:167–170.
8. Graef L, McArthur J. Case 7: a man with shock-like facial pains. http://www.medscape.com/viewarticle/430125 (accessed June 28, 2008).
9. Soyka D. Etiology and therapy of trigeminal neuralgia. Neurochirurgia (Stuttg) 1990; 33(Suppl 1):s11–s13.
10. Haines SJ, Jannetta PJ, Zorub DS. Microvascular relations of the trigeminal nerve: an anatomical study with clinical correlation. J Neurosurg 1980; 52:381–386.
11. Burchiel KJ, Baumann TK. Pathophysiology of trigeminal neuralgia: new evidence from a trigeminal ganglion intraoperative microneurographic recording. Case report. J Neurosurg 2004; 101(5):872–873.
12. Joffroy A, Levivier M, Massager N. Trigeminal neuralgia. Pathophysiology and treatment. Acta Neurol Belg 2001; 101(1):20–25.
13. Rappaport ZH, Devor M. Trigeminal neuralgia: the role of self-sustaining discharge in the trigeminal ganglion. Pain 1994; 56(2):127–138.
14. Devor M, Amir R, Rappaport ZH. Pathophysiology of trigeminal neuralgia: the ignition hypothesis. Clin J Pain 2002; 18(1):4–13.
15. Devor M, Govrin-Lippmann R, Rappaport ZN. Mechanism of trigeminal neuralgia: an ultrastructural analysis of trigeminal root specimens obtained during microvascular decompression surgery. J Neurosurg 2002; 96(3):532–543.
16. Hilton DA, Love S, Gradidge T, et al. Pathological findings associated with trigeminal neuralgia caused by vascular compression. Neurosurgery 1994; 35(2):299–303.
17. Love S, Hilton DA, Coakham HB. Central demyelination of the Vth nerve root in trigeminal neuralgia associated with vascular decompression. Brain Pathol 1998; 8(1):1–11.
18. Love S, Gradidge T, Coakham HB. Trigmeminal neuralgia due to multiple sclerosis: ultrastructural findings in trigeminal rhizotomy specimens. Neuropathol Appl Neurobiol 2001; 27(3):238–244.
19. Chesire WP. Trigeminal neuralgia: diagnosis and treatment. Curr Neurol Neurosci Rep 2005; 5:79–85.
20. Canavero S, Bonicalzi V. Drug therapy of trigeminal neuralgia. Expert Rev Neurotherapeutics 2006; 6(3):429–440.
21. Sindrup SH, Jensen TS. Pharacoptherapy of trigeminal neuralgia. Clin J Pain 2002; 18:22–27.

22. Chesire WP. Defining the role for gabapentin in the treatment of trigeminal neuralgia: a retrospective study. J Pain 2002; 3:137–142.
23. Solaro C, Messmer Uccelli M, Uccelli A, et al. Low-dose gabapentin combined with either lamotrigine or carbamazepine can be useful therapies for trigeminal neuralgia in multiple sclerosis. Eur Neurol 2000; 44:45–48.
24. Khan OA. Gabapentin relieves trigeminal neuralgia in multiple sclerosis patients. Neurology 1998; 51:611–614.
25. Fromm GH, Terrence CF. Comparison of L -baclofen and racemic Baclofen in trigeminal neuralgia. Neurology 37(11):1725–1728.
26. Fromm GTH, Terrence CG, Chattha AS. Baclofen in the treatment of trigeminal neuralgia: double-blind study and long term follow-up. Ann Neurol 1984; 15: 240–244.
27. Obermann M, Yoon MS, Sensen K, et al. Efficacy of pregabalin in the treatment of trigeminal neuralgia. Cephalalgia 2008; 28(2):174–181.
28. Court JE, Kase CS. Treatment of tic douloureux with a new anticonvulsant (clonazepam). J Neurol Neurosurg Psychiatry 1976; 39:297–299.
29. Kanai A, Suzuki A, Osawa S, et al. Sumatriptan alleviates pain in patients with trigeminal neuralgia. Clin J Pain 2006; 22(8):677–680.
30. Kanai A, Saito M, Hoka S. Subcutaneious sumatriptan for refractory trigeminal neuralgia. Headache 2006; 46(4):577–582.
31. Kanai A, Suzuki A, Kobayashi M, et al. Intranasal lidocaine 8% spray for second-division trigeminal neuralgia. Br J Anaesth 2006; 97(4):559–563.
32. Turk U, Iihan S, Alp R, et al. Botulinum toxin and intractable trigeminal neuralgia. Clin Neuropharmacol 2005; 28(4):161–162.
33. Liang YC, Huang CC, Hsu KS. Therapeutic potential of cannabinoids in trigeminal neuralgia. Curr Drug Targets CNS Neurol Disord 2004; 3(6):507–514.
34. Jannetta PJ. Surgical treatment: microvascular decompression. In: Fromm GH, Sessle BJ, eds. Trigeminal Neuralgia Current Concepts Regarding Pathogenesis and Treatment. Boston: Butterworth-Heinemann, 1991:145–157.
35. Elias WJ, Burchiel KJ. Microvascular decompression. Clin J Pain 2002; 18:35–41.
36. Sindou M, Leston J, Decullier E, et al. Microvascular decompression for primary trigeminal neuralgia: long-term effectiveness and prognostic factors in a series of 362 consecutive patients with clear-cut neurovascular conflicts who underwent pure decompression. J Neurosurg 2007; 107(6):1144–1153.
37. Li ST, Want X, Pan Q, et al. Studies on the operative outcomes and mechanisms of microvascular decompression in treating typical and atypical trigeminal neuralgia. Clin J Pain 2005; 21(4):311–316.
38. Mizuno M, Saito K, Takayasu M, et al. Percutaneous microcompression of the trigeminal ganglion for elderly patients with trigeminal neuralgia and patients with atypical trigeminal neuralgia. Neurol Med Chir (Tokyo) 2000; 40(7):347–350.
39. Liu HB, Ma Y, Zou JJ, et al. Percutaneious microballoon compression for trigeminal neuralgia. Chin Med J (Engl) 2007; 120(3):228–230.
40. Barker FG II, Jannetta PJ, Bissonette DJ, et al. The long-term outcome of microvascular decompression for trigeminal neuralgia. N Engl J Med 1997; 334:1077–1083.
41. Fernandez-Carballal C, Garcia-Salazar F, Perez-Calvo J, et al. Management of recurrent trigeminal neuralgia after failed microvascular decompression. Neurocirugia 2004; 15(4):345–352.
42. Scrivani SJ, Keith DA, Mathews ES, et al. Percutaneous sterotactic differential radiofrequency thermal rhizotomy for the treatment of trigmeminal neuralgia. J Oral Maxillofac Surg 1999; 57:104–111.
43. Mathews ES, Scrivani SJ. Percutaneious sterotactic radiofrequency thermal rhizotomy for the treatment of trigeminal neuralgia. Mt Sinai J Med 2000; 67(4): 288–299.
44. Kanpolat Y, Savas A, Bekar A, et al. Percutaneous controlled radiofrequency trigeminal rhizotomy for the treatment of idiopathic trigeminal neuralgia: 25-year experience with 1600 patients. Neurosurgery 2001; 48(3):524–532.

45. Taha JM, Tew JM Jr. Treatment of trigeminal neuralgia by percutaneous radiofrequency rhizotomy. Neurosurg Clin N Am 1997; 8:31–39.
46. Nugent GR. Surgical treatment: radiofrequency gangliolysis and rhizotomy. In: Fromm GH, Sessle BJ, eds. Trigeminal Neuralgia Current Concepts Regarding Pathogenesis and Treatment. Boston: Butterworth-Heinemann, 1991:159–184.
47. Pollock BE. Percutaneious retrogasserian glycerol rhizotomy for patients with idiopathic trigeminal neuralgia: a prospective analysis of factors related to pain relief. J Neurosurg 2005; 102(2):223–228.
48. Cappabianca P, Spaziante R, Graziussi G, et al. Percutaneous retrogasserian glyceral rhizolysis for treatment of trigeminal neuralgia. Technique and results in 191 patients. J Neurosurg Sci 1995; 39:37–45.
49. Bergenheim AT, Hariz MI. Influence of previous treatment on outcome after flycerol shizotomy for trigeminal neuralgia. Neurosurgery 1995; 36:303–309.
50. Peters G, Nurmikko TJ. Peripyheral and gasserian ganglion-level procedures for the treatment of trigeminal neuralgia. Clin J Pain 2002; 18:28–34.
51. McNatt SA, Yu C, Giannotta SL, et al. Gamma knife radiosurgery for trigeminal neuralgia. Neurosurgery 2005; 56(6):1295–1301.
52. Fountas KN, Lee GP, Smith JR. Outcome of patients undergoing gamma knife steroitactic radiosurgery for medically refractory idiopathic trigeminal neuralgia: Medical College of Georga's experience. Stereotact Funct Neurosurg 2006; 84:88–96.
53. Massager N, Murata N, Tamura M, et al. Influence of nerve radiation dose in the incidence of trigeminal dysfunction after trigeminal neuralgia radiosurgery. Neurosurgery 2007; 60(4):687–688.
54. Massager N, Abeloos L, Devriendt D, et al. Clinical evaluation of targeting accuracy of gamma knife radiosurgery in trigmeminal neuralgia. Int J Radiat Oncol Biol Phys 2007; 69(5):1514–1520.
55. Campbell FG, Graham JG, Zilkha KJ. Clinical trial of carbamazepine (Tegretol) in trigeminal neuralgia. J Neurol Neurosurg Psychiatry 1966; 29:265–267.
56. Killian JM, Fromm GH. Carbamazepine in the treatment of neuralgia: use of side effects. Arch Neurol 1968; 19:129–136.
57. Nicol CF. A four year double blind study of Tegretol in facial pain. Headache 1969; 9:545–547.
58. Rockliff BW, Davis EH. Controlled sequential trials of carbamazepine in trigeminal neuralgia. Arch Neurol 1966; 15:129–136.
59. Wiffen P, Collins P, Collins S, et al. Anticonvulsant drugs for acute and chronic pain. Cochrane Database Syst Rev 2005; (3). Art. No.: CD001133. DOI: 10.1002/14651858.CD001133.pub2.
60. He L, Wu B, Zhou M. Non-epileptic drugs for trigeminal neuralgia. Cochrane Database Syst Rev 2006; (3). Art. No.: CD004029. DOI: 10.1002/14651858.CD004029.pub2.

8 Persistent Idiopathic Facial Pain

Bernadette Jaeger

Section of Oral Medicine and Orofacial Pain, UCLA School of Dentistry, Los Angeles, California, U.S.A.

Persistent idiopathic facial pain, formerly known as atypical facial pain and atypical facial neuralgia, is a diagnosis often given to those patients with facial pain that does not fit with other obvious diagnostic categories. These patients typically present with poorly localized, vaguely described, nonanatomic facial pain, and no evidence of a defined organic cause (1). Strictly speaking, these pains are not "atypical" but, rather, idiopathic. These are pains for which we do not yet have sufficient understanding. This realization has lead to the newer term for these disorders, namely persistent idiopathic facial pain.

A retrospective analysis of data collected on 493 consecutive patients who presented to a university orofacial pain clinic was rather enlightening and stressed the importance of careful clinical evaluation and diagnosis (2). In this study a diagnosis of atypical facial pain was made if patients had persistent orofacial pain for more than six months for which previous treatments had been unsuccessful and the diagnosis was unknown on referral to the clinic. Of the 493 patient charts reviewed, 35 (7%) met these criteria. Using the American Academy of Orofacial Pain diagnostic criteria (3), all but one (97%) actually did have diagnosable physical problems and sometimes multiple overlapping physical diagnoses causing the pain. Over half (19 of 35 or 54%) were found to have myofascial pain due to trigger points as the primary cause or significant contributing factor to the pain. Eleven (31%) had periodontal ligament sensitivity, eight had referred pain from dental pulpitis, three had neuropathic pain, and one each had burning mouth from oral candidiasis, burning tongue from an oral habit, pericoronitis, sinus pathology, or an incomplete tooth fracture. A review by Clark suggested that the differential diagnosis in these patients should also include a focal neuropathic pain disorder when no local source of infectious, inflammatory, or other pathology can be found (4).

There is significant debate in the field about the diagnosis and classification of persistent idiopathic facial pains. Myofascial trigger point pain is clearly under-recognized (2,5,6), and trigeminal neuropathies or "dysesthesias," which many believe to be at fault for various atypical facial pains, are still inadequately understood (4,5). Although "persistent idiopathic facial pain" is a more accurate term, the atypical nomenclature is likely to haunt the dental/orofacial pain profession for quite a few years to come.

Two common types of persistent idiopathic facial pain are atypical odontalgia and burning mouth syndrome. Although deafferentation is believed to play a role in both of these pain syndromes, the mechanism and etiology are still largely speculative.

ATYPICAL ODONTALGIA

The Disorder
In 1978, Rees and Harris described a disorder they called atypical odontalgia (7). Synonymous or almost synonymous terms include phantom tooth pain (8), idiopathic orofacial pain (9), vascular toothache (10), and trigeminal dysesthesia. Patients present with pain in a tooth with no obvious pathology (11,12), and the pain may spread to other areas of the face, neck, and shoulder (13). Evidence suggests that 3% to 6% of patients who undergo endodontic treatment, surgical resection of tooth root tips, or tooth extraction may develop atypical odontalgia (7). Peri-menopausal women seem to be disproportionately affected.

Symptoms
The chief complaint is a fairly constant, deep, dull, aching pain in a tooth or tooth site that is unchanging over weeks or months. It has some diurnal fluctuation, and usually worsens as the day progresses. The molars are most commonly involved, followed by premolars. Anterior teeth and canines are less frequently affected (14). The vast majority of patients present with unilateral pain, although other quadrants may become involved and other oral and facial sites may hurt. The pain does not follow the anatomy of the trigeminal nerve and there are no trigger sites as in trigeminal neuralgia (Table 1).

Dental therapies, especially root canal treatment or extraction, trauma, or medical procedures related to the face often, but not always, precede the onset of the pain by a month or so (7). The unrelenting nature of the pain predisposes patients to seek repeated dental therapies that then fail to resolve the problem. Chewing or clenching on painful teeth, heat, cold, and stress are typical but inconsistent aggravating factors.

Diagnosis

Examination
Despite persistent, often severe pain, there are typically no clearly identifiable clinical or radiographic abnormalities associated with atypical odontalgia. If the pain is in a tooth as opposed to an extraction site, responses to percussion, thermal testing, and electric pulp stimulation are variable. Clinically, there is no observable cause, yet thermographic evaluation is always abnormal (15). Initial studies reported that the majority of patients had little or no relief with diagnostic local anesthetic blocks (14,16), although sympathetic blocks seemed to be helpful (14). In a double-blind, multicenter, controlled study, atypical odontalgia patients did get significant, but not complete relief with local anesthetic injection (17).

TABLE 1 Characteristics of Atypical Odontalgia (11)

Pain in a tooth or tooth site
Continuous or almost continuous pain
Pain present for more than 4 months
No sign of local or referred pain
Equivocal response to somatic nerve block

Pathophysiology

The exact pathophysiology of atypical odontalgia remains obscure. Over the years psychogenic, vascular, neuropathic, and idiopathic causes have been entertained. Bell classified atypical odontalgia as a vascular disorder (10), as did Rees and Harris, who postulated a "painful migraine-like disturbance" in the teeth and periodontal tissues, possibly triggered by depression (8). There is little to support a vascular etiology despite the fact that a study using subcutaneous sumatriptan in 19 atypical facial pain patients did show some small, albeit temporary, positive effects (18).

Others have suggested depression or some other psychological disorder as the cause (19,20) since many patients with atypical odontalgia report depressive symptoms on clinical interview (7,21,22). However, these early results were from poor, uncontrolled studies. A more recent case control study (23) found that a majority of atypical odontalgia patients had more comorbid pain conditions and higher scores for depression and somatization than controls. They also had significantly lower scores on quality of life measures. Another study showed that atypical odontalgia patients had moderate to severe mean depression and somatization scores that were similar to patients suffering from temporomandibular disorders (24). Of interest is that a comparison of standard MMPI scores for patients with atypical odontalgia with standard MMPI scores for a chronic headache group (matched for age, sex, and chronicity) showed no significant differences. Furthermore, in this comparison study, the scores for both groups were within normal ranges (14,25), making a psychological cause unlikely.

At this time, the best supported hypothesis is that atypical odontalgia is a focal neuropathic pain disorder (26,4), and is most likely due to deafferentation with or without sympathetic involvement. Atypical odontalgia usually follows a dental procedure, and most dental procedures, including cavity preparation, cause varying degrees of deafferentation. Other causes of direct nerve injury include nerve injection injury, trauma from a fracture or surgical treatment or compression from implants, and osseous or neoplastic growths (4). Studies supporting this theory are also lacking, yet the symptoms and clinical presentation are consistent with posttraumatic neuropathic pain. List et al. found that atypical odontalgia patients did get significant, but not complete relief with local anesthetic injection as compared to placebo (17). This supports the idea that the spontaneous pain of atypical odontalgia is, in part, due to peripheral afferent inputs, but that some of this pain may be due to sensitization of higher order neurons. Many atypical odontalgia cases also respond to sympathetic blocks (14) or phentolamine infusion (27), implying that at least some may be sympathetically mediated or maintained. This theory would also explain why the pain remains even after the painful tooth is extracted. In addition, the preponderance of women suffering from this disorder raises the question of the role of estrogen and other female hormones as a risk factor in atypical odontalgia and related idiopathic orofacial pains (28).

Treatment

Any kind of invasive or irreversible treatments, such as endodontic therapy, exploratory surgery, extraction, or even occlusal adjustments, are contraindicated. This is because, despite possible transient relief, the pain is likely to recur with equal or greater intensity.

The current treatment of choice is the use of tricyclic antidepressant agents such as amitriptyline or imipramine (7,14,16,29). Pregabalin has also shown some promise (30). If the pain has a burning quality, the addition of a phenothiazine, such as trifluoperazine, may be helpful (14,16). Tricyclic antidepressants have analgesic properties independent of their antidepressant effects and often provide good pain relief at a fraction of the dose typically used to treat depression (31,32). Pain relief normally occurs at doses from 50 to 100 mg. Dry mouth is an expected and usually unavoidable side effect. A history of significant cardiac arrhythmias or recent myocardial infarction, urinary retention, and glaucoma are contraindications for the use of tricyclic medications because of their atropine-like action. Patients may need reassurance that the pain is real and not psychogenic but that invasive procedures will not help.

If a patient complains of associated gingival hyperesthesia, use of topical agents such as local anesthetic or capsaicin has been shown to be beneficial (33). Unwanted stimulation of the area can be reduced by construction of an acrylic stent that can also be used to help apply any topical medication.

BURNING MOUTH SYNDROME

The Disorder
Burning mouth syndrome is an intraoral pain disorder that is typically associated with a burning sensation of the tongue and/or palate. Postmenopausal women are most commonly affected. The National Institutes of Dental and Craniofacial Research report on the National Centers for Disease Control household health survey stated that almost 1.3 million American adults (0.7% of the U.S. population), mostly women in the postmenopausal period, are afflicted with this disorder (34). When it primarily affects the tongue, it is referred to as burning tongue or glossodynia. Grushka and her colleagues have conducted several studies to systematically characterize the features of this disorder (35–38).

Symptoms
The patient with burning mouth complains of intraoral burning, the tip and sides of the tongue being the most common sites, followed by the palate. Frequently associated symptoms include dry mouth, thirst, taste and sleep disturbances, headaches, and other pain complaints. Onset is often related to a dental procedure. Patients rate the *intensity* of the pain associated with burning mouth similar to that of toothache, although the *quality* is burning rather than pulsing, aching, or throbbing. The pain increases as the day progresses and tends to peak in early evening. More than two-thirds of patients with burning mouth syndrome have altered taste sensation and may complain of spontaneous tastes or "taste phantoms" (dysgeusia) (39,40).

Diagnosis

Examination
The patient with burning mouth syndrome usually has a negative intraoral examination, but the diagnosis should be established only after all other possible causes such as denture soreness, rough crowns or teeth, xerostomia, candidiasis,

anemia, true vitamin deficiencies, and systemic or rheumatologic disease have been exhaustively ruled out.

Tests

A good diagnostic test for burning mouth syndrome is a local anesthetic rinse. Anesthetizing the oral mucosa will decrease the pain of other conditions such as geographic tongue or candidiasis but *increase* the pain of burning mouth. This increase in pain is thought to be due to further loss of A beta fiber inhibition.

Candidiasis should be tested for even if the mucosa looks normal. Sedimentation rate may be mildly elevated, and in view of the higher incidence of immunologic abnormalities, rheumatologic evaluation should be considered.

Pathophysiology

There are many obvious oral and systemic conditions that cause or are associated with mucogingival and glossal pains. These include candidiasis, geographic tongue, allergies to dental materials, denture dysfunction, xerostomia, various anemias and vitamin deficiencies (iron, vitamin B_{12}, or folic acid), diabetes mellitus, several dermatologic disorders (lupus, lichen planus, erythema multiforme), human immunodeficiency virus, and systemic medications. Certain medications, such as antiretrovirals, antiseizure drugs, hormones, and particularly antihypertensives (particularly those that act on the angiotensin-renin system) have been implicated as causing oral burning directly (41).

Other medications contribute to oral burning indirectly through resultant xerostomia (34,42,43). However, while there is evidence for a higher incidence of immunologic abnormalities in burning mouth syndrome patients than would be expected in a normal population, and several burning mouth syndrome patients have been shown to have Sjögren's syndrome (36), most patients with burning mouth have no obvious organic cause and the oral mucosa appears normal (40,43).

Current research supports a theory that damage to or dysfunction of the chorda tympani branch of CN VII contributes to the dysgeusia and pain of burning mouth (44). The special sense of taste from the tongue is mediated by the chorda tympani (anterior two-thirds) and CN IX (posterior one-third). The chorda tympani innervates the fungiform papillae of the tongue, which, in turn, are surrounded by pain fibers from cranial nerve V. The chorda tympani normally inhibits both cranial nerve V (pain fibers) and cranial nerve IX (taste). Damage or partial deafferentation of the chorda tympani appears to release inhibition of both cranial nerves V and IX, producing both pain and taste phantoms, respectively (42,45).

Burning mouth syndrome is not to be confused with postmenopausal oral discomfort, which has a burning component. In the latter condition, estrogen replacement therapy is effective about half of the time (46).

Psychological factors, although present in some of this population, do not appear to be etiologic (47).

Treatment

There is no satisfactory management approach for burning mouth syndrome that offers efficacy for most patients. Many different families of drugs including antidepressants, antipsychotics, antiepileptic drugs, analgesics, and mucosal protectors, among others, have been tried (48). Studies assessing therapeutic outcome are lacking, and burning mouth syndrome does not appear to remit spontaneously. Topical clonazepam and cognitive therapy have been proven efficacious in some patients (49). Emerging evidence supports the effectiveness of the antioxidant, alpha lipoic acid (49,50), but because burning mouth syndrome is thought to be neuropathic in origin, treatment is typically with medications that may suppress neurologic transduction, transmission, and even pain signal facilitation more centrally (51). Treatment should be tailored to the individual patient and is largely palliative, but few studies report relief without intervention.

REFERENCES

1. Mock D et al. Atypical facial pain: a retrospective study. Oral Surg 1985; 59:472.
2. Fricton JR. Atypical orofacial pain disorders: a study of diagnostic subtypes. Curr Rev Pain 2000; 4:142–147.
3. Okeson JP, editor. Orofacial pain. Guidelines for Assessment, Diagnosis, and Management. American Academy of Orofacial Pain. Chicago: Quintessence, 1996.
4. Clark GT. Persistent orodental pain, atypical odontalgia, and phantom tooth pain: when are they neuropathic disorders? J Calif Dent Assoc 2006; 34(8):599–609.
5. Graff-Radford SB. Facial pain. Curr Opin Neurol 2000; 13:291–296.
6. Pfaffenrath V, Rath M, Pollmann W, et al. Atypical facial pain—application of the IHS criteria in a clinical sample. Cephalalgia 1993; 13(Suppl 12):84–88.
7. Marbach JJ, Raphael KG. Phantom tooth pain: a new look at an old dilemma. Pain Med 2000; 1(1):68.
8. Rees RT, Harris M. Atypical odontalgia. Br J Oral Surg 1978–9; 16:212.
9. Woda A, Tubert-Jeannin S, Bouhassira D, et al. Towards a new taxonomy of idiopathic orofacial pain. Pain 2005; 116(3):396–406.
10. Okeson JP, Bell WE. Bell's Orofacial Pains. 5th ed. Quintessence Publishing, 1995.
11. Graff-Radford SB, Solberg WK. Atypical odontalgia. J Craniomandib Disord 1992; 6(4):260–265.
12. Clark GT, Minakuchi H, Lotaif AC. Orofacial pain and sensory disorders in the elderly. Dent Clin North Am 2005; 49:343–362.
13. Melis M, Lobo SL, Ceneviz C, et al. Atypical odontalgia: a review of the literature. Headache 2003; 43(10):1060–1074.
14. Solberg WK, Graff-Radford SB. Orodental considerations in facial pain. Semin Neurol 1988; 8:318.
15. Graff-Radford SB, Ketelaer MC, Gratt BM, et al. Thermographic assessment of neuropathic facial pain. J Orofac Pain 1995; 9:138.
16. Bates RE Jr, Stewart CM. Atypical odontalgia: phantom tooth pain. Oral Surg 1991; 72:479.
17. List T, Leijon G, Helkimo M, et al. Effect of local anesthesia on atypical odontalgia—a randomized controlled trial. Pain 2006; 122(3):306–314.
18. al Balawi S, Tariq M, Feinmann C. A double-blind, placebo-controlled, crossover, study to evaluate the efficacy of subcutaneous sumatriptan in the treatment of atypical facial pain. Int J Neurosci 1996; 86:301.
19. Marbach JJ. Is phantom tooth pain a deafferentation (neuropathic syndrome)? Part I. Oral Surg 1993; 75:95.
20. Marbach JJ. Is phantom tooth pain a deafferentation (neuropathic syndrome)? Part II. Oral Surg 1993; 75:225.
21. Reik L. Atypical facial pain. Headache 1985; 25:30.
22. Feinman C. Pain relief by antidepressants: possible modes of action. Pain 1985; 23:1.
23. List T, Leijon G, Helkimo M, et al. Clinical findings and psychosocial factors in patients with atypical odontalgia: a case-control study. J Orofac Pain 2007; 21(2): 89–98.

24. Baad-Hansen L, Leijon G, Svensson P, et al. Comparison of clinical findings and psychosocial factors in patients with atypical odontalgia and temporomandibular disorders. J Orofac Pain 2008; 22(1):7–14.

25. Graff-Radford SB, Solberg WK. Is atypical odontalgia a psychological problem? Oral Surg 1993; 75:579.

26. Baad-Hansen L. Atypical odontalgia—pathophysiology and clinical management. J Oral Rehabil 2008; 35(1):1–11.

27. Vickers ER, Cousins MJ, Walker S, et al. Analysis of 50 patients with atypical odontalgia. A preliminary report on pharmacological procedures for diagnosis and treatment. Oral Surg 1998; 85:24.

28. Woda A, Pioncho P. A unified concept of idiopathic orofacial pain: pathophysiologic features. J Orofac Pain 2000; 14:196.

29. Graff-Radford SB, Solberg WK. Atypical odontalgia. J Craniomandib Disord 1992; 6(4):260–265.

30. Backonja MM, Serra J. Pharmacologic management part 1: better-studied neuropathic pain diseases. Pain Med 2004; 5 (Suppl 1):S28–S47.

31. Feinman C. Pain relief by antidepressants: possible modes of action. Pain 1985; 23:1.

32. McQuay HJ, Tramer M, Nye BA, et al. A systematic review of antidepressants in neuropathic pain. Pain 1996; 68:217.

33. Vickers ER, Cousins MJ, Walker S, et al. Analysis of 50 patients with atypical odontalgia. A preliminary report on pharmacological procedures for diagnosis and treatment. Oral Surg 1998; 85:24.

34. Lipton JH, Ship JA, Larach-Robinson D. Estimated prevalence and distribution of reported orofacial pain in the United States. J Am Dent Assoc 1993; 124:115.

35. Grushka M. Clinical features of burning mouth syndrome. Oral Med 1987; 63:30.

36. Grushka M et al. Psychophysical evidence of taste dysfunction in burning mouth syndrome. Chem Senses 1986; 11:485.

37. Grushka M, et al. Pain and personality profiles in burning mouth syndrome. Pain 1987; 28:155.

38. Grushka M, Sessle BJ. Demographic data and pain profile of burning mouth syndrome (BMS). J Dent Res 1985; 64:1648.

39. Mott AE, Grushka M, Sessle BJ. Diagnosis and management of taste disorders and burning mouth syndrome. Dent Clin North Am 1993; 37:33.

40. Bartoshuk LM, Snyder DJ, Grushka M, et al. Taste damage: previously unsuspected consequences. Chem Senses 2005; 30 (Suppl 1):i218–i219.

41. Salort-Llorca C, Mínguez-Serra MP, Silvestre FJ. Drug-induced burning mouth syndrome: a new etiological diagnosis. Med Oral Patol Oral Cir Bucal 2008; 13(3):E167–E170.

42. Grushka M, Bartoshuk LM. Burning mouth syndrome and oral dysesthesia. Can J Diagn 2000; 17:99.

43. Danhauer SC, Miller CS, Rhodus NL, et al. Impact of criteria-based diagnosis of burning mouth syndrome on treatment outcome. J Orofac Pain 2002; 16(4): 305–311.

44. Eliav E, Kamran B, Schaham R,et al. Evidence of chorda tympani dysfunction in patients with burning mouth syndrome. J Am Dent Assoc 2007; 138(5):628–633.

45. Forabosco A et al. Efficacy of hormone replacement therapy in postmenopausal women with oral discomfort. Oral Surg 1992; 73:570.

46. Grushka M, Sessle BJ. Burning mouth syndrome. Dent Clin North Am 1991; 35:171.

47. Bogetto F, Maina G, Ferro G, et al. Psychiatric comorbidity in patients with burning mouth syndrome. Psychosom Med 1998; 60:378.

48. Mínguez Serra MP, Salort Llorca C, Silvestre Donat FJ. Pharmacological treatment of burning mouth syndrome: a review and update. Med Oral Patol Oral Cir Bucal 2007; 12(4):E299–E304.

49. Patton LL, Siegel MA, Benoliel R, et al. Management of burning mouth syndrome: systematic review and management recommendations. Oral Surg Oral Med Oral Pathol Oral Radiol Endod 2007; 103(suppl 39):e1–e13.
50. Zakrzewska JM, Forssell H, Glenny AM. Interventions for the treatment of burning mouth syndrome. Cochrane Database Syst Rev 2005; (1):CD002779.
51. Suarez P, Clark GT. Burning mouth syndrome: an update on diagnosis and treatment methods. J Calif Dent Assoc 2006; 34(8):611–622.

9 Orofacial Pain Syndromes and Other Facial Neuralgias

Gary. W. Jay

Clinical Disease Area Expert-Pain, Pfizer, Inc., New London, Connecticut, U.S.A.

Organic causes of headache account for about one half of one percent of all headache problems. While they are rare, they can be devastating (1). Some common etiologies of intra-oral pain include the following:

1. Infection, abscess
2. Viral infection (herpetic)
3. Inflammation (pulpitis)
4. Trauma
5. Bruxism
6. Referred myofascial pain
7. Atrophic candidiasis
8. Ulcerative mucositis (includes Bechets syndrome)
9. Benign mucus membrane pemphigoid (an erosive/desquamative disorder)
10. Erythema multiforme

To evaluate pulpal pain, the use of electovitalometers, thermal tests, and periodontal ligament diagnostic anesthetic blocks may supplement clinical and radiological examinations.

Referred pain from specific trigger points can radiate to normal teeth as well as from the mouth to the temporomandibular joint. If that is suspected, palpate the lateral pterygoid muscle. If it is extremely tender, inject using a tuberculin syringe about a half cc of lidocaine without epinephrine.

Other myalgic pain syndromes may originate in the medial pterygoid, the buccinator, the mylohyoid, the omohyoid muscle, and the short and long head of the temporal muscle tendons and the temporalis muscle (2).

Ligamentous pain syndromes can include the hyoid bone syndrome, Eagle's syndrome (stylohyoid ligament insertion tendinitis), stylomandibular and sphenomandibular ligamentous pain, and capsular ligament pain.

These craniomandibular pain syndromes may be best diagnosed and dealt with by a dentist or oral surgeon who has experience in the differential diagnosis of these problems, as well as the ability to perform a differential neural blockade.

FACIAL NEURALGIAS AND OROFACIAL PAIN SYNDROMES

It should be noted first that with the possible exception of postherpetic neuralgia, the entities noted below are considered uncommon if not rare.

Postherpetic neuralgia is secondary to herpes zoster viral infection. It follows the distribution of the involved trigeminal nerve division. It may be associated with odontalgia. It may also produce excessive scarring and fibrosis at nerve terminals. There is a peripheral loss of afferent inhibition: specifically, the loss of large diameter sensory nerves such as the A-delta nerves. It may be difficult to control the pain. Treatment should start early with burst steroids. Follow-up treatment may include capsaicin and anticonvulsants, with carbamazepine being the drug of choice (3–6).

GLOSSOPHARYNGEAL NEURALGIA

The Disorder
Glossopharyngeal neuralgia is an electrical-like, excruciating paroxysmal lancinating pain in the throat—the lateral and posterior pharynx, tonsillar fossa, soft palate, and the base of the tongue with frequent radiation to the ear. The pain may be set off by swallowing, coughing, yawning, or chewing. It may last seconds to minutes (7,8). The association of this ninth cranial nerve neuralgia with cardiac syncope is rare, but may be identified by brief periods of bradycardia, hypotension, and asystole (8,9).

Diagnosis
Other than by history, high-resolution MRI of the brain stem with three-dimensional visualization may allow a diagnosis of neurovascular compression (10).

Pathophysiology
GPN is typically idiopathic. It may occur secondary to neurovascular compression. The anterior, inferior cerebellar artery usually is commonly found to be compressing cranial nerves IX and X at the root entry zones. One study of 30 adult cadavers with a history of GPN found 10 subjects to have glossopharyngeal nerves compressed by the posterior inferior arteries. Eight of twenty patients were found to have their glossopharyngeal nerve compressed by the posterior inferior cerebellar arteries (11).

Other pathophysiological entities can be unusual and/or more rare. A report of GPN secondary to a pontine lesion has been noted, showing a single hyperintense signal in the left pons, without other pathology on MRI. Ephaptic transmission occurring between the central pain fibers and the trigeminal or glossopharyngeal fibers, both of which enter the spinal trigeminal nuclear tract, inducing both conventional and "referred" GPN was postulated (12).

Four multiple sclerosis patients were reported to have GPN (7). One patient was found to have GPN after trauma to the neck (13). GPN may also be associated with laryngeal carcinoma. Many of these patients may also have trigeminal neuralgia (14).

Treatment
Conservative treatment is tried first. Carbamazepine has long been considered the drug of choice. Several authors more recently reported pharmacological treatments which included gabapentin and pregabalin (15,16). Of interest is the fact that gabapentin did not help patients who had previously undergone neurosurgical nerve decompression (15).

If conservative treatment fails, neurosurgical decompression (a Jannetta procedure) may be performed. The other treatment is sectioning of the ninth cranial nerve (10,11).

CAROTIDYNIA

The Disorder
Carotidynia is an episodic, throbbing, deep, dull neck pain with occasional neck swelling. The pain over the neck may project to the ipsilateral side of the head. It is self-limiting, usually less than two weeks. Carotidynia is thought by many to be nothing more than a unilateral neck pain associated with local tenderness that can be secondary to a number of vascular and nonvascular etiologies (including fibromuscular dysplasia, giant cell arteritis, lymphadenitis, local aphthous ulcers, and malignant infiltration) (17–23).

Diagnosis
There has been a major shift in thought. The first edition of the International Headache Society gave diagnostic criteria for this entity (24). The second edition in 2004 took Carotidynia out of the IHS diagnostic criteria (25). This was felt to invalidate the diagnosis. A number of authors have since evaluated the disorder with clinically effective tools and found it to have associated abnormalities.

Basically, the disorder is neck pain association with palpatory tenderness over the carotid bifurcation. For years it was thought that there were no radiologic or pathologic findings.

Pathophysiology
Burton et al. (26) noted, using MRI, abnormal enhancing tissue surrounding the symptomatic carotid artery at the level of the distal common carotid and carotid bifurcation. In one patient, repeat imaging after symptom resolution was associated with an absence of the previous abnormality. A more recent study (27) using ultrasonographic investigation shows poor echoic wall thickening of the carotid bulb, in the area of tenderness, associated with mild lumen narrowing and large outward extension of the vessel. Using CAT scan and ultrasonography, another group (28) noted in two cases that there was abnormal soft-tissue infiltration surrounding the symptomatic carotid artery, which surrounded the symptomatic distal common carotid and carotid bifurcation. Repeat CAT and ultrasonography after resolution of symptoms was associated with an absence of the prior abnormality.

Several other studies can be found which demonstrate the presence of an abnormality at the carotid in the region of pain, using MRI and Doppler sonography (29–31). The final conclusion of all of these authors is that the disorder is probably a distinct entity, possibly caused by inflammation.

Carotidynia is thought to be associated with migraine; the differential diagnosis would also include pseudotumor of the carotid sheath (32), pharyngitis, otitis, bruxism, neuralgia, myalgia, temporal arteritis, thyroiditis, head and neck neoplasms, and temporomandibular joint syndrome (33,34).

Still other parts of the differential diagnosis include dissecting aneurysm of the internal carotid artery, intramural clots with incomplete vessel obstruction of the internal carotid artery, spontaneous aneurysm of the common carotid bifurcation, and giant cell arteritis. While the other parts of the differential are essentially benign, these etiologies are most likely not (35).

Treatment
Clark et al. also note that carotidynia may be split into three distinct classifications: migrainous, nonmigrainous (classic), and arteriosclerotic. Ergotamine, propranolol, and tricyclic antidepressants have been used for the migrainous form, while steroids and nonsteroidal anti-inflammatory medications have been used successfully for the classic type of carotidynia (33). Both dihydroergotamine (36) and almotriptan (37) have been used to treat carotidynia.

NECK–TONGUE SYNDROME

The Disorder
The neck–tongue syndrome (NTS) is an uncommon problem characterized by attacks of occipital pain precipitated by sudden rotation of the head and associated with a subjective sensation of numbness in the ipsilateral side of the tongue (38). The prevalence in one study of 1835, 18- to 65-year-old parishioners in Norway was 4 patients (0.22%). There was also a variant among these cases in that one young man had "spasm" of the tongue instead of numbness (39). The authors of the latter study also postulated a possible relationship between NTS and cervicogenic headache.

Diagnosis
The diagnosis is primarily one of history. In one chiropractic case, it was noted that radiographs showed a narrowing of the left para-odontoid space, with mildly painful restriction on rotation at C1–2 with no muscular hypertonicity (40).

There has also been a familial aspect to the disorder, with suggestions of an autosomal dominant inheritance pattern (41).

Pathophysiology
The disorder is explicable by compression of the second cervical root in the atlantoaxial space on sharp rotation of the neck; afferent fibers stemming from the lingual nerve and traveling via the hypoglossal nerve to the second cervical root give a pertinent anatomical explanation for compression of that root inducing numbness of half the tongue (38).

Treatment
Treatment may be via immobilization by a soft collar. In some cases, atlantoaxial fusion or resection of the C2 spinal nerves has been performed (42–45).

TOLOSA–HUNT SYNDROME

The Disorder
Patients with Tolosa–Hunt syndrome (THS), an uncommon disorder, may present with typically severe retro-orbital or periorbital pain which begins acutely. It can be described as constant and "boring." It is associated, typically

after the pain begins, and although it may be the first issue- with diplopia associated with opthalmoparesis. Visual loss may occur if inflammation extends to and affects the optic nerve. If the first division of the trigeminal nerve is involved, the patient may also experience paresthesias along the forehead. The problem is most commonly unilateral (46).

The THS is an idiopathic disorder of exclusion.

Diagnosis

Painful ophthalmoplegia may be secondary to a variety of problems, including superior orbital fissure syndrome, orbital apex syndrome, cavernous sinus syndrome, parasellar syndrome, and the THS. It is unilateral, with an associated paralysis of one or more cranial nerves: III, IV, or VI. There is an associated parasympathoplegia or sympathoplegia of the eye. There may also be supra- and retro-orbital pain indicating participation of the V cranial nerve (47).

Differential diagnosis includes other causes of painful ophthalmoplegia, including migraine, aneurysms, collagen vascular disease, specific infections, mucoceles, tumors, and benign granulomas of unknown etiology (48).

Pathophysiology

Most commonly, the painful ophthalmoplegia of THS is secondary to an idiopathic granulomatous inflammation of the cavernous sinus/superior orbital fissure (49). Unspecific granulomatous tissue has also been found around the intracavernous aspects of the carotid artery as well as the dura mater in the region of the cavernous sinus (47).

Cohn et al. found among three subjects with THS no abnormalities on CAT scan in two cases, and right optic nerve enlargement and an abnormal area round the orbital apex in the third case. MRI showed an abnormal soft tissue area in the cavernous sinus which diminished postcorticosteroid therapy (50). Another study investigated MRI features of 11 patients with THS. Nine had abnormal signal and/or mass lesions in the cavernous sinuses, two did not. In six of nine cases, the affected cavernous sinus was enlarged. One patient had a thrombosed cavernous sinus and superior ophthalmic vein in addition to a cavernous soft-tissue mass (51).

Carotid arteriography may show stationary waves of the carotid artery, with narrowing of its intracavernous section (47). One report showed four patients with THS secondary to a parasellar tumor. All four were responsive to steroids and had normal radiologic and medical investigations (52).

The question of THS *versus* recurrent cranial neuropathy was noted in a report of two cases detailing patients with 12-year histories of episodes of painful ophthalmoplegia consistent with THS which alternated with palsies of cranial nerves other than the fifth and seventh bilaterally (53).

THS has also been reported in association with a peripheral facial paralysis (54), as well as Horner's syndrome (1). As the diagnosis of THS is one of exclusion, lab and CSF testing may be useful to rule out other primary diagnoses.

Treatment

Corticosteroids are the treatment of choice: a 10-day course of prednisone may be satisfactory. However, if no response is seen after 72 hours, the diagnosis must be re-evaluated (1,47,51). If the patient cannot tolerate steroids, other immuno-suppressants may be used, including chlorambucil (0.1–0.2 mg/kg daily) or methotrexate (7.5–15 mg/week). These treatments are empiric (55). The disorder (THS) should always be part of a differential diagnosis (56–59).

RAMSEY–HUNT SYNDROME

The Disorder
Patients with Ramsey–Hunt syndrome (RHS) have otalgia, which on examina-tion, is associated with herpes zoster vesicles on/in the external ear (herpes zoster oticus) as well as on the exterior of the neck. Complications including hearing loss and vertigo are not uncommon (60). Diplopia from skew deviation secondary to RHS has been seen (61).

A case of RHS with multiple cranial nerve paralysis and acute respiratory failure has also been documented (62).

Necrotizing arteritis has been seen in a woman who died, after suffer-ing from herpes zoster oticus, 7th and 10th nerve paralysis, vertigo and hear-ing loss. Postmortem showed significant inflammation on the pons and medulla oblongata and necrotizing arteritis in the cerebello-pontine angle, with associ-ated damage to the adjacent facial nerve (63).

Diagnosis
The diagnosis is made from both history, and visualization of the internal and external ear canals. Vesicles from the herpes zoster are evident there, as well as, possibly, on the anterior tongue and soft palate (1).

Pathophysiology
Irritation by the zoster infection may be associated with geniculate neuralgia, which may be seen in association with the RHS: this consists of irritation of facial nerve sensory fibers, which can correspond to the pain sensation within the auricle. The pain can be paroxysmal and centered directly in the ear. It can have a gradual onset and be dull and persistent, or it can be sharp and stabbing (64). Sphenopalatine and vidian neuralgias (some feel this is the same as cluster headache) can induce similar pain via crossing fibers of the greater superficial petrosal nerves and facial nerves. Glossopharyngeal neuralgia can induce otal-gia by simulating excitation of the Jacobson nerve.

Treatment
Treatment, typically conservative at first, consists of medications: antivirals (acy-clovir), and if the attack is severe, the addition of corticosteroids. An anticon-vulsant such as carbamazepine (200 mg bid–tid) may be used. Analgesics, even narcotics, may not be effective.

If there is no relief over time, a surgical option may be needed. The nervus intermedius and geniculate ganglion may be excised (64). Computer-guided per-cutaneous trigeminal tractotomy-nucleotomy or nucleus caudalis dorsal root entry zone operation may be used (65).

RAEDER'S (PARATRIGEMINAL) NEURALGIA

The Disorder

Raeder's syndrome consists of severe unilateral frontal headache with an ipsilateral full or partial Horner's syndrome (ptosis, miosis, and with/without anhidrosis). >It usually affects men in the fifth decade. Raeder first looked at patients with mixed features of trigeminal nerve pathology and oculosympathetic impairment, with or without other affected cranial nerves (66). This constellation of symptoms first drew Raeder's attention to the area that may induce, secondary to a lesion in the middle cranial fossa, trigeminal nerve involvement, neuralgic pain or sensory change, and ptosis, miosis or both, but no anhidrosis. That is, by definition, any painful postganglionic Horner's syndrome (67).

Not all subjects have the same lack of sweating diathesis as sweating may be preserved, which is distinct from Horner's syndrome, since some third-order sympathetic fibers may be spared.

Diagnosis

The diagnosis is historical. Men are affected fairly exclusively with the onset in middle to old age. Blood work may be done to rule out underlying pathology such as inflammatory and infectious etiologies. MRI and/or CAT scans are called for in patients with the typical Raeder's syndrome to rule out any other occult cause such as tumor or arterial dissection. Indeed, Raeder's syndrome has been noted to be the presenting symptom of internal carotid artery dissection (68,69).

Pathophysiology

Patients with this syndrome have been divided into three groups: first, those with the painful postganglionic Horner's syndrome (the unilateral headache in association with interruption of postganglionic oculosympathetic fibers which run along the course of the internal carotid artery) that can be associated with multiple parasellar cranial nerve involvement which necessitates a full workup of the middle cranial fossa. The second and third groups do not have multiple cranial nerve damage and have benign prognoses (67).

Benign Raeder's syndrome has been called a manifestation of carotid artery disease (70), while tumor in the middle cranial fossa has also been seen (71). >Raeder's syndrome with postganglionic Horner's syndrome has also been associated with Lyme's disease (72). Finally, there is a report of a patient with cluster headache who progressed to Raeder's syndrome, with a marked response to corticosteroid therapy (73).

The attendant paratrigeminal oculosympathic syndrome (POSS) should remind clinicians to carefully investigate the middle cranial fossa. Goadsby also notes that it raises the question of keeping the eponym for this syndrome or calling it what it is, via the anatomical description, POSS (66).

Treatment

Steroids, oral or IV, may be used if there is no proven parasellar pathology.

For pain management, gabapentin, pregabalin, carbamazepine, other anticonvulsants, or baclofen may be effective (74). Anti-inflammatory agents can also be effective, and at times, narcotic analgesics may be necessary. The efficacy of tricyclic antidepressants has been demonstrated in controlled trials for idiopathic facial pain and appears to be independent of the antidepressant effect. Steroids, as noted, may also be effective in some patients.

NASOCILIARY NEURALGIA

The Disorder
This neuralgia (also called Charlin's neuralgia) is rare. It is seen when one touches the outer aspect of one nostril and receives stabbing/lancinating, electrical-like pain radiating to the medial frontal region.

It is seen most commonly in middle-aged women.

Diagnosis
The pain lasts seconds to hours only on one side of the nose. It can radiate upward to the medial frontal region. It can be started by touching the lateral aspect of the ipsilateral nostril (25). The disorder appears similar to ethmoid sinusitis and frontal sinusitis, but there is no rhinorrhea (75).

Pathophysiology
The pain in this disorder is in the territory of the nasociliary nerve and the ciliary ganglion. The etiology appears to be idiopathic (76).

Treatment
Carbamazepine may be tried. Otherwise, a block or section of the nasociliary nerve may be performed. In the past, cocaine was applied to the nostril on the ipsilateral side (25).

NERVOUS INTERMEDIUS NEURALGIA

The Disorder
Nervous intermedius neuralgia is a rare disorder in which paroxysmal pain is felt deep in the auditory canal. It may also be of gradual onset of a dull persistent nature with occasional sharp, stabbing pain (77). It has also been called geniculate neuralgia or "tic douloureux of the nervus intermedius."

Diagnosis
The pain is intermittent, lasts for seconds to minutes and is deep in the ear (otalgia). There is a trigger area in the posterior wall of the auditory canal. This disorder, NIN (geniculate ganglion), may induce the pain deep in the ear and not have any signs of atypical trigeminal neuralgia nor deep face or throat pain (78).

Disorders of salivation, lacrimation, and/or taste may accompany the pain. There may be an association with herpes zoster. In some patients, because of the sparse innervation of the region of the nervus intermedius, there may be an otalgic variant of glossopharyngeal neuralgia (25).

Pathophysiology
The pain of NIN affects a sensory branch of the facial nerve. Temporomandibular joint pathology must be ruled out (79). Afferent sensory nerve fibers pass not

only through the nervus intermedius, but also through the main motor trunk of the facial nerve.

Treatment
Conservative treatment with carbamazepine or other ACMs may be tried initially. If the patient fails pharmacological treatment, then surgical considerations must be entertained.

Excision of the nervus intermedius and/or of the geniculate ganglion using a middle cranial fossa approach has been reported (77). Surgery on the middle turbinate and nasal septum has also been found to be effective, and, unlike the first surgery noted, avoid the possible complication of dysosmia (75).

SUPERIOR LARYNGEAL NEURALGIA

The Disorder
The pain of this rare neuralgic disorder is characterized by severe antalgia in the lateral aspect of the throat, submandibular region, and under the ear. It is precipitated by shouting, swallowing, or turning the head (25).

Diagnosis
The pain is paroxysmal and lasts for seconds to minutes in the throat, submandibular area and/or under the ear. The pain is triggered by swallowing, straining the voice, or turning the head. There is a trigger point present on the lateral aspect of the throat overlying the hypothyroid membrane (25). It is not attributed to another disorder, structural or otherwise.

Pathophysiology
It has been suggested that the superior laryngeal nerve is affected by specific characteristics of the neuralgia: pain along the anterior cervical triangle; hoarseness; and paralysis of the ipsilateral cricothyroid muscle on laryngoscopy (80). There is a reported case of the neuralgia being secondary to a deviated hyoid bone (81).

Treatment
The typical conservative treatment is with carbamazepine (82,83). Blockade of the superior laryngeal nerve with high doses of lidocaine in patients who were resistant to carbamazepine has also been successful (82).

SUPRAORBITAL AND INFRAORBITAL NEURALGIA

The Disorder
These neuralgias are characterized by pain in the region of the supra- or infra-orbital notch and medical aspect of the forehead in the region supplied by the supraorbital nerve, or the region lateral to the nose and up to and on occasion including the lower eyelid in the region of the infra-orbital nerve.

Supraorbital neuralgia has also been called the "swimmer's headache," secondary to its relationship to wearing goggles that impact on the supraorbital foramen (84).

Diagnosis

The pain is paroxysmal or constant in the areas of the supraorbital or infraorbital nerves. There is tenderness over the nerve in either supra- or infraorbital notch. The disorder may be associated with chronic sinusitis. The headache in sinusitis patients may be caused or aggravated by supraorbital neuralgia. In other words, this may be coincidental or both entities coexist (85).

Pathophysiology

Most typically, the nerves may be injured via posttraumatic entrapment at the foramen (86). The supraorbital nerve is part of the first division of the trigeminal nerve, while the infraorbital nerve is part of the second division of the trigeminal nerve. Both nerves can be injured years before the pain manifests, by trauma to the face. The headache may not present initially until the scar cicatrix tightens around the nerve at the foramen and entrapment ensues.

In both neuralgias, headaches may be triggered by bright lights that cause squinting. Supraorbital neuralgia can be mistaken for frontal sinusitis as well as cluster headache. The infraorbital neuralgia can present as menstrual headaches or migraine.

Treatment

Treatment, along with diagnosis, can be achieved by injecting small amounts of local anesthetic, with or without steroid, into the region of the supra- or infra-orbital foramen. There is typically little or no help with carbamazepine and/or indomethacin. Cryoablation can be used (freezing the nerve at the supra- or infra-orbital notch). Decompressive surgery is also an excellent alternative (86,87).

OCCIPITAL NEURALGIA

The Disorder

Occipital neuralgia is a paroxysmal jabbing pain in the distribution of the greater or lesser occipital nerves or of the third occipital nerve. It may be accompanied by decreased sensation or dysesthesias in the affected areas. It may also be associated with tenderness over the nerve causing the difficulty.

Diagnosis

The headache secondary to occipital neuralgia is characterized by piercing, throbbing, or electric-shock-like chronic pain in the upper neck, back of the head, and behind the ears, usually on one side of the head. Frequently, the pain of occipital neuralgia begins in the neck and then spreads upward. A patient can also experience pain in the scalp, forehead, and behind their eyes. Their scalp may also be tender to the touch, and their eyes especially sensitive to light. The location of pain is related to the areas supplied by the greater and lesser occipital nerves, which run from the area where the spinal column meets the neck, up to the scalp at the back of the head.

In one prospective study in an emergency department, lasting a year, the patients had unilateral aching pain of the head, associated with pain in the distribution of the occipital nerve, Tinel's sign, and relief of pain after local injection of anesthetic. Associated clinical features included tinnitus in 33%; scalp paresthesias in 33%, nausea in 42%, dizziness in 50%, and visual disturbances in 67% of patients (88). ON may also present as orofacial pain (89).

Pathophysiology
Most commonly, the pain of ON is idiopathic in nature.

The pain may be caused by irritation or injury to the occipital nerves, which can be secondary to trauma to the neck or back of the head; pinching of the nerves by overly tight neck muscles; compression of the nerve as it leaves the spine due to osteoarthritis, or tumors or other types of lesions in the neck. Localized inflammation or infection, gout, diabetes, blood vessel inflammation (vasculitis), and frequent lengthy periods of keeping the head in a downward and forward position are also associated with occipital neuralgia. Finally, physical and emotional tension can be contributing factors to the condition.

Parts of the differential diagnosis to rule out, prior to making a final diagnosis, include occipital pain referred from the atlantoaxial or upper zygapophyseal joints for from active trigger points in neck muscles (25).

Treatment
Conservative medication treatment may include anti-inflammatories, antidepressants, anticonvulsants, or antispasmodics. Drug treatment, when useful, frequently loses its effectiveness within months. The most common diagnostic and treatment procedure for ON is greater occipital nerve blocks performed with local anesthetic (90).

As ON is well localized, it is possible to consider various surgical treatments including ablation, decompression and electro-modulation of the C2 nerve (91). The C2 dorsal root ganglionectomy has also been used successfully (91). Patients who do not tolerate conservative treatments as well as occipital nerve blocks or other invasive procedures may, if the nerves have not been ablated, be candidates for occipital nerve stimulation. Electrical stimulation of the occipital nerve engenders both peripheral and central nervous system effects that modulate nociception (92). It has also been noted that response to occipital nerve block is not, in and of itself, a good predictor of success or failure of occipital nerve stimulation (93).

Evidence-Based Medicine
Because of the rarity of the majority of facial neuralgias, there has been a paucity of published evidence-based medicine information. One evidence-based medicine study evaluated the strength of evidence that occipital nerve stimulation was an effective treatment for benign headache. The authors located only 10 observational studies, of which 4 were prospective, and a number of case series, case reports, and reviews. No RCTs were found. The conclusion was that the use of occipital nerve stimulators was Level IV, or limited, in nature (94).

Burning tongue and mouth may be related to hormonal status, chronic depression, denture irritation, or vitamin B deficiency (see chap. 8). Atypical odontalgia or neurovascular odontalgia may be possible variants of cluster headache. A painful toothache with no local pathological process in or around the tooth or gums may be secondary to referred pain from myofascial trigger points (1,2).

REFERENCES

1. Jay GW. Headache Handbook. Boca Raton, FL: CRC Press, 1999:171–172.
2. Jay GW. Chronic Pain. New York: Informa Healthcare, 2007:193–222.
3. Watson CPN, Deck JH, Morshead C, et al. Postherpetic neuralgia: further post-mortem studies of cases with and without pain. Pain 1991; 44:105–117.
4. Mathew NT, Chandy J. Painful opthalmoplegia. J Neurol Sci 1970; 11:243–256.
5. Portenoy RK, Duma C, Foley KM. Acute herpetic and postherpetic neuralgia: clinical review and current management. Ann Neurol 1986; 20:651–664.
6. Hatangdi VS, Boas RA, Richards EG. Postherpetic neuralgia: management with antiepileptic and tricyclic drugs. In: Bonica JJ, Albe-Fessard D, eds. Advances in Pain Research and Therapy. Vol. 1. New York: Raven Press, 1976:583–587.
7. Minager A, Sheremata WA. Glossopharyngeal neuralgia and MS. Neurology 2000; 54(6):1368–1370.
8. Korkes H, de Oliveira EM, Brollo L, et al. Cardiac syncope induced by glossopharyngeal "neuralgia": a rare presentation. Arq Bras Cardiol 2006; 87(5):e189–e191.
9. Esaki T, Osada H, Nakao Y, et al. Surgical management for glossopharyngeal neuralgia associated with cardiac syncope: two case reports. Br J Neurosurg 2007; 21(6): 599–602.
10. Gaul C, Hastreiter P, Duncker A, et al. Improvement of diagnosis and treatment of glossopharyngeal neuralgia. Schmerz 2008; 22(Suppl 1):41–46.
11. Han J, Han N, Faz Z. The pathogeny and treatment of glossopharyngeal neuralgia. Lin Chuang Er Bi Yan Hou Ke Za Zhi 2002; 16(6):259–260.
12. McCarron MO, Bone I. Glossopharyngeal neuralgia referred from a pontine lesion. Cephalagia 1999; 19(2):115–117.
13. Webb CJ, Makura ZG, McCormick MS. Glossopharyngeal neuralgia following foreign body impaction in the neck. J Laryngol Otol 2000; 114(1):70–72.
14. Rushton JG, Stevens C, Miller RH. Glossopharyngeal (vagoglossopharyngeal) neuralgia. Arch Neurol 1981; 38:201–205.
15. Garcia Callejo FJ, Marco Algarra J, Talamantes Esceriba F, et al. Use of gabapentin in glossopharyngeal neuralgia. Acta Otorrinolaringol Esp 1999; 50(2):175–177.
16. Kitchener JM, Guido M, Specchio LM. Glossopharyngeal neuralgia responding to pregabalin. Headache 2006; 46(8):1307–1308.
17. Raskin NH, Prusiner S. Carotidynia. Neurology 1977; 27:43–46.
18. Vijayan N, Watson C. Raeder's syndrome, pericarotid syndrome and carotidynia. In: Vinken PJ, Bruyn GW, eds. Handbook of Clinical Neurology. Vol. 4(48). Headache. Amsterdam: Elsevier Publishing Co., 1986:329–341.
19. Roseman DM. Carotidynia. N Y State J Med 1963; 63:2651–2653.
20. Lovshin LL. Vascular neck pain—a common syndrome seldom recognized. Cleve Clin A 1960; 27:5–13.
21. Roseman DM. Carotidynia: a distinct syndrome. Arch Otolaryngol 1967; 85:81–84.
22. Pearce HE, Hinshaw JR. Bilateral arteritis simulating carotid body tumors. Surg Gynecol Obstet 1956; 103:263–266.
23. Hilger JA. Carotid pain. Laryngoscope 1949; 59:829–838.
24. Headache Classification Committee of the IHS. Classification and diagnostic criteria for headache disorders, cranial neuralgias and facial pain. Cephalalgia 1988; 8:1–96.
25. Headache Classification Subcommittee of the International Headache Society. The international classification of headache disorders, 2nd ed. Cephalalgia 2004; 24(Suppl 1):1–151.
26. Burton BS, Syms MJ, Petermann GW, et al. MR imaging of patients with carotidynia. AJNR Am J Neuroradiol 2000; 21(4):766–769.
27. Arning CH. Ultrasonographic imaging of carotidynia: syndrome or entity. Nervennartzt 2004; 75(12):1200–1203.
28. Maruyama Y, Endo K, Tsukatani T, et al. CT and ultrasonographic findings in patients with carotidynia. Nippon Jibiinkoka Gakkai Kaiho 2005; 108(2):168–171.
29. Kuhn J, Harzheim A, Horz R, et al. MRI and ultrasonographic imaging of a patient with carotidynia. Cephalalgia 2006; 26(4):483–485.

30. Kosaka N, Sagoh T, Uematsu H, et al. Imaging by multiple modalities of patients with carotidynia syndrome. Eur Radiol 2007; 17(9):2430–2433.
31. Tardy J, Pariente J, Nasr N, et al. Carotidynia: a new case for an old controversy. Eur J Neurol 2007; 14(6):704–705.
32. Farage L, da Motta AC, Goldenberg D, et al. Idiopathic inflammatory pseudotumor of the carotid sheath. Arq Neuropsiquiatr 2007; 65(4B):1241–1244.
33. Clark HV, Kind DE, Yow RN. Carotidynia. Am Fam Physician 1994; 50(5):987–990.
34. Cannon CR. Carotidynia: an unusual pain in the neck. Otolaryngol Head Neck Surg 1994; 110(4):387–390.
35. Chambers BR, Donnan GA, Riddell RJ, et al. Carotidynia: aetiology, diagnosis and treatment. Clin Exp Neurol 1981; 17:113–123.
36. White JR, Bell WL. Dysphonia associated with carotidynia and migraine responding to dihydroergotamine. Headache 2003; 43(1):69–71.
37. Valle N, Gonzalez-Mandly A, Aterino A, et al. A case of carotidynia with response to almotriptan. Cephalalgia 2003; 23(2):155–156.
38. Lance JW, Anthony M. Neck–tongue syndrome on sudden turning of the head. J Neurol Neurosurg Psychiatry 1980; 43:97–101.
39. Sjaastad O, Bakketeig LS. Neck–tongue syndrome and related (?) conditions. Cephalalgia 2006; 26(3):233–240.
40. Borody C. Neck tong syndrome. J Manipulatibe Physiol Ther 2004; 27(5):E8.
41. Lewis DW, Frank LM, Toor S. Familial neck–tongue syndrome. Headache 2003; 43(2):132–134.
42. Bogduk N. An anatomical basis for neck–tongue syndrome. J Neurol Neurosurg Psychiatry 1981; 44:202–208.
43. Bertoft ES, Westerberg CE. Further observations on the neck–tongue syndrome. Cephalalgia 1985; 5(Suppl 3):312–313.
44. Fortin CJ, Biller J. Neck–tongue syndrome. Headache 1985; 25:255–258.
45. Elisevich K, Stratford J, Bray G, et al. Neck–tongue syndrome: operative management. J Neurol Neurosurg Psychiatry 1984; 47:407–409.
46. Taylor DC, Mankowski K. Tolusa–Hunt syndrome. http://www.emedicine.com/neuro/TOPIC373.HTM.
47. Cohn DF, Carasso R, Streifler M. Painful opthalmoplegia: the Tolosa–Hunt syndrome. Eur Neurol 1979; 18(6): 373–381.
48. Hunt WE. Tolosa–Hunt syndrome: one cause of painful opthalmoplegia. J Neurosurg 1976; 44L544–44L549.
49. Kline LKB. The Tolosa–Hunt syndrome. Surv Othalmol 1982; 27(2):79–95.
50. Goto Y, Hosokawa S, Goto I, et al. Abnormality in the cavernous sinus in three patients with Tolosa–Hunt syndrome: MR and CT findings. J Neurol Neurosurg Psychiatry 1990; 53(3):231–234.
51. Yousem DM, Atlas SW, Grossman RI, et al. AJR Am J Roentgenol 1990; 154(1): 167–170.
52. Spector RH, Fiandaca MS. The "sinister" Tolosa–Hunt syndrome. Neurology 1986; 36(2):198–203.
53. Barontini F, Maurri S, Marrapodi E. Tolosa–Hunt syndrome versus recurrent cranial neuropathy. Report of two cases with a prolonged follow-up. J Neurol 1987; 234(2):112–115.
54. Vallat JM, Vallat M, Julien J, et al. Painful ophthalmoplegia (Tolosa–Hunt) accompanied by peripheral facial paralysis. Ann Neurol 1980; 8(6):645.
55. Bakshi R. What is the best immunosuppressant regimen for Tolosa–Hunt syndrome? http://medscape. com/viewarticle/413768.
56. Mathew NT, Chandy J. Painful opthalmoplegia. J Neurol Sci 1970; 11:243–256.
57. Hunt WE, Meagher JN, Lefever HE, et al. Painful ophthalmoplegia: its relation to indolent inflammation of the cavernous sinus. Neurology 1961; 11:56–62.
58. Takeoka T, Gotoh F, Fukuchi V, et al. Tolosa–Hunt syndrome: arteriographic evidence of improvement in carotid narrowing. Arch Neurol 1978; 35:219–223.
59. Hannerz J. Recurrent Tolosa–Hunt syndrome. Cephalalgia 1992; 12:45–51.

60. Hyden D, Roberg M. Diagnosis of Ramsey Hunt syndrome is both simple and diffi-cult. The viral attack is more extensive than expected earlier. Lakaertidningen 2000; 97(10):1114–1120.
61. Verhulst E, Van Lammeren M, Dralands L. Diplopia from skew deviation in Ramsey–Hunt syndrome. A case report. Bull Soc Belge Ophtalmol 2000; 278:27–32.
62. Sato K, Nakamura S, Koseki T, et al. A case of Ramsey–Hunt syndrome with multiple cranial nerve paralysis and acute respiratory failure. Nihon Kyobu Shikkan Gakkai Zasshi 1991; 29(8):1037–1041.
63. Pilz P. Herpes zoster oticus—neuropathologic contribution to the genesis of concomi-tant facial paralysis (author's transl). Wein Klin Wochenschr 1981; 93(24):753–755.
64. Pulec JL. Geniculate neuralgia: long-term results of surgical treatment. Ear Nose Throat J 2002; 81(1):30–33.
65. Kanpolat Y, Savas A, Batay F, et al. Computed tomography- guided trigeminal tractotomy–nucleotomy in the management of vagoglossopharyngeal and geniculate neuralgias. Neurosurgery 1998; 43(3):484–489.
66. Goadsby PJ. Raeder's syndrome [corrected]: paratrigeminal paralysis of the oculop-upillary sympathetic system. J Neurol Neurosurg Psychiatry 2002; 72(3):297–299.
67. Grimson BS, Thompson HS. Raeder's syndrome. A clinical review. Surv Ophthalmol 1980; 24(4): 99–210.
68. Dihne M, Block F, Thron A, et al. Raeder's syndrome: a rare presentation of internal carotid artery dissection. Cerebrovasc Dis 2000; 10(2):159–160.
69. Schmidt F, Dihne M, Steinbach J, et al. Raeder and Collet-Siccard-Syndrome. Acute pareses of cranial nerves symptomatic of a dissection of internal carotid artery. Ner-venarzt 2000; 71(6):502–505.
70. Solomon S, Lustig JP. Benign Raeder's syndrome is probably a manifestation of carotid artery disease. Cephalalgia 2001; 21(1):1–11.
71. Salvesen R. Raeder's syndrome. Cephalalgia 1999; 19(Suppl 25):42–45.
72. Murphy MA, Szabados EM, Mitty JA. Lyme disease associated with postganglionic Horner syndrome and Raeder paratrigeminal neuralgia. J Neuroophthalmol 2007; 27(2):123–124.
73. Ikeuchi T, Tokutake T, Sakamaki Y, et al. Progressuin if cluster headache to Raeder's syndrome with marked response to corticosteroid therapy: a case report. Rinsho Shinkeigaku 2005; 45(4):321–323.
74. Schechter SH. Raeder paratrigeminal syndrome. http://www.emedicine.com/neuro/topic331.htm on July 13, 2008.
75. He C, Dai X, Jian J, et al. Analysis of clinical manifestations in nasociliary neuralgia. Lin Chuang Er Bi Yah HYou Ke Za Zhi. 2004; 18(11):653–654.
76. Strupler W. Styloid syndrome; Sluder's syndorme; Charlin's syndrome. SSO Schweiz Monatsschr Zahnheilkd 1979; 89(2):106–111.
77. Pulec JL. Geniculate neuralgia: diagnosis and surgical management. Laryngoscope 1976; 86(7):955–964.
78. Lovely TJ, Jannetta PJ. Surgical Mangement of geniculate neuralgia. Am J Otol 1997; 18(4):512–517.
79. Figueiredo R, Vazquez-Delgado E, Okeson JP, et al. Nervus intermedius neuralgia: a case report. Cranio 2007; 25(3):213–217.
80. O'Neill BP, Aronson AE, Pearson BW, et al. Superior laryngeal neuralgia: carotidynia or just another pain in the neck. Headache 1982; 22(1):6–9.
81. Kodama S, Oribe K, Suzuki M. Superior laryngeal neuralgia associated with deviation of the hyoid bone. Auris Nasus Larynx 2008; 35(3):429–431.
82. Takahashi Sato K, Suzuki M, Izuha A, et al. Two cases of idiopathic laryngeal neural-gia treated by superior laryngeal nerve block with a high concentration of lidocain. J Clin Anesth 2007; 19(3):237–238.
83. Schmidt D, Strutz I. Superior laryngeal neuralgia. J Neuralgia 1981; 225(3): 223–225.
84. O'Brien JC. Swimmer's headache, or supraorbital neuralgia. Proc Bayl Univ Med Cent 2004; 17(4):416–419.

85. Talmi YP, Finkelstein Y, Wolf M, et al. Coincidental supraorbital neuralgia and sinusitis. Am J Rhinol 1999; 13(6):463–468.
86. Adant JP, Bluth F. Endoscopic supraorbital neurolysis. Acta Chir Belg 1999; 99(4): 182–184.
87. Sjaastad O, Sotlt-Mielsen A, Pareja JA, et al. Supraorbital neuralgia. On the clinical manifestations and a possible therapeutic approach. Headache 2002; 39(3):204–212.
88. Kuhn WF, Kuhn SC, Gilberstadt H. Occipital neuralgias: clinical recognition of a complicated headache. A case series and literature review. J Orofac Pain 1997; 11(2): 158–165.
89. Sulfara MA, Gobetti JP. Occipital neuralgia. Oral Surg Oral Med Oral Pathol Oral Radiol Endod 1995; 80(6):751–755.
90. Ward JB. Greater occipital nerve block. Semin Neurol 2003; 23(1):59–62.
91. Wang MY, Levi AD. Ganglionectomy of C-2 for the treatment of medically refractory occipital neuralgia. Neurosurg Focus 2002; 12(1):E14.
92. Schwedt TJ. Occipital nerve stimulation for medically intractable headache. Curr Pain Headache Rep 2008; 12(1):62–66.
93. Schwedt TJ, Dodick DW, Trentman TL, et al. Response to occipital nerve block is not useful in predicting efficacy of occipital nerve stimulation. Cephalalgia 2007; 27(3):271–274.
94. Jasper JF, Hayek SM. Implanted occipital nerve stimulators. Pain Physician 2008; 11(2):187–200.

10 Psychological Aspects of Chronic Noncancer Pain

Gary W. Jay

Clinical Disease Area Expert-Pain, Pfizer, Inc., New London, Connecticut, U.S.A.

Richard H. Cox

Private Practice, Chapel Hill; Duke University Medical Center, Durham, North Carolina; Georgetown University Medical Center, Washington DC, U.S.A.

"Pain, the barking watchdog of our health, is normally temporary. It immobilizes the damaged muscle, tendon, or ligament so that healing can occur. This acute or subacute pain usually passes quickly and is completely forgotten after it has" (1).

There are psychological aspects of all forms of pain, particularly when the pain becomes chronic. The neurochemical changes associated with chronic myofascial pain have been adequately discussed elsewhere. However, to further clarify, the changes in the serotonergic tonus, for example, do appear to play a role in depression, as well as other affective changes found in the chronic pain patient. This may help explain why the chronic pain patient may have at least a subclinical depression, many have a more profound depression, and why serotonergic medications are often helpful.

On the other hand, pain has *meaning* to some patients. For some, this *meaning* is temporary and for others it takes on an existential nature. For some, it is interpreted in the light of present and past culture, religious thought, and even legal considerations. Pain becomes a constant companion in some chronic pain patients. It directs and runs, and sometimes ruins, their lives. It takes on a life of its own, irrespective of its etiology. It can be an acceptable reason for a patient *not* to do things. It is also a potential "reason" for doing the unusual, gaining extra attention, obtaining special favors and exceptions from normally executed daily activities. It is a socially acceptable reason for obtaining prescription, nonprescription medications, and opiates. It can be many things. It can, and most often does, make life-altering changes in virtually every facet of human existence.

Part of the job of a pain management specialist is to determine exactly what it *means* to a *specific* patient. This is not an easy task since frequently, in fact, usually, the patient does not know either. A careful review of family dynamics, patient history, work history, religious beliefs, and even psychological personality testing is required to help determine the nature and value of the hidden meaning. Once the meaning is determined, and validated by the patient and/or patient's family, the task of introducing it to the patient in healing terms is critical. That which is hidden to our consciousness is usually either considered not important or as too threatening to allow into conscious thought. In either case, careful therapeutic intervention is required. Later it will be seen that cognitive behavioral therapy offers the best and most time-efficient approach for dealing with personality and behavioral factors in the chronic pain patient.

Chronic pain can mean so much to a patient that the pain specialist, if he or she does not understand exactly what it entails, may do a significant disservice to a patient by quickly eradicating his or her pain. Pain specialists, like others in the human helping professions, tend to measure their own personal success against rapid positive results. Early gained "positive results" in pain management may, in the long run, be less than positive. The elimination of pain, i.e., a positive result may only produce an emotional or even physical invalid for life, or worse, i.e., "the patient was relieved of back pain and died of a malignancy"! This is a particular concern when nonmedically trained personnel are involved, i.e., psychologists, social workers, and others who may not have adequate grounding in medical conditions that camouflage as emotional disorders and vice versa. This chapter is specifically meant to refer to chronic noncancer pain secondary to chronic soft tissue pain, but it can certainly be generalized.

The *specificity theory* of pain still prevails in today's medical education. This theory suggests that pain is a *specific* sensation and that its intensity is initially proportional to the degree of peripheral tissue damage. This concept has been gradually modified in that the perception of pain, in addition to the degree of peripheral tissue damage, is influenced by attention, anxiety, suggestion, prior conditioning, learning, and other variables (2). This change in thinking in no way demeans the newer neurophysiologic, neurohormonal, pharmacologic, and mechanical aspects of soft tissue injury, but does significantly influence the approaches to pain management.

Pain is not considered merely sensory because it has motivational affective consequences (3). Behavioral and physiologic studies (4) have proposed the following sequence in appreciating pain:

1. A precise evolution of neurophysiologic aspects of the mechanism of pain.
2. Activation of the reticular and limbic systems through ascending neuropathways that involve emotional aspects of neurophysiology by studying these neurological sites which are anatomically linked.
3. Involvement of higher centers implicating powerful motivational drives such as suggestion, learned responses, anxiety, and fears that exert control over physiologic activities.

Acute pain is usually responsive to a specific treatment approach, but chronic pain is a totally different matter. The presence of pain with no discernible *organic* etiology presents a dichotomy. The "benign" aspect of pain (while there is nothing benign about chronic noncancer pain) is a term that denotes the enigma of disabling pain proceeding from a relatively innocuous etiology. Individual treatments often fail to diminish such pain and may even enhance it. Disruptions of the nerve tracts that are recognized as mediators of pain may not relieve pain. Patients who fail to respond to a *specific* treatment may become depressed, resentful, and suffer further from being dismissed as *malingerers,* or *neurotics,* rather than being fully diagnosed. Further, chronic pain sufferers who do not respond in the expected fashion frequently become the victims of polypharmacy. They also become "doctor-shoppers" and unproven alternative treatment seekers, thus often rendering themselves even more confused and sometimes suffering with additional iatrogenic disorders.

A major reason for this kind of failure is often due to the type of treatment that is utilized. Treating the chronic noncancer pain patient without utilizing an inter/transdisciplinary approach that deals with the psychological aspects of a patient's pain, in addition to simultaneously treating the organic aspects, is typically doomed to failure. This, in turn, increases a patient's emotional and physical discomfort as well as their fears that the "system" is not out to help them. It also makes the physicians frustrated and less likely to be amenable to viewing the patient's problem as one entity with various parts. It is easier to label the patient as having a major psychological problem and ignore the reality of any concurrent physical/organic aspects of their pain.

Responses to placebo therapy have also further categorized patients in this manner (5). Placebo responses were initially discredited, but now that study design flaws have been eliminated, it may be proven to be an effective tool in evaluating and controlling pain. The use of suggestion is one example of this enhancement (6), and it is now recognized that multiple approaches are more effective (7). About one-third of placebo users muster a definite endogenous opiate system response. This is absolutely not to say that patients should receive "placebo" medications, *versus* "real" pain medications while in treatment. Nothing erodes trust in the physician faster than the patient feeling "tricked."

Chronic pain has frequently grown progressively worse when the inferred pathologic cause has been removed. It persists day after day and night after night leading to an endless circle of sleeplessness, depression, "agony," and social isolation. Pain, formerly considered merely a symptom, has now become a distinct disease entity. Scientific attempts to explain chronic pain are incomplete. Although many claims have been advanced regarding the liability of specific personality traits and genetic hereditary factors, none have withstood the test of time and subsequent studies.

One hypothesis (8) is that muscular responses of an injured part persist due to a psychophysiological mechanism. This learned cortical process (memory) responds to stressful events that trigger the latent increased state of muscular tension (9,10). Muscles that undergo prolonged muscular tension are those in the region of the initial tissue injury site.

Moderate levels of muscle tension may induce pain in both healthy subjects and patients with chronic pain (11). In people prone to reactive stress, these muscles fail to relax to baseline levels in a normal time, which causes them to become the site of pain (12,13). This implies a central mechanism, as evidenced in both electrophysiological and imaging studies that have demonstrated (experimentally) that pain activates cortical and other central nervous system (CNS) structures (14,15).

Psychophysiological reactivity is a major contributing and confounding problem in the persistence of chronic soft tissue pain. The term itself indicates that the patient's physiological etiology of pain (muscle spasm in the upper trapezius musculature, for example) may be increased and/or reinforced by psychological aspects such as stress, anxiety, and depression. It has long been postulated, and clinically demonstrated, that there are unique, highly individualized body styles for sequestering tension-induced pain. Some are said to "carry it in the lower back," others to "shoulder it," and various other descriptions of body-part pathology in relation to stress-induced pain. This pathological, yet not at all unusual, presentation of pain may obscure other salient factors in the overall pain syndrome.

A supporting study (16) has shown electromyographically that patients with carpal tunnel syndrome and low back pain initiate co-contraction of the agonist and antagonist muscles simultaneously and that the antagonists fail to reciprocally relax. This may well explain the onset and persistence of low back pain in individuals prone to it. This *proneness*, however, remains unclear in terms of neurophysiologic causes. Psychophysiological aspects play an important role here. The cascade of emotional pain, physical discomfort, social and/or employment dysfunction, familial and domestic issues, memories from previous injuries, and much more, all produce results that do not lend themselves to easy unraveling.

Each individual appears to have (or have had) a breaking point under stress, after which his or her coping mechanisms have failed. Learned maladaptive coping mechanisms have emerged, both consciously and unconsciously. This pathology is often referred to in the psychiatric literature as the "learned helplessness" syndrome. Although it does not always render one "helpless," it always renders one maladaptive, thus at time, allowing treatment to be of no value, which under other conditions would be highly successful.

It is good to remember that early in the history of the subspecialty of pain medicine, a major disagreement between its originators was whether pain was "peripheral" or "central." The peripheralists perceived pain as originating specifically from the site of peripheral injury. When that area healed, the pain was terminated. The centralists felt that pain may have begun in the periphery but was perceived and perseverated centrally. Some of us felt that acute and chronic pain has both peripheral and central components. A strong argument for this connection is frequently seen in the emergency room. Patients with acute pain from (soft tissue) injury can perceive a reduction in their pain from the early use of an anxiolytic, a reminder that the fear and acute anxiety postinjury occurs immediately and simultaneously.

Brena (17) postulated the five consequences of chronic pain in what he termed the Five "D" syndrome:

1. Drug misuse and abuse
2. Dysfunction
3. Dependency
4. Depression
5. Disability

The importance of psychosocial factors as determinants of low back pain and resultant disability has become increasingly prominent in the literature (18). Frymoyer (19) developed a model based on the experience of numerous experts in determining the resulting disability from low back pain. He concluded that the following factors had equal weight: physical requirements and job satisfaction were equal to stress, Minnesota Multiphasic Personality Inventory (MMPI) scores, and psychological symptoms. The Boeing study made the relationship between job satisfaction and recovery after a soft tissue, low back injury equally clear (20).

In those patients with chronic low back problems who do not respond to rehabilitation efforts, there was evidence of depression, anxiety, distress, and pain behaviors (21–25). To rehabilitate work-injured patients, studies discerning pertinent factors needing correction have been produced (26). Physical work load reduction has been accepted, but recent studies emphasize avoidance of sick leaves of long duration, and the early initiation of rehabilitation measures in poorly educated injured people is more effective.

The old technique of "days off" after a simple, uncomplicated, work-related soft tissue injury has been rejected. Keeping injured workers at work in a light duty job has become a much more appropriate treatment strategy. The latter four stages of the Brena "Five D syndrome" are thus avoided, i.e., *dysfunction*—the injured worker continues to function; *dependency* is also avoided by continuing to allow the injured worker to earn his or her wages rather than depend upon workmen's compensation or other nonearned income; *depression* is frequently avoided by continuing a positive cognitive framework and feeling of self-worth; and finally, *disability* is avoided by disallowing atrophy of mind, body, and spirit. There have proven to be no guaranteed methods for preventing Brena's first stage, i.e., drug misuse and abuse.

A qualitative study (27) emphasized the fact that people sustaining a low back injury perceive their back problem as being a lifelong one to which they remain susceptible. This indication highlights the need to indoctrinate and educate the injured person, as early as possible, about the cause, significance, and prognosis of the given musculoskeletal problem using meaningful and easily understood terminology.

PANIC AND ANXIETY DISORDERS

Undoubtedly chronic pain is prevalent in patients who develop acute pain and panic secondary to the threatening symptoms. Anxiety disorders are among the most prevalent forms of psychiatric illness in the United States. They are more prevalent in women and in both genders in lower socioeconomic groups.

Differentiation must be made between significant anxiety and everyday normal episodic anxiety associated with upsetting life experiences ("daily hassles"). A clinically significant anxiety reaction literally interferes with a person's ability to function and thus should be considered an illness.

The biologic basis of anxiety is an abnormality in chemical neurotransmission. Presynaptic neurons normally transmit impulses both electrically and chemically. These neurotransmitters are both fast signal and slow signal. Fast signals are mediated by glutamate ("on") and gamma-amino butyric acid (GABA) ("off"). The slow signals are mediated by monoamines and peptides.

Effective chemical treatment of anxiety disorders, in recent decades, has clarified much of this chemical interplay. The discovery of benzodiazepine receptors and delineation of reciprocal relationships between benzodiazepines and GABA have evolved. Their effect on the locus coeruleus has been postulated.

Besides GABA and norepinephrine, current evidence shows that serotonin, which is significantly involved in pain perception, is also intrinsic to mood disorders and anxiety disorders, as well as in obsessive–compulsive disorders. Anxiety has been considered as a disorder caused by serotonin excess. At least one of the newer antianxiety medications is a specific serotonin (5HT-IB) receptor antagonist. Higher levels of serotonin have also been found in most obsessive–compulsive disorders, whereas aggressive impulsive patients may suffer from lower serotonin levels.

The uses of specific medications which help to obviate psychological problems with the help of psychotherapy are an integral part of an appropriate interdisciplinary treatment approach (28).

PAIN BEHAVIOR

The evaluation of pain behavior to indicate the presence and severity of pain has been the starting point for behavioral psychologists in their management of pain (29). Such patient behaviors have been verbal, nonverbal, related to medications, emotional attitudes and postures, and evidence in facial expressions (30). In an attempt to document behavior objectively, electromechanical devices are being developed to record activity and gait patterns (31).

Pain behaviors are most frequently observed directly and are then recorded. Observations can be modified depending on whether the action is being performed in a natural situation or a regulated one, which may simulate the natural production of pain and may be videotaped for further clinical evaluation (32).

Objectivity is a challenge to the trained observer. Most criteria are considered too simplistic and focus on behavior that denies the presence of pain and questions whether such behavior is an expression of pain or merely a mechanism for coping (33).

In the 1980s, Waddell described five nonorganic signs (34). These five types or categories of signs are tenderness, simulation, distraction, regional disturbances, and overreaction.

Tenderness is not related to a particular skeletal or neuromuscular structure. It is nonspecific and diffuse. Examples include superficial tenderness such as skin tenderness to light pinch over a large area not the specific dermatome associated with pain. Also, there may be a nonanatomic sign of deep tenderness over a wide area not localized to one structure and which often extends to areas other than the lumbar spine.

Simulation tests give the patient the impression that a particular examination is being carried out when it really is not. These tests must be nonpainful. Then, if pain is reported, a nonorganic influence is suggested. These may include axial loading, where a patient is asked to sit straight and a quick downward pressure is applied to the top of the patient's head and the patient then reports low back pain. Another, the rotational test, may be performed by passively rotating the shoulders and pelvis in the same plane in which the patient stands relaxed with his or her feet together and low back pain may be described.

Distraction tests are used after a positive physical finding is demonstrated in a routine manner. This finding is then rechecked while the patient's attention is distracted. The testing should be nonpainful, nonemotional, and nonsurprising. A simple example is to perform the plantar reflex (Babinski) while the patient is in a sitting position. If the patient is able to fully extend the lower extremity, without significant pelvic tilting, and the patient complains of significant pain and a very positive straight leg-raising test when prone, an obvious lack of consistency is noted.

Regional disturbances are indicated by a divergence from neuroanatomically established motor and sensory distributions. First, however, multiple nerve root involvement must be ruled out, as well as a history of multiple spinal surgeries and spinal stenosis. An example would be "give-way" weakness of an extremity that involves multiple muscle groups.

Overreaction to stimulation includes disproportionate verbalization, facial grimacing, muscle tension, and tremor, collapsing, or sweating during a nonpainful examination. This sign mandates that the clinician takes into consideration observations and judgments made over the entire patient contact, including how they were reacting to sitting and answering historical questions.

Waddell noted that the presence of three or more types of nonorganic signs correlated with abnormal psychological profiles and was, therefore, considered "positive."

Other techniques include performing a simple vibratory stimulation test, looking for changes in perception of vibration on similar areas, bilaterally. The examination ends when the tuning fork is placed in the middle of the sternum and the patient is asked if there is a sensory difference on either side. Neurophysiologically, the answer should be no. A positive answer also adds suspicion that the patient may not be fully forthcoming.

It is extremely important to note that patients with positive inorganic signs may also have true organic findings. There are many reasons for this, including the fact that patients in the Workers' Compensation system, or those who have experienced a motor vehicle accident, may have already seen numerous physicians who, they feel, discounted their complaints and did not find any organic pathology at all. This is not uncommon in contested cases where the patient is forced to attend any number of insurance company-mandated Independent Medical Examinations (IMEs) from clinicians being paid by the insurance company.

The patients may develop a somatoform disorder in which their complaints are magnified, at least in part, as a cry for help from a patient who feels helpless and feels that no one is listening or trying to help. They feel that if they can "up the physical ante," someone, sometime, somewhere along their medical odyssey will listen to them and/or find some organic pathology.

Over exaggeration of pain/discomfort may exist because a patient has a real, albeit not necessarily medically serious, injury. For this reason, it is imperative that patients be fully examined for organic pathology, even simple muscle spasm, in spite of overexaggeration of pain or the finding of nonorganic signs.

PSYCHOLOGICAL TESTING IN PATIENTS WITH CHRONIC PAIN

It must be made clear from the start that there is no reliable measurement of pain, psychologically or otherwise. Valiant attempts have been made to correlate the physical dimensions of perceived anatomical distress against resultant personality and or psychologically measured factors, but such has been impossible to date. There are, however, relatively reliable measurable psychological traits that have been shown to have a positive relationship in clinical settings. Also, since pain clearly alters one's thinking, and thought can be reliably measured in terms of specific brain functions, psychological testing is usually valuable in treating the whole person and understanding the larger context of chronic pain. Attention span, memory, thought processes, computational skill, right/left hemispherical function, and many other neuropsychological functions, as well as alterations in personality functioning, can be reliably measured. Psychological testing must not be viewed as a measurement of intelligence for the purposes of dealing with chronic pain. There is no reliable measurement regarding the relationship of pain to IQ. Although persons with varying degrees of intelligence tend to philosophize, rationalize, or otherwise deal with pain intellectually, higher or lower IQs have not shown to be reliable indicators of experiential phenomenon. At best, possessing average or above intelligence may give one the tools for greater understanding, better results from psychotherapy, and a more efficient use of resources for coping with the ramifications and residua of pain. Such ability may also allow one more sophisticated and even devious method of dealing with anticipated financial gains as a result of employment injury.

Pain has traditionally been considered a stimulus-evoked response with the response being equivalent to the stimulus. Relief of pain should, therefore, follow removal of the noxious stimulus. Repeated stimuli over time, however, modify, diminish, or eliminate the relationship of time to stimulus, and the response becomes dependent upon other factors (2).

Through generalized stimuli, sensations similar to the original noxious stimulus acquire the ability to elicit a pain response. These stimuli are then considered to be *conditioned* and *learned*. The pain response loses its correspondence with the original stimulus, which was *unconditioned* and becomes a response to a variety of stimuli (35) not necessarily similar to the original.

There is a large difference between pain and *suffering*. The former is secondary to nociception while the second is an emotional response. Many times, the clinician sees more evidence of suffering than pain in the chronic noncancer pain patient. This can be, in many cases, the only thing noted on an examination. It should be noted, but in the context of the patient as a "whole." There are patients who have pain and relatively little suffering, and there are those who have great suffering and very little pain. Patients rarely differentiate the two, but clinicians must be alert to the often subtle yet profound differences and drastically different results of each.

In many patients, pain may have a specific meaning. That is, there may be a direct, transcendent relationship between a patient's pain and another experience. An example of this may include patients who see their pain as a result of something they have done wrong and feel that the pain is their punishment. Giving up that pain, or punishment, may create an even more untenable situation for the patient than continuing to have the pain. The pain may be, on an unconscious level, a reminder of something exceptionally potent in their consciousness.

The phenomenon of pain can be conceptualized as a *behavior* controlled by the initial unconditioned (pathologic) stimulus and the conditioned stimuli that follow (36). Tissue pathology initiates the noxious stimuli that are transmitted throughout all neural mechanisms, or the entire neuromatrix, following which a given pain behavior evolves.

Unfortunately, physical pain cannot be measured. A patient's verbal pain measurement may be subject to any number of contravening factors. While it is certainly important, if not mandatory, to obtain this patient data, it is best associated or correlated with the patient's level of function, before, during and at the end of treatment. Physical function is typically a much better measure of a patient's physical gain and possible diminution of pain.

It is obvious that the chronic noncancer pain patients have both physical as well as emotional aspects to their pain. While a good neurological or musculoskeletal examination can give a clinician a great deal of information, additional information is needed to treat the entire person. Psychological testing can be used to provide a good part of the remaining, necessary information needed to treat the chronic benign pain patient.

Psychological testing can be used for a number of things. It is a good screening tool for determining the level of psychopathology a patient may have. It can determine specific psychiatric diagnoses. These aspects are mandatory in determining an appropriate, individualized interdisciplinary treatment protocol for a chronic benign pain patient.

Numerous tests for substantiating and quantifying pain have been reported in the literature. Only a few of these tests will be discussed here because most have validity, level of acceptance, and worth as outcome assessments. Any test must be used carefully to diagnose a patient with pain. The initial assumption of the existence of a psychological aspect, not necessarily a basis, which may then be therapeutically pursued, must be validated; treatment, as well as diagnosis, must not be based solely on the outcome of such a test. Patients, not test results, must be treated. Further, regardless of the psychological or scientific validity of a given psychological test, the only truly valid measurement is the *competence of the clinician*. The education, training, experience, and competence of the chosen psychologist cannot be over emphasized. Doctoral-level psychologists with the letters ABPP (Board Certification from the American Board of Professional Psychology) behind their name and degree usually provide the most reliable level of competence.

Treatment that ensues from the interpretation of any test must also be based on the age, sex, cultural background, educational level, and potential secondary gains, including economic (e.g., litigation), as well as acceptance by the patient. The competence of the therapist must be measured as well, as previously stated.

The Melzack or Melzack–McGill Pain Questionnaire consists of three major classes of word descriptors: sensory, affective, and evaluative. Reviewing the total score and the categories selected by the patients to describe their pain can give a good, initial indication of the presence or absence of a mild, moderate, or large affective component to the patient's pain complaints (37).

A test that has had acceptance for many years is the MMPI (38). This test has a self-administered true-and-false format. It consists of either a 550–question form or an abbreviated 399-question form. The test, in its original form, had statements requiring an answer of "true or false." The test is computer scored and may be computer interpreted. It is a checklist of physical and emotional symptoms, both at the time of examination and in the past.

Scores vary in patients with acute pain and those with chronic pain. In the latter, patients score lower in hypochondriasis (HS), depression (D), and hysteria (Hy), whereas patients in acute pain score higher in hypochondriasis (Hs) and hysteria (Hy). Because patients with both acute and chronic pain are preoccupied with the significance of their pain, they may express agitation [i.e., elevated Ma (mania) score], which mitigates when the pain becomes chronic, and depression (D) rises.

Rejection of the MMPI test was based on the fact that the study group used to determine normal or average behaviors was not a good cross-section of the general public. The original group had 700 men and women, all white and all residents of Minnesota. The average members of the group interviewed were semiskilled workers or farmers with an eighth grade education. The phrasing of the statements was considered awkward and unclear. Many topics such as drug abuse, alcoholism, and suicidal tendencies were not addressed. The revised MMPI-2 corrected these flaws and now consists of 567 items, which include a posttraumatic stress scale and a gender role scale; this revision has been evaluated to determine its efficacy.

In evaluating a MMPI-2 scale, the physician cannot determine whether the scores were elevated before or after the onset of chronic pain (39). Another disadvantage is the length of time needed for the patient to take the test and the differing interpretation placed on its scores by psychologists.

The MMPI-2 results, or the actual configuration of the results, were looked at as a possible diagnostic indicator for specific pain types. The "Conversion V," with elevations of scales 1, 2, and 3, with 1 and 3 more elevated than scale 2 was felt to be diagnostic for tension-type headache (40). Other work showed that the configuration noted was seen in many other chronic benign pain syndromes (41).

The Eysenck Personality Test (EPI) measures mental stability *versus* neurosis and introversion *versus* extroversion (42). This test primarily indicates the stability of the patient's reaction to stress and the tendency for the patient to break down. A direct relationship of susceptibility to the N score exists. A high N score does not indicate neurosis but merely susceptibility; it indicates an introverted person. Extroverts allegedly complain more freely than introverts but have a higher threshold to pain. The EPI test is not as much help in therapy as it is in evaluating the patient's susceptibility to decompensate under stress.

The Beck Depression Inventory (43) test consists of 21 items, is self-administered, and can be taken in five minutes. Each item relates to a factor connected with depression but not to other psychological factors that may aggravate pain.

The Hospital Anxiety and Depression Scale (HADS) has been found to be a useful screening tool for the detection of comorbid depression and anxiety disorders in patients with musculoskeletal pain disorders, and cardiovascular disorders (44,45).

More specific tests, such as the Behavioral Assessment of Pain (BAP) have emerged and are useful in the evaluation of the chronic benign pain patient (46).

The Fibromyalgia Impact Questionnaire (FIQ) was developed by Bennett and first published in 1991. It has been modified twice since that time and translated into eight languages (47). It measures physical functioning, work status, depression, anxiety, sleep, pain, stiffness, fatigue, and well-being (47,48).

Hendler (49,50) proposed a test validating the complaint of chronic pain but it has been used mainly for low back pain. Its value to substantiate other types of chronic pain, such as that likely to result from surgical intervention in low back pain, remains untested (51).

The strong emotional component of any significant pain and the proportion of the emotional component frequently remains obscure, often to the detriment of the patient and to the frustration of the clinician. Cultural and educational factors in today's society imply potential ominous sequelae of any pain with possible mitigating psychological involvement.

Considering these claims and implications, it is evident that many soft tissue pains, as subjective complaints, with little, if any, confirmatory, objective findings, especially to those clinicians who do not know how to evaluate for these problems, tend to be labeled psychogenic. Failure of the patient to respond to what is considered appropriate treatment lends further support to a psychogenic basis for the pain, rather than an organic basis. Accusation, rather than diagnosis, ensues. Pain becomes chronic, resistant, and intractable. Inappropriate exotic treatments may be pursued by the patient in search of another solution that fails and, thus, further frustrates them.

Patient–physician rapport and communication are the cornerstones of appropriate examination, diagnosis, and treatment. Actively listening to a complaint and interpreting it properly is the initial basis of diagnosis and the beginning of effective treatment. The examiner should have knowledge of the presence of the underlying psychological aspect of any, if not all pain complaints, especially when evaluating soft tissue pain.

The use of understandable "words" in explaining the cause and effects of a patient's pain is mandatory. It can never be denied that a patient's cooperation in receiving benefit from any treatment begins with the patient's clear understanding of the problem. The presence of a psychological component to the acceptance of pain—either causative or as an aggravation—can and must be conveyed to the chronic noncancer pain patient. Its acceptance is the beginning of relief and even, in extremely rare situations, a "cure".

One relatively simple way of doing this in a manner that will not alienate patients who may feel that the clinician thinks their pain is "all in their head" is to explain that many common psychological problems such as depression and anxiety are (neuro)chemical in nature and are very common *effects* of chronic pain and, thus, out of their control.

The validity of psychological testing has not been demeaned but its proportion of etiology needs clarification before a treatment protocol is initiated and evaluated. In too many chronic pain centers, the psychological aspect is stressed even where it is not used to the exclusion of other modalities. *The* exact psychological test remains to be accepted and management of *the* psychological abnormality needs to be outcome assessed. Use of a standardized test and conventional "one size fits all" treatment protocol, regardless of any "specific" diagnosis for the individual patient, will inevitably lead to failure.

SECONDARY GAIN

Nowhere is the term secondary gain so rampantly used than in therapy for pain and disability resulting from soft tissue disorders. Fishbain (52) noted in 1994 that the term "secondary gain" was mentioned in 163 articles by authors of various specialties and disciplines.

The definition of secondary gain, however, remains unclear. Whether it is consciously or unconsciously motivated remains objectively undetermined; its relationship with malingering needs clarification.

Gain was first noted as a psychoanalytic concept by Freud in 1917 (53), who described two types of gain from illness: primary and secondary. He defined primary gain "as a decrease in anxiety brought about through a defensive operation that had resulted in the production of the symptom of the (an) illness." He termed this *intrapsychic*. Freud considered secondary gain as "an interpersonal (social) advantage attained by the patient as a consequence of the illness." Although Freudian psychotherapy, i.e., psychoanalysis, offers little for the chronic pain sufferer, the basic concept of intrapsychic phenomenon helps us to understand the complicated mechanisms that join mental processes with anatomical expression.

Barsky (54) also defined primary gain as "a reduction in intrapsychic conflict and the partial gratification accomplished by the defense operation." He defined secondary gain as "acceptable or legitimate interpersonal advantages that result when one has the symptoms of a physical disease." It must be understood that there are two kinds of secondary gain. Some secondary gain benefits the patient's intrapsychic needs but always within a biopsychosocially respectable framework. A second kind is more pathological and benefit is gained for intrapsychic needs irrespective of help or hurt to others. It is the second type that is more commonly encountered.

Tertiary gains were described and defined by Dansak (55) as gains sought or attained by someone other than the patient from the patient's illness.

The operant conditioning concept claimed that "reinforcers" enhanced the concept of gain (30,56). Operant behaviors were considered as "rewards" that maintained and promoted chronic pain behavior. Some of these behaviors included rest, excessive, and inappropriate; relief from pain including narcotic medications taken as needed; avoidance of responsibility; compensation, including financial compensation; avoidance of sexual activities; approval and justification from physician; pending litigation and its rewards; little job satisfaction before injury and consequent avoidance of work; and a poor relationship with an employer.

The relationship between the secondary gain concept and operant reinforcers has never been clearly defined. Fordyce (56) believed that although reinforcers can maintain pain behavior, they did not necessarily produce that behavior and he further believed that reinforcers did not necessitate real or imaginary pain. Fordyce's theory was that observed behavior is merely a response to reinforcers, whereas psychodynamic gains have an unconscious meaning and motivation. Cameron (57) claimed that secondary gains are the result of a neurotic process and not its cause. It is apparent that the relationship between secondary gains and reinforcers remains unclear.

If a patient responds because of secondary gains, the subsequent behavior generally results in secondary losses (58). Some of these losses may include earnings; meaningful social relationships; recreational activities; community approval; guilt over disability; and the perception of social stigma. The psychophilosophical basis is easy to understand. When one receives that which he/she has extracted from an unwilling donor, neither can benefit in the end. This is particularly true of secondary gain within the context of chronic pain. The unwilling donor cannot experience the chronic pain or its unique individualized meaning to the painful person, and the person in pain becomes a donor usually out of guilt for not being able to adequately identify and/or change the plight of the one in pain. The secondary pain is, then, not a pure gain but, rather, the proceedings from a hostile relationship.

The secondary gain concept has been associated, unfortunately, with malingering. According to recent definitions, the presence of unconscious secondary gain is a somatoform disorder and not an example of malingering. Also confusing the issue is the fact that financial rewards are often associated with disability (59). The mere presence of litigation or disability benefits can be considered by some as secondary gain.

Chronic pain patients are usually only *sick* for a short time, after which they develop their subsequent impairment and disability, which becomes a *disability role*. The *sick-role* concept now differs from the disability concept. Studies have not been published to determine whether secondary gain necessarily has an etiologic or a reinforcing effect on the chronic pain.

The conscious–unconscious dichotomy regarding secondary gain is critical to establishing a clear definition. This is particularly true of patients involved in litigation (60,61).

Another form of secondary gain may be seen to have an acceptable etiology. Pain fear is another problem, where in the patient does not want to do anything, or perform any task that will increase or re-establish his or her pain. The secondary gain seen by a patient's not working must also be evaluated in terms of pain fear.

Secondary gain may help or harm the patient (62) because there are unanswered terms of insinuation such as unfulfilled dependency or unconscious motivation, which may be difficult to define.

Observed reinforcers are suggested to represent "rewards for secondary gain behaviors or perceptions" (63), which seemingly rewrites the definitions of operant psychology (30).

The relationship between a patient's emotional and physical difficulties must be determined and used, together, to determine an individualized treatment program. It is therefore imperative to have a psychologist experienced in working with chronic noncancer pain patients as part of the interdisciplinary treatment team. Without this input and treatment, the ability to help the chronic noncancer pain patient is markedly, negatively impacted.

Another empirical clinical point is that, particularly in the lower socioeconomic classes, the concept of emotional or psychological distress is not considered pertinent or possibly even real. As the clinician's job is to help the patient, despite his or her feelings, it may best benefit the patient to utilize some physical treatment along with any necessary psychological care, with the patient therefore understanding that a primarily "physical" problem is being dealt with, in spite of the extreme importance of certain aspects of the work being done in the psychologist's office.

Unfortunately, the importance of individual and group psychotherapy has been discounted by the insurance companies who typically "authorize" an inappropriately small number of sessions to be used by the psychologist and the patient, if any are authorized at all. The majority of these companies will not authorize or pay for group psychological therapy. This is very unfortunate as the chronic noncancer pain patients may learn more about how to help themselves from their peers, who have moved along the road to improved health and decreased pain, than from the clinicians alone.

In considering the relationship between soft tissue pain and disability, which may lack objective definition and acceptance, much abuse and argument has come from physicians, insurers, attorneys, and claims adjusters. Only the patient, however, is experiencing pain and continues to suffer until all aspects of his or her diagnoses are made and treated.

PSYCHOLOGICALLY BASED TREATMENTS FOR NONCANCER CHRONIC PAIN

There are many psychotherapeutic techniques that have proven beneficial for the treatment of chronic pain. There is no "one size fits all" therapy. In spite of their zealot devotees, nearly every kind of psychotherapy has *some* value for *some* patients. Further, the literature has repeatedly demonstrated that the "kind" of psychotherapy is less important than the relationship between patient and therapist. Further, even when psychotherapy or medication has proven helpful alone, the benefits are much greater when provided together.

It is of value to consider a few of the more utilized approaches through the lens of the chronic pain patient. Chronic pain alters one's perception of self, the world, and frequently diminishes hope. These factors tend to change the cognitive base from which a patient may respond to any kind of therapeutic approach. For this reason, cognitive behavioral therapy (CBT) has proven to be the most successful method of psychotherapy. CBT is not a singular modality. It encompasses many ideological and methodological components. Rarely is "pure" CBT utilized; rather, the philosophical concept of CBT is coupled with other individualized adjunctive approaches. The CBT therapist may combine relaxation therapy, guided imagery, biofeedback, hypnosis, or even marital and family therapy, depending upon unique patient need. It was found that CBT alone was effective 48% of the time, while CBT combined with other forms of therapy, especially pharmacotherapy, was effective 73% of the time (64).

As such, CBT is considered a framework from which the patient translates, endures, or ameliorates pain. The basis of CBT combines cognition with behaviorism and emphasizes the role of perceptions and interpretations as determinants in consequences, including pain. The examination of coping skills, problem solving, hardiness, and other factors in relation to the here and now is essential. Little, if any, attention is given to one's memory, the past, childhood experiences, and other factors that might be considered within the psychoanalytic framework. Introspection is critical, but the microscope of CBT is on the present, not the past. As a result, therapies that depend upon memory, such as psychoanalysis, offer little value. Further, memory tends to become altered over time through the lens of one's perceptions, history, and current state of emotional well-being, and therefore, unreliable.

Since the here and now is the focus of CBT, adjunctive therapies are sometimes required to deal with the social, domestic, employment, academic, or other issues that prevent making positive cognitive choices that could impact the furtherance of pain, or the hindrance of treatment toward health.

Aaron Beck, one of the fathers of CBT postulated that erroneous thinking causes erroneous interpretations, hence, erroneous choices, thus producing ineffectual and/or harmful results. His basic thesis has been expanded and varied by multiple leaders in the field; however, the basis is the same, i.e., faulty thinking produces ineffectual dealing with life's problems and, most often, contributes to the development of other problems. We must include in this litany both the perception of and the dealing with pain, particularly chronic pain. He theorized, and therapists have continued to validate, that a negative schema made up of the patient's past and present, including a negative triad schemata (made up of the negative schema and one's cognitive biases) produce a framework which must be confronted (65). The underlying framework which initiates the domino reaction, although beneath the patient's immediate awareness, must be challenged. Such a process does not usually require intensive psychoanalytic-type therapy. The more reliable memories are preconscious, thus available to the immediate consciousness with therapeutic support, and non-judgmental acceptance. The process by which one thinks eventuates into the framework, which is cognitive and becomes the underlying foundation for neuropathological, neuroanatomical, and neurochemical abnormalities. CBT recognizes that by the time thought produces action, it becomes "naturalized" in the psyche and is no longer considered suspect. CBT produces a questioning environment in which the mind can examine itself subjectively within a relatively neutral field, yet with some degree of objectivity, as mirrored, repeated, questioned, and interpreted by the therapist.

Human behavior, particularly that which is socially determined, is largely mediated through the frontal cortex. However, this system acts at the behest of anatomical functioning in the limbic, thalamus, hypothalamus, amygdala, and other key brain structures. Since the manifestation of pain-mediated perceptions are filtered through these and other brain anatomies, psychological intervention must begin with the assumption that "how one thinks directly effects how one feels." This is especially where the theory and practice of CBT is useful. To the extent that one can alter feelings by thought, chronic pain can be ameliorated by thought transformation. To this end, although not distinctive therapies in and of themselves, some of the newer approaches of "positive psychology" (66) and the "mindfulness" movement may be of value. Although certainly not new in the philosophical sense, the application of believing that negative thinking abets a more acute awareness of chronic pain is clinically valuable.

The "hope factor" can be critical for patients suffering from chronic pain. To them, it seems, and is sometimes truly the case, that the future will be a continuous repeat of painful stimuli from morning until night until death intervenes. The concept of hope has proven to be a valuable friend, all the way from the concentration camps, as reported by Viktor Frankl (67), to psychotherapists treating everything from poverty to grief. Patients who give up hope lose the will to live, hence, obviously and necessarily the will to heal, to recover, and certainly, the will to thrive. The loss of this basic instinct for self-preservation produces an untreatable patient from any psychological perspective.

At this point, a word of caution is prudent. Adjunct therapies that have the ability to alter thought processes without sufficiently taking into account the underlying physical pathologies may be very destructive. Hypnosis, for example, which can minimize or even alleviate pain, may produce thought patterns that ignore life-threatening pathology. Biofeedback, while helpful in visualizing the extent of one's capacity for altering autonomic functioning, may lead to faulty thinking, thus preventing the patient from seeking additional diagnosis and treatment.

CBT in competent hands, i.e., persons adequately medically trained, allows for a safe integration of the most prudent of all therapies while monitoring it through what might be considered "real behavior" and measurement by validated laboratory findings. This is not to suggest that only physicians (MDs, DOs) should treat persons with chronic pain. It is to state emphatically that psychologists, social workers, and other team members must be thoroughly trained in the physiological aspects of chronic pain as well as the competencies of their specific discipline; just as those medically trained must be biopsychosocially knowledgeable.

The downside of CBT is that it is time and cost dependent. Although many patients improve in a relatively short time, frequently 6 to 15 sessions, (controlled studies of 13 sessions) (68), in many cases, protracted visits are required. On the other hand, Guzman et al. (69) found that anything short of three months of intensive, multidisciplinary, biopsychosocial rehabilitation did not show improvements. Professionals most likely to provide such one-hour segments of time are psychologists. The Cochrane Back Review group reported that "Behavioral treatment seems to be an effective treatment for patients with chronic low back pain, but it is still unknown what type of patients benefit most from what type of behavioral treatment" (70).

Herein lies both a benefit and a caution. While board-certified (ABPP) psychologists are trained in CBT, they may have neither the ability nor the availability of physicians for the prescription of medication. Simply having two professionals seeing the same patient is not "team treatment." It is required that they know what each is doing, monitor medications in concert with current treatment gains (or losses) and treatment plans, and tailor both the cognitive challenges and the pharmacological changes in tandem.

The great advantage of CBT over other kinds of psychotherapy is that it is reality based; thus, the alert, astute therapist always has an accurate measurement of both thinking and behavior. CBT when combined with marital, family, and/or group therapy also offers a reality-based measurement. Patients in pain are not often able to objectively report the extent of their daily dysfunction (71,72). They are caught up in either stoicism or secondary gain. In either case, a third-party measurement tool, that is, family or external observers, is most useful. There are several valuable aids to understanding the larger context of the chronic pain patient within the family context (73,74). The trained CBT professional is able to incorporate the quality of life experienced by, interpreted by, and reported by others, as part of the reality-based thinking required of a patient as an aid toward healthy thinking.

The final concern is not the pain but the person as a whole. Since pain is subjective, has many meanings, and is inextricably interwoven with suffering, the well-being of the patient must take precedent over the professional's evaluation of success in patient care. Healers who rush to alleviate their own perception of pain, as has been pointed out, may only induce greater overall patient dysfunction in the form of more suffering, additional pathology, and/or the exacerbation of perceived pain by the patient. The value of a team-oriented approach with committed, compassionate, competent, care offers the best hope for help for the chronic pain patient. Since patients have a brain and mind as well as body, it is only prudent that the brain as a neurological organ, and the mind as a human attribute be given their rightful attention.

REFERENCES

1. Brom B. Corticalization of chronic pain. Am Pain Soc J 1994; 3:131–135.
2. Melzack R. The Puzzle of Pain. New York: Basic Books, 1973.
3. Melzack R. Psychological concepts and methods for the control of pain. In: Advances in Neurology. Vol. 4. New York: Raven Press, 1974:275–280.
4. Melzack R, Casey KL. In: Thomas CC, ed. The Skin Senses. Springfield, IL: Charles C. Thomas, 1968:423.
5. Beecher HK. Measurement of Subjective Response. New York: Oxford University Press, 1959.
6. Turk DC, Wack JT, Kerns RD. An empirical examination of the "pain behavior" construct. J Behav Med 1985; 8:119–130.
7. Sternbach RA. Acute versus chronic pain. In: Wall PD, Melzack R, eds. Textbook of Pain. London: Churchill Livingstone, 1984:606.
8. Flor H, Birbaumer N. Acquisition of chronic pain: psychophysiological mechanisms. Am Pain Soc 1994; 3:119–127.

9. Flor H, Birbaumer N, Turk DC. A diathesis—stress model of chronic back pain: empirical evaluation and therapeutic implications. In: Gerber WD, Miltner W, Mayer K, eds. Behavioral Medicine: Results and Perspectives of Empirical Research. Weinheim: Edition Medizin, 1987.

10. Flor H, Turk DC, Birbaumer N. Assessment of stress—related psychophysiological reactions in chronic back pain patients. J Consult Clin Psychol 1985; 53:354–364.

11. Borgeat F, Hade B, Elie R, et al. Effects of voluntary muscle tension increases in tension headaches. Headache 1983; 24:199–202.

12. Christensen LV. Physiology and pathophysiology of skeletal muscle contraction: part 1. Dynamic activity. J Oral Rehabil 1986; 13:451–461.

13. Christensen LV. Physiology and pathophysiology of skeletal muscle contraction: part II. Static activity. J Oral Rehabil 1986; 13:463–477.

14. Backonja M, Miletic G. Somatosensory cortical neurons on mononeuropathy model. Soc Neurosci Abst 1983; 19:1074.

15. Kenshalo DR Jr, Willis WD Jr. The role of the cerebral cortex in pain sensations. In: Peters A, Jones EG, eds. Cerebral Cortex. New York: Plenum, 1991:153–212.

16. Donaldson S, Romney D, Donaldson M, et al. A single blind randomized study of the application of SMU training principles to chronic low back pain personal contact. 1994; 4(1):23–37.

17. Brena SF. Chronic Pain: America's Hidden Epidemic. New York: Atheneum, 1978.

18. Linton SJ, Althoff B, Melin L, et al. Psychological factors related to health, back pain, and dysfunction. J Occup Rehabil 1994; 4:1–10.

19. Frymoyer JW. Predicting disability from low back pain. Clin Orthop Rel Res 1992; 279:101–109.

20. Bigos SJ, Spengler DM, Martin NA, et al. Back injuries in industry: a retrospective study III. Employee-related factors. Spine 1986; 11:252–256.

21. Jensen MP, Karoly P. Pain—specific beliefs, perceived symptoms severity, and adjustment to chronic pain. 1992; 8:123–130.

22. Keefe FJ, Williams DA. Assessment of pain behaviors. In: Turk DC, Melzack R, eds. Handbook of Pain Assessment. New York: Guilford Press, 1992:275–294.

23. Truner JA, Robinson J, McCreary CP. Chronic low back pain: predicting response to nonsurgical treatment. Arch Phys Med Rehabil 1983; 64:560–563.

24. Jensen MP, Turner JA, Romano JM, et al. Coping with chronic pain: a critical review of the literature. Pain 1991; 47:249–283.

25. Feuerstein M, Thebarge RW. Perceptions of disability and occupational stress as discriminators of work disability in patients with chronic pain. J Occup Rehabil 1991; 1:185–195.

26. Kemmlert K, Lundholm L. Factors influencing ergonomic conditions and employment rate after an occupational musculoskeletal injury. J Occup Rehabil 1994; 4: 11–21.

27. Tarasuk V, Eakin JM. Back problems are for life: perceived vulnerability and its implications for chronic disability. J Occup Rehabil 1994; 4:55–64.

28. Keltner NL, Folks DG. Psychotropic Drugs. 2nd ed. St. Louis: Mosby, 1997.

29. Keefe FJ, Dunsmore J. Pain behavior: concepts and controversies. Am Pain Soc J 1992; 1:92–100.

30. Fordyce WE. Behavioral Methods for Chronic Pain and Illness. St. Louis: Mosby, 1976.

31. Keefe FJ, Hill RW. An objective approach to quantifying pain behavior and gait patterns in low back pain patients. Pain 1985; 21:153–161.

32. Follick MJ, Ahern DK, Aberger EW. Development of an audio—visual taxonomy of pain behavior: reliability discriminate validity. Health Psychol 1985; 4:555–568.

33. Turk DC, Wack JT, Kerns RD. An empirical examination of the "pain behavior" construct. J Behav Med 1985; 8:119–130.

34. Waddell G, et al. Low back pain: a framework for clinical decision making. Drug Therapy 1983; 8(3):92–96.

35. Fordyce WE, Fowler RS, Lehman JF, et al. Some implications of learning in problems of chronic pain. J Chronic Dis 1968; 21:179.

36. Brena SF, Koch DL. A "pain estimate" model for quantification and classification of chronic pain states. Anesth Rev 1975; 2:8–13.
37. Melzack R. The McGill Pain Questionnaire: major properties and scoring methods. Pain 1975; I:277–299.
38. Dahlstrom WG, Welsh GS, Dahlstrom, LE. An MMPI Handbook. Vol. 1. Minneapolis: University of Minnesota Press, 1960.
39. Naliboff BD, Cohen MJ, Yellen AN. Does the MMPI differentiate chronic illness from chronic pain? Pain 1982; 13:333–341.
40. Kudrow L. Muscle contraction headaches. In: Rose FC, ed. Handbook of Clinical Neurology. Vol. 48. Amsterdam: Elsevier Science, 1986:343–352.
41. Jay GW, Grove RN, Grove KS. Differentiation of chronic headache from non-headache pain patients using the Millon Clinical Multiaxial Inventory (MCMI). Headache 1987; 27:124–129.
42. Bond MR. Personality and Pain. Edinburgh: Churchill Livingstone, 1984:45–50.
43. Beck AT, Ward CH, Mendelson M, et al. An inventory for measuring depression Arch Gen Psychiatry 1961; 4:561–571.
44. Harter M, Reuter K, Gross-Hardt K, et al. Screening for anxiety, depressive and somatoform disorders in rehabilitation—validity of HADS and GHQ-12 in patients with musculoskeletal disease. Disabil Rehabil 2001; 23(16):737–744.
45. Bambauer KZ, Locke SE, Aupont O, et al. Using the Hospital Anxiety and Depression Scale to screen for depression in cardiac patients. Gen Hosp Psychiatry 2005; 27(4):275–284.
46. Jay GW. Headache Handbook: Diagnosis and Treatment. Boca Raton, FL: CRC Press, 1999:89.
47. Bennett R. The Fibromyalgia Impact Questionnaire (FIQ): a review of its development, current version, operating characteristics and uses. Clin Exp Rheumatol 2005; 23(5 Suppl 39):S154–S162.
48. Buskila D, Neumann L. Assessing functional disability and health status of women with fibromyalgia: validation of a Hebrew version of the Fibromyalgia Impact Questionnaire. J Rheumatol 1996; 23(5):903–906.
49. Hendler NH. The four stages of pain. In: Hendler NH, Long DM, Wise TN, eds. Diagnosis and Treatment of Chronic Pain. Boston: John Wright, PSG Publishing, 1982: 1–8.
50. Hendler N, Viernstein M, Gucer P, et al. The Hendler Ten Minute Screen Test for chronic back pain patients. Baltimore, MD: Chronic Pain Treatment Center, Johns Hopkins Hospital, 1978.
51. Mersky H. Classification of chronic pain descriptions of chronic pain syndromes and definitions of pain terms. Pain 1986; 3(Suppl): S1–S225.
52. Fishbain DA. Secondary gain concept: definition problems and its abuse in medical practice. Am Pain Soc J 1994; 3:264–277.
53. Freud S. Introductory lectures on psychoanalysis (1917). London: Hogarth Press, 1959:378–391.
54. Barsky AJ, Klerman GL. Overview: hypochondriasis bodily complaints and somatic styles. Am J Psychiatry 1983; 140:273–282.
55. Dansak D. On the tertiary gain of illness. Compr Psychiatry 1973; 14:523–534.
56. Fordyce WE, Fowler RS, Lehmann JF, et al. Some implications of learning in problems of chronic pain. J Chronic Dis 1968; 21:179–190.
57. Cameron N. Personality Development and Psychopathology. Boston: Houghton Mifflin, 1963:273–274.
58. Bienoff J. Traumatic neurosis of industry. Ind Med Surg 1946; 15:109–112.
59. Finneson BE. Modulating effect of secondary gain on the low back pain syndrome. Adv Pain Res Ther 1976; 1:949–952.
60. Thompson DL. Secondary gain, a second look: issues in counseling the industrially injured worker. NARPPS J News 1991; 6:59–63.
61. Weissman FIN. Distortions and deceptions in self-presentation: effects of protracted litigation in personal injury cases. Behav Sci Law 1990; 8:67–74.

62. Gallagher RM. Secondary gain in pain medicine. Am Pain Soc J 1994; 3:274–278.
63. Whitehead W, Kuhn WF. Chronic pain: an overview. In: Miller TW, ed. Chronic Pain. Vol. 1. Madison, WI: International Universities Press, 1990:5–48.
64. Keller MB, McCullough JP, Klein DN, et al. A comparison of nefazodone, the cognitive behavioral-analysis system of psychotherapy, and their combination for the treatment of chronic depression. N Engl J Med 2000; 342(20):1462–1470.
65. Neale JM, Davison GC. Abnormal Psychology. 8th ed. New York: Wiley, 2001:247.
66. Seligman M, Steen TA. Positive psychology progress: empirical validation of interventions. Am Psychol 2005; 410–421.
67. Frankl V. Man's Search for Meaning. Boston, MA: Beacon Press, 1997.
68. Deale A, Chalder T, Wessely S. Cognitive behavior therapy for chronic fatigue syndrome: a randomized controlled trial. Am J Psychiatry 1997; 154:408–414.
69. Guzman J, Esmail R, et al. Multidisciplinary rehabilitation for chronic low back pain: systematic review. Br Med J 2001; 322:1511–1516.
70. Van Tulder MW, et al. Behavioral treatment for chronic low back pain: a systematic review within the framework of the Cochrane Back Review Group. Lippincott Williams & Wilkins, 2000, as reported by Spine 2000; 25(20): 2688–2699.
71. Briere J, Scott C (eds). Cognitive interventions. In: Principles of Trauma Therapy. Thousand Oaks, CA: Sage, 2006; chap 7, 109–119.
72. Dobson KS, Dozois DJA. Historical and philosophical bases of the cognitive-behavioral therapies. In: Dobson KS, ed. Handbook of Cognitive-Behavioral Therapies. 2nd ed. New York: Guilford, 2001:3–39.
73. Roy R. Chronic Pain and Family: A Clinical Perspective. New York: Springer, 2006.
74. Silver JK. Chronic Pain and the Family: A New Guide. Cambridge: Harvard University Press, 2004.

11 Neuropsychological Aspects of Neuropathic Pain

Richard H. Cox

Private Practice, Chapel Hill; Duke University Medical Center, Durham, North Carolina; Georgetown University Medical Center, Washington DC, U.S.A.

The *neuropsychological* aspects of pain are herein considered as distinct from other psychological diagnoses in that only conditions arising primarily or secondarily from *neuropathic* pain are discussed. Neuropathic pain is that which results from damage and/or dysfunction of the peripheral and/or central nervous system. Whereas "pain," per se, is a necessary protective mechanism, neuropathic pain is that which has escalated to a pathological level, thus becoming an entity in and of itself.

By definition and solid clinical and laboratory findings, *neuropathic* pain must be addressed by those especially educated and trained in a combination of the neurological and psychological fields. Although neurologists, neuropsychiatrists, and others in the health field also have interdisciplinary training, the neuropsychologist is particularly and specifically educated and trained for this integrated multidisciplinary task. The neuropsychologist is one who has an earned doctorate in clinical psychology, which provides a broad base of knowledge in both normal and abnormal psychological functioning and, in addition, has doctorate and postdoctorate studies ranging from two to four or more years in neuroanatomy, neuropharmacology, neuropathology, and related studies, in clinical settings, training with a team of interdisciplinary professionals from general medicine, rehabilitation, neurology, psychiatry, neurosurgery, and neuroimaging. Typically, the thoroughly competent neuropsychologist will be board certified by the American Board of Professional Psychology (ABPP) with a specialization in neuropsychology and/or rehabilitation psychology. Their armamentarium of skills, therefore, includes a range of abilities from diagnostic interviewing to clinical examination to an extremely broad variety of neuropsychological assessment instruments which render objective measurements of brain and the normal and abnormal functioning as a result, thereof.

Neuropsychology recognizes and integrates both the actual bodily changes as well as the emotional concomitants, thus, arriving at reasonable approaches to both diagnoses and treatments. Since neuropathic pain is the end result of chronic severe pain, neuropsychologists are essential in the rehabilitative aspects of pain medicine. Constant vigilance to the visible and invisible physiological changes in individual patients is necessary since many persons, even health care professionals, still tend to consider pain, even neuropathic pain, as primarily emotional in origin and continuance. Careful neuropsychological examination helps to determine which is primarily peripheral nervous system and/or central nervous system related and which is rooted in the emotions, either primary or secondary to the pain manifestations.

The uniqueness of this professional allows for a kind of interdisciplinary leadership and teamwork that no other discipline offers. The academic and experiential armamentarium of a neuropsychologist is impressive, indeed, and allows such a person to utilize both the emotional and physical aspects of chronic pain. While neuropsychologists are knowledgeable regarding scans, MRI, etc., their particular diagnostic expertise is in the utilization of specialized neuropsychological testing, a kind of testing that is well validated for distinguishing the locus of brain pathology, establishing a baseline and assisting in rehabilitation. Further, such professionals are uniquely equipped to assist with costs for rehabilitation, daily living activities, and other behavioral and "real-life" concerns.

Neuropatich pain is real, not imaginary, or simply an emotive perception as some would see it; we must look at the pathophysiological etiology of such perceptions that otherwise could, often are, and historically were considered simply as products of "the mind." That which is "in the mind" has demonstrable neuroanatomical, neurochemical, and neuropathophysiological bases. It has often been said that, "pain is a friend, for without such one could die without knowing one were ill," and surely this is true. However, when pain becomes neuropathic, life is disheveled, thinking is blurred, behavior is dysfunctional, and the body often accommodates in unhealthy ways, even to the degeneration of brain tissue!

The neuropsychological implications of neuropathic pain are myriad. When the brain can localize, hence, identify causality, it is often able to adjust, rationalize, accommodate, and tolerate even serious noxious stimuli; however, ambiguity and unidentifiable stimuli are much less well tolerated and set the brain into an interminable search for causality. In the absence of reasonable answers, psychopathology is the result (1–5). Patients with neuropathic pain often migrate from one health care professional to another seeking relief because the pain has been either labeled "emotional" or the health care providers could not "explain" it. Understanding the causes of neuropathic pain seldom relieves it, but it goes a long way in relieving the patient from the stigma that it is "imaginary" and all in "one's mind."

It will be helpful first to visit the relationship of pain with specific brain anatomy. While done only cursorily, to understand the role of neuropsychology in pain, we must understand the dimension of neuropsychological factors that are based in anatomy. Through fMRI and phfMRI, it has been conclusively demonstrated that chronic pain produces demonstrable temporary and permanent physiological changes. These changes present resultant thought and behavioral disorders both of a temporary and permanent nature. Classical diagnostic procedures of brain function and the fMRI and phfMRI "... are not sufficient to provide an understanding of the operational principles of a dynamic system such as the brain ..." (6). Not only is the brain dynamic in the moment but also related to many known factors, such as age, environment, concomitant disease states, and other factors unidentified and unidentifiable. While behavior is related to specific brain function(s), individual psychological factors are also involved. It is in the understanding of this relationship that often brings answers.

While all nervous systems are involved, recent experimental studies (7–10) indicate that sufficient neuroplasticity exists so as to greatly confuse the primary afferent mechanisms in neuropathic pain patients (11). Changes include the calcitonin gene-related peptide, substance P, isolectin B4, as well as glutamate, galanin, neuropeptide Y, vasoactive intestinal peptide, and dynorphin, and also numerous other neurochemical substances including a marked reduction of μ-opioid receptors resulting in an insensitivity to opioid analgesics (12,13). When a patient does not respond to narcotics, it is often assumed that the pain is, therefore, "psychosomatic," when in fact it is very real and the body has developed insensitivity to the narcotics.

Concurrently, and plasticity related, there are changes caused by variations in peripheral input, resulting in spinal processing changes, hence, followed by changes transmitted to the cortex via thalamic nuclei (14,15). These are only a few of the currently known neuroanatomical changes resultant from neuropathic pain. The neurophysiological and neuropsychological changes are equally as numerous and will be discussed later.

Until recently, pain was perceived as a temporary physical causality for emotional discomfort. The very few illustrations stated herein show that such is not the case. Structural changes of both a temporary and permanent nature occur with great variation within the same patient with age-related, disease-related, and morbidity-related factors.

The classical approaches to brain anatomy and mind function are not adequate for today's expanded knowledge of neuropsychological systems. The brain is not a static organism with the same anatomical changes resulting from neuropathic pain from patient to patient. Neither is it static in relation to its function as a mind. Mind functions result from a combination of anatomy, physiology, neurochemistry, neuropsychology, and unique individual cognitive processes not easily understood and as yet unmeasurable by any valid instrument. The combination of brain and mind make for a complex, dynamic system.

Brain is herein differentiated from *mind*. The philosophical discussion of whether the brain has a mind or does the mind have a brain, while esoteric, may be important from the standpoint of neuroplasticity and our ability to diagnose and treat *brain and behavioral* dysfunction. Without doubt, brain + mind is more than anatomy and thinking. The *person* is more than the whole of anatomy and thought processes. The neuropsychological understanding of this complex human conundrum may give us a better tool by which we can see the functions of mind on brain and the structural aspects of brain on mind. There is no *mind* without anatomical structure; however, anatomical structure alone does not guarantee a *mind* that can assist in brain plasticity. Those who seek to treat an illness as an entity rather than a person with an illness mistakenly view *brain* and *mind*.

Two physiological illnesses, postherpetic neuralgia (PHN) and chronic back pain (CBP) illustrate the subtleties of changes that can originate from very different origins and produce very different yet similar neurophysiological changes. In PHN patients, "... the main regions that were activated and responded most robustly to long-term treatment were the amygdala and ventral striatum ... in the CBP (chronic back pain) patients, ... both the ventral striatum and amygdala were active but at a lower statistical significance ... the brain regions associated with spontaneous pain in both CBP show similarities and preferentially engage various components of the same circuitry" (16). While various pathologies involve similar, or even the same anatomical structures, the subtleties of anatomy, neurochemistry, and neurological systems make it difficult to identify target sites for treatment. While pharmacological agents may excite one site, the same medication may depress a site nearby, thus, voiding the benefits, or vice versa.

These neurophysiological and cortical changes, combined with mind functions (mind as differentiated from brain), result in a disease. Thus neuropathic pain is not the pain that results from chronic severe pain but, rather, an illness, a pathology, a syndrome, an identifiable disease state in and of itself.

The phenomenon of neuroplasticity allows that the brain is not a fixed, static organ. It postulates, and increasingly demonstrates that the brain has the capacity for regeneration. Neuroplasticity is bivalent and, therefore, allows for brain remodeling following the disruption of membrane neurochemistry, probably due to altered gene or protein expression, channelopathies that induce aberrant calcium concentration, and other neurochemical and neuroelectrical factors. By the same token, degeneration may also occur as a result of excessive calcium influx, excitotoxicity and the engagement of apoptotic mechanisms. Neuroplasticity, is a much more recently recognized phenomenon, and is often responsible for brain circuitry and brain functions, which can be either degenerative or regenerative. The brain is paradoxically constantly growing, changing, and deteriorating at the same time. Additionally, neuroplasticity augments the electrophysiological abnormalities, afferent responses to stimuli, and often results in abnormalities in spontaneous firing rates and bursting activities.

Since temporary and permanent changes occur, time and expertise are of the essence. Early diagnosis and treatment have proven effective in slowing degeneration and, in many cases, reversing dysfunction. While the brain "will do what the brain will do," in most cases, positive plasticity is promoted with early, aggressive intervention. Neuropsychological "brain training," often with neuropharmacological support, has proven effective.

However, without adequate remediation, neuropathic pain results in permanent dysfunction. "... when neurons fire too much, they may change their connections with other neurons or even die, because they can't sustain high activity for so long ..." (17). It is understandable, even to the layperson, that when one is constantly in pain the nervous system is working overtime, the stress system is in overdrive, and the emotional sequelae are multitudinous.

It is clear from volumetric studies that neuropathic pain affects both the volume and function of brain matter, particularly gray matter. There is accumulating evidence that neuropathic pain actually results in permanent pathophysiology secondary to specific and actual anatomical changes in the thalamic gray matter.

Chronic back pain, for instance, actually reduces the volume of gray matter (1,2,18). Gray matter is distributed on the surface of the cerebral cortex; the cerebellar cortex; the thalamus; hypothalamus; subthalamus; basal ganglia, including the putamen, globus pallidus, nucleus accumbens, septal nuclei, nucleus, and the brainstem, which includes the substantia nigra, red nucleus, olivary nuclei, cranial nerve nuclei, and also the spinal white matter including the anterior horn, lateral horn, and posterior horn. This litany of anatomy is listed, and overly simplified at that, to demonstrate the ubiquity of potential neuropsychological sequelae that may accompany and/or result from neuropathic pain. Further, since gray matter is the route for both sensory and motor stimuli to the interneurons of the CNS in order to develop responses to the stimuli through chemical synaptic activity, the potential for life-changing neuropsychology is profound.

There is increasing evidence that not only gray matter is decreased but that there are white matter changes as well. "There appears to be an association between migraine and white matter lesions in the brain on structural MRI . . . there are specific disorders that result in prominent white matter changes in addition to migraine . . . it is postulated that ischemic damage causes white matter abnormalities as a result of microvascular processes such as hypoglycemia, oxidative stress, transient ischemia, or platelet hyperaggregability" (19).

It must be emphasized that the demonstration of loss of both white and gray matter within the brain is a profound consideration in any and all neuropsychological studies and in the diagnosis and treatment of persons with neuropathic pain. Apart from neuroplasticity, of which we now know only very little, these patients are at the mercy of palliative treatment and are in need of a tremendous amount of professional care, if only to sustain their current level of functioning. In cases of posttraumatic pain, sustaining current functioning levels and rehabilitation offer greater possibilities. In the case of repeated trauma, such as migraine, continuing brain destruction may occur, thus, rendering a greater challenge for rehabilitation.

Chronic back pain and PHN are only two illustrations of continuing neuropathic pain and the potential for actual anatomical brain changes. Neuropathic pain differs in ultimate anatomical and neuropsychological manifestations from patient to patient. Anatomically, the ventral striatum, amygdala, and portions of the prefrontal cortex are inextricably interconnected, thus, becoming a part of the deepest, emotionally hedonic aspects of perception and, thus, also of memory. Further, greatly differing pathologies may eventuate in a similar kind of neuropathic pain. For instance, PHN and chronic back pain most likely involve similar and, at times, even the same neural circuitry, while originating in very different neural pathways.

The concept of neuropathic pain cannot be discussed apart from stress factors and the impact of such factors upon cognitive functioning and memory. Chronic pain sets into firing the lateral occipital cortex which is known to override one's ability to concentrate, remember, and rationally function (20). Chronic pain alters the way in which a patient with neuropathic pain processes information of all kinds: that which is related to the pain syndrome itself and that which is not. One's focus is understandably on the pain, hence, not on the immediate attention to any other function, rendering the patient at risk for most tasks of daily life. It is known that when nonpain patients settle to perform a task, neural networks tend to focus on the specific sensory and motor requirements for that task; however, in the neuropathic pain patient, such is not the case. In these patients, focus is on the pain, and the cortex that is closely associated with emotion becomes overactive giving rise to disequilibrium.

Fibromyalgia serves as a particularly demonstrable model of neuropathic pain culminating in debilitating neuropsychology. Age-dependent differences as well as cultural and emotional differences, polypharmacy, and polypathology no doubt contribute to the chronicity of severe pain in producing a depletion, degeneration, and/or dysfunction of gray matter in the cortices and, particularly, in the area of the thalamus (1,2,21).

Migraine headache patients are reported to have "subtle but persistent cerebral dysfunction" (22). It has already been mentioned that migraineurs may well have decreased gray and white matter as a result of chronic severe headaches. While most pain syndromes may be assessed via various medical and neuropsychological means simultaneously with the pain, the migraine patient presents in a particularly complicated neuropsychological fashion in that the pain, itself, renders the patient unable to be evaluated by neuropsychological tests during the episodes. Testing done in the postictal state is not necessarily representative of the mental state while in the excruciating pain of migraine. Neuropsychologically, this is very important in that, although it is often most uncomfortable, a patient in most neuropathic states can be evaluated to determine the effect of his or her pain on mental performance; but such is not the case in migraine.

Even though stress is a universally accepted etiology of pathology, it is still not fully understood. Since its introduction by Hans Selye, stress has been increasingly recognized as an entity in and of itself, capable of producing both temporary and permanent changes in the human body. The "stress circuit" is undoubtedly implicated in the neuropsychological manifestations of neuropathic pain. "Their theory explains the complex interplay between the nervous system known as the hypothalamic-pituitary-adrenal (HPA) axis . . . the HPA axis is a feedback loop by which signals from the brain trigger the release of hormones needed to respond to stress. Because of its function, the HPA axis is also sometimes called the 'stress circuit'" (23).

Stress factors, particularly conditions that perpetuate chronic stress states, such as sexual abuse, emotional harassment, and physical torture, are doubtless the foundation for some patients' neuropathic pain. With the prevalence of reported sexual abuse victims, one must consider the possible relationship between sexual abuse history and an increased incidence of neuropathic pain. There are studies that indicate a relationship between sexual abuse and fibromyalgia, in particular those by Boisset-Pioro et al. (24). The authors concluded, "A high frequency of sexual abuse was identified in control patients and in FMS patients." The problems resulting are not only seen in the fibromyalgia syndrome but also in the neuropsychological functioning. In addition to severe and unrelenting pain, the patient may also present with depression, guilt, fear, withdrawal, or anxiety related to anything within a sexual context including literature, films, TV, both same and other gender relationships, purposeful self-bodily harm, eating disorders, regressive behaviors, insomnia, and overt attempts both to avoid and to perpetuate revictimization, and numerous other complaints as well as vague and indescribable sensations (25).

The following are only a few of the problems a clinician may expect to find in the patient with neuropathic pain: cognitive functioning, executive skills, attentional capacity, processing speed, psychomotor speed, figure and ground perception, language skills, both receptive and expressive communication, computational skills, emotional lability including the characteristics of a bipolar disorder, and other commonly diagnosed psychiatric syndromes.

Physical conditions leading to neuropathic pain are far too numerous to list and such are not appropriate for this paper. However, the neuropsychological sequelae are particularly prominent in the following commonly encountered pathologies: traumatic injury to brain and spinal cord, phantom limb, type 1 and 2 diabetes, migraine, fibromyalgia, chronic allergy, and anatomical degenerative syndromes.

We have demonstrated changes in neurochemistry, neuroelectricity, and neuroanatomy resultant from neuropathic pain. It is now safe to assume and await further investigation as to the extent of the invasiveness and permanency of the many pain-state syndromes. Since neuropathic pain is not solely an emotional condition, psychotherapy and other neuropsychological modalities are doubtless helpful but best utilized in conjunction with pharmacologic agents and other medical interventions. Probably no other disorder of human suffering better demonstrates the need for treating the whole person with the most massive armamentarium we can muster.

We can hope for neuroplasticity to work naturally toward neuroregeneration and neurorehabilitation and for continued discovery into ways both pharmacologically and psychodynamically to assist in that direction. Just as the heart develops collaterals and the brain learns transfer of hemispherical abilities, perhaps we can encourage the whole anatomical, neuromolecular, and neurodynamic mechanisms to develop patterns to better mediate pain.

When one considers the magnitude of actual anatomical changes, with concomitant thought process and behavioral changes, it is obvious that the neuropsychological sequelae of neuropathic pain are enormous. Consider that gray matter decreases; white matter changes; and hypoglycemia, oxidative stress, transient ischemia, platelet hyperaggregability, cortex changes, and cerebellar changes occur. It would be impossible to list the resultant structural, electrical, hormonal, neurochemical, and behavioral changes.

Neuroanatomical changes lead to neurophysiolgical changes which lead to *neuropathological* changes which lead to *neurofunctional* changes which lead to *neuropsychological* changes which lead to *perceptual dysfunction;* hence, *behavioral accommodations* to those mistaken cues that result in *neuropsychological syndromes,* which then become a *cycle* of neuropathic pain to emotional and anatomical dysfunction and back to neuropathic pain, inevitably lead to severe physical and emotional disease.

REFERENCES

1. Apkarian AV, Sosa Y, Krauss BR, et al. Chronic pain patients are impaired on an emotional decision-making task. Pain 2004; 108:129–136.
2. Apkarian AV, Sosa Y, Sonty S, et al. Chronic back pain is associated with decreased prefrontal and thalamic gray matter density. J Neurosci 2004; 24:10410–10415.
3. Apkarian AV, Bushnell MC, Treede RD, et al. Human brain mechanisms of pain perception and regulation in health and disease. Eur J Pain 2005; 9:184–188.
4. Baliki M, Apkarian AV. The neurological effects of chronic pain. Pain Europe 2006; 2:4–5.
5. Geha PY, Apkarian AV. Pain and neuroanatomical effects: evidence for cortical reorganization. Psychiatric Times 2006; 23:22–24.
6. Marshall JC, Morris-Kay GM. J Anat 2004; 205:415.
7. Abbadie C et al. Spinal cord substance P receptor immunoreactivity increases in both inflammatory and nerve injury models of persistent pain. Neuroscience 70:201–209.
8. Mantyh PW et al. Molecular mechanisms of cancer pain. Nat Rev Cancer 2:201–209.
9. Gardell LR et al. Enhanced evoked excitatory transmitter release in experimental neuropathy requires descending facilitation. J Neurosci 23:8370–8379.
10. Haines et al. Central representation of chronic on-going neuropathic pain studied by positron emission tomography. Pain 1995; 63:225–236.
11. Woolf CJ, Salter MW. Neuronal plasticity: increasing the gain in pain. Science 2000; 288:1765–1769.
12. Narita et al. 2000. High expression of high-affinity receptor for immunoglobulin, nih.gov/pbmed15196280.
13. Narita et al. 2004. High expression of high-affinity receptor for immunoglobulin, nih.gov/pbmed15196280.

14. Coderre et al. 1993. High expression of high-affinity receptor for immunoglobulin, nih.gov/pbmed15196280.
15. Hsieh JC, Belfrage M, Stone-Elander S, et al. Central representation of chronic ongoing neuropathic pain studied by positron emission tomography. Pain.1995; 63:225–236.
16. Baliki M, Geha Y, Apkarian AV. Spontaneous pain and brain activity in neuropathic pain: functional MRI and pharmacologic functional MRI studies. Curr Pain Headache Rep 2007; 11:171–177.
17. Chialvo, D. Chronic pain harms brain's wiring. Medline Plus, Friday, February 8, 2008.
18. Apkarian AV. 2008.
19. Afridi SK, Goadsby PJ, Neuroimaging of migraine. Curr Headache Rep 2006; 10: 221–224.
20. Dick BD, Rashiq S. Disruption of attention and working memory traces in individuals with chronic pain. Anesth Analg 104:1223–1229.
21. Bushnell MC et al. Pain perception: is there a role for primary somatosensory cortex? Proc Natl Acad Sci USA 96:7705–7709.
22. Bell BD, Pimeau M, Sweet J, et al. Neuropsychological functioning in migraine headache, nonheadache chronic pain, and mild traumatic brain injury patients. Abstract. Arch Clin Neuropsychol 1999; 14(4):389–399.
23. Chrousos G, Gold P. Stress System Malfunction Could Lead to Serious, Life Threatening Disease. National Institutes of Health and Human Development; Silver Spring, MD, September 9, 2002.
24. Boisset-Pioro MH, Esdaile JM, Fitzcharles MA. Sexual and physical abuse in women with fibromyalgia syndrome. Arthritis Rheum 1995; 38(2):235–241.
25. Newton CJ. Child abuse: an overview. *Ment Health J.* April 2001; IV, 46–49.

12 Interdisciplinary Treatment of Chronic Noncancer Pain

Gary W. Jay

Clinical Disease Area Expert-Pain, Pfizer, Inc., New London, Connecticut, U.S.A.

Interdisciplinary pain treatment programs were in existence before the advent of the subspecialty of Pain Medicine/Management. They worked well, by EBM standards, and then were "over-taken" by other insurer preferred pain treatment methods. Even though pain is a biological–psychological–sociological phenomenon, insurers would refuse to pay for interdisciplinary pain programs stating "I won't cover psych" or psychological treatment for a chronic pain patient. This may be one reason that the subspecialty has become so dependent on narcotic usage and interventional treatment, as the later could be demonstrated to insurers by a picture from a C-arm. Whether the insurer could read these X-rays correctly to determine that they were what they were claimed to be may be another story. But the interdisciplinary treatment of chronic noncancer has become too expensive to do secondary to insurance refusals to pay, in spite of the weight of the evidence.

Acute pain may last days to weeks, even two to three months or so. Chronic pain, in existence for three to six months or more, is in itself a disease. It is the cause of a great deal of financial distress secondary to increased medical system utilization, loss of work, and familial disintegration coupled with significant costs to insurers and patients for both medical services and medications.

The treatment of pain is relatively straightforward in the acute pain patient. Once the cause of the symptom of pain is identified, it may be treated in a rather straightforward manner. The problems involved in the treatment of the chronic pain patient increase substantially, as chronic pain is biological (organic)–psychological and sociological in nature, making treatment far more complex and of necessity more significantly encompassing.

While medication and possibly a modality (such as a short course of physical therapy) may be all that is necessary to treat an acute pain patient (who is not suffering from a significant primary problem such as cancer or a specific disk herniation), the 15% of acute pain patients who go on to become chronic pain patients need an integrated treatment paradigm.

The pain treatment armamentarium includes medication; physical therapy; occupational therapy; interventional anesthesiological procedures ("nerve blocks"); psychological treatment; neuropharmacological treatment; work hardening and much more.

What has been learned over the past several decades is that "shot-gunning" a patient with various treatments given by different providers at different places or over-reliance on narcotic pain medication will not help the patient to obtain more than a temporary "fix."

To treat only one aspect of a chronic pain patient's problem, such as using pain medication and physical therapy for a chronic soft-tissue (muscle) injury and ignoring the patient's depression, anxiety, loss of self esteem and his/her inability to return to work, may typically do more harm than good. It only potentiates the problem and makes the patient's chronic pain harder to treat. It becomes more costly in time, services and money to help these problems, and enable the patient to return to a normal life.

The International Association for the Study of pain (IASP) has defined four levels of pain treatment facilities (1). The first, the lowest level, is the single or dual modality-oriented facilities. These organizations provide treatment limited to a specific intervention, such as nerve blocks, physical therapy or biofeedback. These are the most common types of pain treatment facilities, mostly run by Interventional Anesthesiologists, who utilize nerve blocks and pain medications, on occasion with physical therapy. These health care facilities do not manage the pain condition or evaluate the patient with a comprehensive interdisciplinary approach.

The second defined entity is a "syndrome-oriented" facility, such as a headache clinic or a low back pain center; they specialize in a particular diagnosis or pain associated with a specific area of the body.

The third level, the interdisciplinary pain clinic, is a facility containing a diverse group of health care specialists and which offers evaluation and treatment of both acute and chronic pain disorders. Multiple therapeutic assessments and interventions/treatments are available, with the health care providers working as a team.

The fourth and "highest" level, the interdisciplinary pain center, is similar to the interdisciplinary pain clinics. These centers treat both acute and chronic pain disorders using a variety of health care specialists, lead by a physician pain specialist; they have the added components of research and teaching as an operating feature. Unlike the term "multidisciplinary pain clinic," where members of various disciplines may work in different locations, a key feature of the interdisciplinary pain center is that all members of the pain treatment team work "under one roof." This enhances the ability to communicate and work as a true team to help patients.

INEFFICIENCIES IN CURRENT TREATMENT METHODS

Generally speaking, pain is first encountered by the family physician who will attempt to treat it within their frame of expertise. If they need to, they may send the patient to a mono- or bimodality facility or a syndrome-oriented clinic, which treats only one form of pain problem, i.e., a "back pain" clinic, or uses one modality, such as nerve blocks. Over the course of years, the chronic pain patient may have been seen at three to six such facilities.

In terms of chronic pain patients (patients with pain for three to six months or longer), these forms of pain treatment may initially help up to 60–80% of them, leaving, in the rest, a continuous drain on health resources—insurance, workers' compensation insurance and personal finances, which will typically go on for years.

Only 6% of chronic pain patients find their way to obtain treatment at a tertiary care center for pain—a comprehensive, interdisciplinary pain management/neurorehabilitation center. As noted above, such a center is constructed around the ability to diagnose and treat all aspects of all forms of acute and chronic pain under one roof. These centers have at least one physician who is the "Captain of the Medical Ship." He/she is able to obtain the correct diagnosis, and treat with appropriate neuropharmacological medications (not typically narcotic analgesics) and design a specific treatment plan for a specific patient. The other members of the center's treatment team typically consist of a psychologist (Ph.D. or Psy.D) or psychiatrist (MD); physical therapists; occupational therapists; and nurse specialists, all on a full time basis, and any other necessary clinicians on a full or part time basis. The center most typically begins treatment by detoxifying or weaning patients off of unnecessary medications and obtaining a complete and correct diagnosis.

In a large Comprehensive Interdisciplinary Pain Management/ NeuroRehab Center (the author's), patient outcome data were kept for seven years, placing it on the Center's web site; the average patient had suffered from pain for over 5.6 years on average; 63% of the patients seen were incorrectly and or incompletely diagnosed; and 85% needed to be taken off of unnecessary medications including narcotics and barbiturates. These were significant factors in the patients' being seen at the Center. Essentially, all of the other treating clinicians had given up on these patients.

Aside from pain reduction and decreasing or eliminating inappropriate/ unnecessary opioid medications, the major outcome data from this form of treatment should also include increased physical activity; return to work where possible; closure of disability claims; stopping unnecessary medications; and reduction in health-care (over)utilization.

Patients, all too commonly, when they initially develop pain—low back pain for example (low back pain is a description, not a real diagnosis, but is frequently seen as a patient diagnosis)—become labeled with the diagnosis; physicians may rarely reevaluate the patient to ascertain if the initial diagnosis is correct. With the development of chronicity, the initial pain-related diagnosis becomes only one of several diagnoses—including, possibly, depression, anxiety disorder, and iatrogenic substance abuse—all of which must be identified and treated for the patient to achieve some return to function, wellness/work or reduction in symptomatology.

A study performed in 1995 (2) found that only 6% of all patients treated by "pain specialists" (6% = 176,850 patients) were treated at an interdisciplinary pain center. These patients were sent to these facilities almost as a "last resort," as they had already had a mean 7-year history of pain and pain treatments, with $13,284/patient/year being spent on nonsurgical pain-related health care costs. These patients also had an average of 1.7 surgeries performed at an average cost (1994–1995 dollars) of $15,000/surgery.

The cost of health care for these patients (only 6% of the pain patients seen in that year) was greater than $20 billion.

The cost of treatment at the interdisciplinary centers was greater than $1.4 billion (1995 average cost of $8100 × 176,850). The medical cost savings after one year (posttreatment at the interdisciplinary centers) was greater than $1.87 billion, an 86% reduction in health care costs (3).

Chronic pain is a biological–psychological–sociological phenomenon. If all aspects of a patient's pain are not dealt with appropriately, and simultaneously, the overall effectiveness of treatment is poor. A number of published studies go further, stating that it is the inclusion of treatment of the chronic pain patients' psychological and sociological (including economic factors—return to work) problems that enables the interdisciplinary pain centers to successfully treat these patients (4–6).

The full focus of the biological–psychological–sociological aspects of chronic pain (as well as return to work) is not dealt with in the mono- or dual-modality pain treatment facilities, or in the typical "syndrome-oriented" pain treatment facilities.

CHRONIC NONCANCER PAIN SYNDROME TREATMENT

The fact that the interdisciplinary pain center is clinically effective, cost effective and provides clinical relief that lasts during the first year posttreatment has been well documented (2,7–9).

In one systematic review, it was concluded that patients could be returned to work with nonsurgical, interdisciplinary pain center treatment (37 controlled and noncontrolled studies were evaluated) (7). In another systematic review (8), 65 controlled and noncontrolled studies were evaluated. The reviewed studies supported the effectiveness of interdisciplinary treatment but noted methodological problems existed in some of these studies.

The costs of chronic pain, particularly in the workers' compensation environment have been well documented. In 1994, the direct costs (medical costs, disability payments) and indirect costs (training substitute workers, paying them, legal costs) for injured workers equaled $171 billion. In 1999, the total financial impact of workers' compensation injuries (direct and indirect) equaled more than $240 billion. A day lost from work equals 1 day's salary times 3.75, a significant cost when one looks at over 20 million days a year lost from work, just from headache.

Another study found that treatment at an interdisciplinary center was more clinically effective and more cost effective than the traditional treatment methods, including medication; surgery; interventional procedures (nerve blocks); noninvasive treatment modalities such as physical therapy; and implantable devices such as spinal cord stimulators and medication pumps (10).

It was also found that the cost to return one injured worker after treatment at an interdisciplinary pain center was $11,913, while the cost to return one patient to work after back surgery was $75,000. The cost to return patients to work indicates that treatment at an interdisciplinary pain center is 6.3 times more cost effective than surgery (3).

As medicine is starting to be driven by cost and outcome data, such information is extremely important. Also, as noted earlier, the myofascial pain syndrome is one of the, if not the, most common cause of chronic noncancer pain syndrome patients. Research has noted that there is "overwhelming, consistent meta-analytic evidence that pain facilities provide effective treatment for a wide range of outcome variables for such patients" (11). The same study notes that referring physicians should be aware of the type of pain treatment facility to which they send their patients, as not all facilities use the same treatment methods.

An EBM review (from the Cochrane Database) entitled "Multidisciplinary rehabilitation for FMG and musculoskeletal pain in working age results" which used a different definition of multidisciplinary pain management than pain specialists use, found all poor studies and stated the level of scientific evidence regarding multidisciplinary pain rehabilitation for "these diagnosis (sic) is limited" (12).

When utilizing more commonly accepted criteria, another systematic review (from the Cochrane Database) entitled "Multidisciplinary Bio-psycho-social rehabilitation for chronic low back pain" (13) concluded that evidence showed intensive (>100 hours of therapy) interdisciplinary bio-psycho-social pain rehabilitation programs with a functional restoration approach engendered greater improvements in pain and function for patients with "disabling chronic low back pain," then did non-multidisciplinary rehabilitation or "usual care."

Please note that some utilize the terms "interdisciplinary" and "multidisciplinary" synonymously—as is done here, while others use them differently. Of interest, the term "multidisciplinary" predated and in some ways, has been "updated" to "interdisciplinary."

Finally, dual diagnosis multidisciplinary pain programs which deal with chronic noncancer pain and substance abusing patients are also found to work well (14).

Turk and Burwinkle (15) note an "epidemic of 'Mural Dyslexia'," the "inability to read the handwriting on the wall." They note that outcome data are necessary and important to have for the sake of the payers as well as the patients. They reiterate that there is a large cohort of published information indicating that the interdisciplinary pain centers are clinically effective, cost effective and via their treatment paradigm, able to provide significant savings in health care and disability payments.

In an important study, Robbins et al. (16) noted that patients in their interdisciplinary pain management programs who were forced by insurance company "carve outs" to have physical therapy elsewhere experienced negative treatment outcomes at one year, in comparison to those patients who were able to participate in the full, intact program.

The restoration of function must be a primary goal of all interdisciplinary treatment programs. Rehabilitation, while it focuses on function and not specifically pain, is associated with decreased pain and improvements in psychological status as function improves (17).

A recent study looking at a more abbreviated "comprehensive pain management programme" including education, cognitive and behavioral interventions for patients experiencing neuropathic pain status—post spinal cord injury were considered an important and valuable complement to the patients' treatment (18).

FIBROMYALGIA TREATMENT STUDIES

A half-day treatment program for FMS was done by Kaiser Permanente and evaluated by patient questionnaires (19). It was found to be helpful in both mental health and functional measures.

Another FMS study (20) found that when interdisciplinary treatment was customized, based on patients' individualized psychosocial needs, outcomes are enhanced.

Davidson (21) indicates that a multidisciplinary treatment approach to FMS patients offers the best method to achieving effective pain relief.

Other studies also show the efficacy of interdisciplinary pain management programs for FMS patients (22,23).

MORE RECENT DATA

The Swiss have noted that there are high-quality randomized controlled trials which indicated that multidisciplinary pain programs represented the best therapeutic option in the treatment of complex chronic pain issues, as well as the lack of work being done to appropriately treat chronic pain and deal with both the direct and indirect costs of chronic pain. Further, they note the need for more well-designed, interdisciplinary and internationally comparable studies to help contribute to the prevention of some future pain states (24).

The Japanese have also noted the efficacy of interdisciplinary treatment for chronic noncancer pain patients (25).

Turk et al. (26) also note that while none of the most commonly prescribed pain treatment regimens are by themselves sufficient to eliminate pain, a more realistic approach, they felt, would most likely combine pharmacological, physical and psychological components tailored to individual patient needs.

That both multidisciplinary and interdisciplinary pain management programs deal with the biopsychosocial model of chronic pain, one of the most important aspects of these programs are felt to be the collaborative communication among the various clinical team members, the patient and the case manager (27,28). It is important to note here that the chronic pain patient is also a member of the interdisciplinary pain management team.

The military, which had one of the first interdisciplinary pain programs established at Walter Reed Hospital, also notes the importance and efficacy of such programs for treating currently returning veterans with polytrauma injuries as well as a high prevalence of brain injuries, cognitive impairment as well as emotional distress (29,30).

It has also been noted that interdisciplinary biopsychosocial models of pain management treatment are effective in the treatment of pain-associated disability in children and adolescents (31).

TECHNIQUE

In over a quarter century of private practice, the author has found that neurological and musculoskeletal examination and diagnosis come first—then, if the patient has chronic pain and needs an interdisciplinary treatment program, the physical therapist, the psychologist and the occupational therapist perform evaluations. The entire team then meets and discusses diagnoses and examination findings.

An individualized interdisciplinary treatment program is then determined, if found to be appropriate.

The team meets weekly to discuss the patient's progress or lack of progress in each individual treatment modality. In many cases, the patient may join the staff to discuss how his/her treatment is progressing. During the weekly team staff meeting, each clinician who is treating a specific patient gives his/her report of the patient's progress or lack of progress during the past week.

The interdisciplinary team is the most important treatment tool available to the chronic pain patient. Each member of the team should be "cross trained" regarding the basics of each other's discipline. It is not unusual for a patient to tell the physical therapist, rather than the physician or the psychologist, of his or her feelings of suicidality. The physical therapist would need to understand how to deal with this information without abreacting, and know how to deal with the patient while waiting for the physician who they immediately notify, to come to talk to the patient.

The clinic's nurse specialists should be the patients' internal case managers, who make certain that all orders from the physician and/or the rest of the treatment team have been carried out. The nurse also serves as each patient's primary liaison with the physician and the team. The nurse's role is of extreme importance. They must have a good degree of knowledge about pain medicine, and medication. For one thing, some physicians never give medication refills—patients must call each month for refills, and the nurse is responsible for determining if the patient has been taking their medications on a timely fashion, and discussing any problems with the physician. Training is well worth the time and effort for the nurse and the entire team.

The weekly team staffings are also the best time to have appropriate third party visitors come to the clinic. This would include outside nurse case managers or, if they can get away, adjustors. The patient's attorney may desire to attend such a staff meeting.

Interdisciplinary pain management programs have been the most medically efficacious, time and cost-effective treatment paradigm for the chronic non-cancer pain patients with a chronic MPS or FMS. Unfortunately, there is a very limited number of this type of treatment facility. Many excellent programs at prestigious medical institutions have been forced to close secondary to poor insurance reimbursement.

The dwindling number of these programs bodes poorly for the chronic pain patient, and their insurers, for the reasons—both clinical and financial—noted above.

REFERENCES

1. Loeser JD. Desirable characteristics for pain treatment facilities: report of the IASP taskforce. In: Bond MR, Charleon JE, Woolf CJ, eds. Proceedings of the Sixth World Congress on Pain. Seattle: International Association for the Study of Pain, 1991: 411–415.
2. Marketdata Enterprises. Chronic pain management programs: a market analysis. Tampa, FL: Marketdata Enterprises, 1995.
3. Turk DC, Loeser JD, Monarch ES. Chronic pain: purposes and costs of interdisciplinary pain rehabilitation programs. Trends Evidence-Based Neuropsychiatry 2002; 4(2):64–69.
4. Roy R. Pain clinics: reassessment of objectives and outcomes. Arch Phys Med Rehabil 1984; 65(8):448–451.
5. Rosomoff HL, Rosomoff RS. Comprehensive multidisciplinary pain center approach to the treatment of low back pain. Neurosurg Clin N Am 1991; 2:877–890.
6. Becker N, Hojsted J, Sjogren P, et al. Sociodemographic predictors of treatment outcome in chronic non-malignant pain patients. Do patients receiving or applying

for disability pension benefit from multidisciplinary pain treatment? Pain 1998; 77: 279–287.

7. Cutler RB, Fishbain DA, Rosomoff HL, et al. Does nonsurgical pain center treatment of chronic pain return patients to work? A review and meta-analysis of the literature. Spine 1994; 19(6):643–652.

8. Flor H, Fydich T, Turk DC. Efficacy of multidisciplinary pain treatment centers: a meta-analytic review. Pain 1992; 49:221–230.

9. Chapman SL, Brena SF, Bradford LA. Treatment outcome in a chronic pain rehabilitation problem. Pain 1981; 11:155–268.

10. Turk DC, Okifuji A. Treatment of chronic pain patients: clinical outcomes, cost-effectiveness and cost-benefits of multidisciplinary pain centers. Crit Rev Phys Med Rehabil 1998; 10:181–208.

11. Fishbain DA, Cutler R, Rosomoff H, et al. Pain facilities: a review of their effectiveness and referral selection criteria. Curr Headache Pain Rep 1997; 1(2):107–115.

12. Karjalainen K, Malmivaara A, van Tulder M, et al. Multidisciplinary rehabilitation for fibromyalgia an musculoskeletal pain in working age adults (Cochrane Review). In: The Cochrane Library, Issue 4. Oxford: Update Software, 2002.

13. Guzman J, Esmail R, Karjalainen KI, et al. Multidisciplinary bio-psycho-social rehabilitation for chronic low back pain (Cochrane Review). In: The Cochrane Library, Issue 4. Oxford: Update Software, 2002.

14. Mahoney ND, Devine JE, Angres D. Multidisciplinary treatment of benign chronic pain syndrome in substance abusing patients. Curr Rev Pain 1999; 3:321–331.

15. Turk D, Burwinkle T. Treatment of chronic pain sufferers—an antidote to mural dyslexia. The Pain Practitioner (American Academy of Pain Management) 2004; 14(3):20–25.

16. Robbins H, Gatchel RJ, Noe C, et al. A prospective one-year outcome study of interdisciplinary chronic pain management: compromising its efficacy by managed care policies. Anesth Analg 2003; 97(1):156–162.

17. Schofferman J. Restoration of function: the missing link in pain medicine? Pain Med 2006; 7(Suppl 1):S159–S165.

18. Norrbrink Budh C, Kowalski J, Lundeberg T. A comprehensive pain management programme comprising educational, cognitive and behavioural interventions for neuropathic pain following spinal cord injury. J Rehabil Med 2006; 38(3): 172–180.

19. Beck A, Breth G, Ellis J, et al. Multidisciplinary group intervention for fibromyalgia: a study of psychiatric symptom and functional disability outcomes. Permanente J 2002; 6(2). Available at www.kaiserpermanente.org/medicine/permjournal/spring02/fibromyaglia.html.

20. Turk DC, Okifuji A, Sinclair JD, et al. Differential responses by psychosocial subgroups of fibromyalgia syndrome patients to an interdisciplinary treatment. Arthritis Care Res 1998; 11(5):397–404.

21. Davidson P. Fibromyalgia: a painful and treatable illness. San Francisco Medical Society. Available at www.sfms.org/sfm/sfm202b.htm.

22. Bennett RM, Burckhardt CS, Clark SR, et al. Group treatment of fibromyalgia: a 6 month outpatient program. J Rheumatol 23(3):521–528.

23. Bennett RM. Multidisciplinary group programs to treat fibromyalgia patients. Rheum Dis Clin North Am 1996; 22(2):351–367.

24. Scascighini L, Sprott H. Chronic nonmalignant pain: a challenge for patients and clinicians. Nat Clin Pract Rheumatol 2008; 4(2):74–81.

25. Kitahara M, Kojima KK, Ohmura A. Efficacy of interdiscilinary treatment for chronic nonmalignant pain patients in Japan. Clin J Pain 2006; 22(7):647–655.

26. Turk DC, Swanson KS, Tunks ER. Psyhological approaches in the treatment of chronic pain patients—when pills, scalpels and needles are not enough. Can J Psychol 2008; 53(4):213–223.

27. Stanos S, Houle TT. Multidisciplinary and interdisciplinary management of chronic pain. Phys Med Rehabil Clin N Am 2006; 17(2):435–450, vii.

28. Stanos S, McLean J, Rader L. Physical medicine rehabilitation approach to pain. Anesthesiol Clin 2007; 25(4):721–759, v–vi.
29. Clark ME, Scholten JD, Walker RL, et al. Assessment and treatment of pain associated with combat-related polytrauma. Pain Med 2009; 10(3):456–469.
30. Gatchell RJ, McGeary DD, Peterson A, et al. Preliminary findings of a randomized controlled trial of an interdisciplinary military pain program. Mil Med 2009; 174(3): 270–277.
31. Maynard CS, Amari A, Wieczorek B, et al. Interdisciplinary behavioral rehabilitation of pediatyric pain-associated disability: retrospective review of an inpatient treatment program. J Pediatr Psychol Advance Access published on May 22, 2009; doi:10.1093/jpepsy/jsp038.

13

Interventional Pain Medicine in the Treatment of Chronic Noncancer Pain—An Update

Gary W. Jay

Clinical Disease Area Expert-Pain, Pfizer, Inc., New London, Connecticut, U.S.A.

DIFFERENT WAYS OF LOOKING AT EVIDENCE-BASED MEDICINE

Strength of Recommendations[a]

The U.S. Preventive Services Task Force (USPSTF) grades its recommendations according to one of five classifications (A, B, C, D, I) reflecting the strength of evidence and magnitude of net benefit (benefits minus harms).

A. —The USPSTF strongly recommends that clinicians provide [the service] to eligible patients. The USPSTF found good evidence that [the service] improves important health outcomes and concludes that benefits substantially outweigh harms.

B. —The USPSTF recommends that clinicians provide [this service] to eligible patients. The USPSTF found at least fair evidence that [the service] improves important health outcomes and concludes that benefits outweigh harms.

C. —The USPSTF makes no recommendation for or against routine provision of [the service]. The USPSTF found at least fair evidence that [the service] can improve health outcomes but concludes that the balance of benefits and harms is too close to justify a general recommendation.

D. —The USPSTF recommends against routinely providing [the service] to asymptomatic patients. The USPSTF found at least fair evidence that [the service] is ineffective or that harms outweigh benefits.

I. —The USPSTF concludes that the evidence is insufficient to recommend for or against routinely providing [the service]. Evidence that the [service] is effective is lacking, of poor quality, or conflicting and the balance of benefits and harms cannot be determined.

QUALITY OF EVIDENCE

The USPSTF grades the quality of the overall evidence for a service on a three-point scale (good, fair, poor):

---

[a]U.S. Preventive Services Task Force Ratings: Strength of Recommendations and Quality of Evidence. *Guide to Clinical Preventive Services, Third Edition: Periodic Updates*, 2000–2003. Agency for Healthcare Research and Quality, Rockville, MD. http://www.ahrq.gov/clinic/3rduspstf/ratings.htm. Accessed Aug 22, 2008.

Good: Evidence includes consistent results from well-designed, well-conducted studies in representative populations that directly assess effects on health outcomes.

Fair: Evidence is sufficient to determine effects on health outcomes, but the strength of the evidence is limited by the number, quality, or consistency of the individual studies, generalizability to routine practice, or indirect nature of the evidence on health outcomes.

Poor: Evidence is insufficient to assess the effects on health outcomes because of limited number or power of studies, important flaws in their design or conduct, gaps in the chain of evidence, or lack of information on important health outcomes.

Systems to stratify evidence by quality have been developed, such as this one by the U.S. Preventive Services Task Force for ranking evidence about the effectiveness of treatments or screening:

- Level I: Evidence obtained from at least one properly designed randomized controlled trial.
- Level II-1: Evidence obtained from well-designed controlled trials without randomization.
- Level II-2: Evidence obtained from well-designed cohort or case–control analytic studies, preferably from more than one center or research group.
- Level II-3: Evidence obtained from multiple time series with or without the intervention. Dramatic results in uncontrolled trials might also be regarded as this type of evidence.
- Level III: Opinions of respected authorities, based on clinical experience, descriptive studies, or reports of expert committees.

OXFORD CENTRE FOR EVIDENCE-BASED
MEDICINE LEVELS OF EVIDENCE (MAY 2001)[b]

The UK National Health Service uses a similar system with categories labeled A, B, C, and D. The above levels are only appropriate for treatment or interventions; different types of research are required for assessing diagnostic accuracy or natural history and prognosis, and hence different "levels" are required. For example, the Oxford Centre for Evidence-based Medicine suggests levels of evidence (LOE) according to the study designs and critical appraisal of prevention, diagnosis, prognosis, therapy, and harm studies (1):

- Level A: Consistent randomized controlled clinical trial, cohort study, all or none (see the note below), clinical decision rule validated in different populations.
- Level B: Consistent retrospective cohort, exploratory cohort, ecological study, outcomes research, case–control study, or extrapolations from level A studies.
- Level C: Case-series study or extrapolations from level B studies.
- Level D: Expert opinion without explicit critical appraisal, or based on physiology, bench research or first principles.

---

[b]http://www.cebm.net/index.aspx?o = 1025. Accessed Aug 22,2008.

The use of interventional pain medicine techniques continues to grow, with encouragement from insurance companies. Unfortunately, the published evidence-based medicine remains unconvincing. It is the stakeholders of this form of pain treatment who write for other stakeholders, sometimes contradicting each other.

The majority of Pain Medicine specialists remain interventional anesthesiologists; a decade or so ago, this was not the case.

The majority of Interventional Pain Medicine specialists are anesthesiologists, many of whom have done a fellowship for additional certification in interventional pain medicine. There are currently an increasing number of physiatrists and neurologists who can take a pain fellowship which gives them the ability to perform interventional procedures.

Much or most of this treatment, according to interventional anesthesiologists (multiple private communications), is based on finding an abnormality on the CAT scan or MRI.

This appears to ignore the literature demonstrating that many people with abnormalities that can be found on MRI or CAT scan are pain free (2,3–5).

Boden et al. (2) found that out of 67 pain-free individuals, who had no history of low-back pain, sciatica, or neurogenic claudication, about one-third had substantial abnormalities on lumbosacral MRIs. Of the patients with age less than 60 years, 20% had a herniated nucleus pulposis, and one had spinal stenosis. In the patients who were 60 years of age or older, 57% had abnormal MRIs, with 36% having herniated nucleus pulposus (HNP) and 21% having spinal stenosis. Thirty-five percent of the subjects between 20 and 39 years of age had degeneration or bulging of a disk at least one level.

Jensen's study in the NEJM (3) looked at the MRI of the lumbar spine in 98 asymptomatic subjects. Fifty-two percent had a disk bulge at least one level; 27% had a disk protrusion; and 1% had an extrusion. Thirty-eight percent had abnormalities in more than one intervertebral disk. Annular defects were found in 14% of patients, and facet arthropathy was found in 8% of patients. No substantial differences were seen between men and women. The authors commented that the discovery by MRI of bulges or disk protrusions in people with low back pain may "frequently be coincidental."

Stadnik et al. (4) found that annular tears and focal disk protrusions on MRI images were frequently found in an asymptomatic population. Savage et al. (5) found that 32% of asymptomatic subjects had "abnormal" lumbar spines and 47% of subjects with complaints of LBP had "normal" lumbar MRIs ($n = 149$ subjects; 78 aged 20–30 and 71 aged 31–58 years).

The majority of physicians with a patient in pain will gladly send their patients to the interventionalist, many of whom will also use pain medications too often while they are doing their injections. Patients who show improvements may do so secondary to pain medications. This solves the referring physician's problems: they don't want to prescribe pain medications in today's fear-ridden atmosphere regarding opioid use.

Another issue is that the proliferation of interventionalists along with insurance companies that do not want to pay for anything else (except possibly two to four physical therapy treatments prior to a two-week stop to get more treatments approved, and definitely not psychotherapy) makes other types of treatment difficult to access.

Also, pain medication, for the most part, is far cheaper than neurorehabilitative treatment.

An evaluation of the interventional pain medicine literature, using an evidence-based medicine (EBM) approach is extremely interesting. There are four basic levels (some consider five) of EBM:

Level 1—strong research-based evidence—several high-quality RCTs (randomized controlled trials); high-quality scientific studies done well with homogeneous results; one or more meta-analyses

Level II—moderate research-based evidence—at least ONE relevant RCT or several adequate studies

Level III—limited research-based evidence—no RCT; at least one adequate scientific study

Level IV—no scientific evidence—expert panel evaluations; other published case studies

Evidence-based medicine is commonly defined as "The conscientious, explicit, and judicious use of current evidence in making decisions about the care of individual patients. The practice of evidence based medicine means integrating individual clinical expertise with the best available external clinical evidence from systematic research" (6).

There is a lack of scientific evidence regarding the value of interventional procedures secondary, at least in part, to significant and unnecessary variation in the provision of interventional pain procedures (6,7). Further, a review of the literature shows that in spite of unclear criteria and "uncertain long-term value" (8) regarding facet injections, Medicare was billed $60 million for these procedures in 2001. The Medpac (9) study shows different rates of usage of the various interventional procedures which were geographically based. This poses the question: if these therapies are the most up-to-date and efficacious procedures for pain in the hands of physicians of adequate and equivalent training, why should such geographic barriers/variations occur?

Friedly et al. (7,10) published several times after reviewing Medical Physician part B claims for 1994–2001. During that time, there was a 271% increase in lumbar epidural steroid injections (ESIs) and a 231% increase in facet injections. They noted that while lumbosacral injections increased significantly, less than half were performed for sciatica or radiculopathy, indicating, they felt, a lack of consensus regarding the indications for ESIs, as well as a cause for concern regarding large increases in costs for these procedures, from $24 million to more than $175 million, generally, and individual costs increased from $115 to $227 per injection (7).

A year later, Friedly et al. published on geographic variation in ESI use in Medicare patients, noting a substantial geographic variation in the USA, with the Southern states having the highest procedure rates, and the northeast the lowest (10).

In 2001, Medicare paid physician charges of over $370 million for interventional pain procedures, not including facility fees (10). The national bill in 2001 for physician charges, alone, for interventional pain procedures for acute, chronic, and cancer-related pain would be higher than $1.8 billion (as Medicare pays on average 21% of the total national bill for physician charges) (11).

The question of the efficacy of interventional pain procedures and the EBM used to determine such efficacy is, therefore, markedly important, as an enormous amount of medical fees is paid on a yearly basis for interventional pain procedures by such national programs.

There are multiple treatment guidelines for the same clinical problem. The question is which guideline should be/must be used, and why.

Such treatment guidelines are based on expert opinion, systematic reviews, and meta-analyses. Ioannidis et al. (1) note that significant problems may exist between the findings of large trials and meta-analyses including significant discrepancies secondary to heterogeneity of study populations and treatment protocols and bias. Another group (8) noted that at least 90% of meta-analyses of interventional pain management studies had serious flaws in methodology. This would create an amplification of the negative effect of a poor-quality RCT by its inclusion in a meta-analysis, inducing a 30% to 50% overestimation of the value of the intervention being evaluated (12–14).

Merrill (12), an anesthesiologist, notes that interventional pain medicine is based on the belief in the "value of acute, invasive interventions in chronic disease." He further notes that "EBM has befallen interventional pain therapy early in the development of both and has found that the scientific underpinnings of these invasive therapies are as yet unprepared for scrutiny."

Boas (8) noted that when nerve blocks are used for diagnostic rather than treatment purposes, they are "only as good as the detailed clinical examinations which precede and follow the block itself." This would necessitate performing a thorough neurological examination, as well as, possibly, a neuromuscular evaluation.

One of the questions here is whether acute invasive intervention can effectively intervene in a chronic disease process. Chronic pain is considered by many to be a chronic disease; these individuals think that it should be treated as one, and they are doubtful that a few epidural steroid injections (ESIs) (i.e., one to three series of three ESIs) will stop a chronic biological–psychological–social disease process. Proponents of interventional pain medicine appear to disagree with this issue.

There is apparent chaos in the ranks. A recent study found that there is no clear consensus as to the best or ideal method to use in the performance of an epidural steroid injection (ESI): whether fluoroscopy should or should not be used, or a transforaminal approach should be taken or not (15).

Smuck et al. recommends the use of live fluoroscopy to observe dynamic contrast flow during transforaminal ESIs (16). Barre et al. stated that a caudally placed, fluoroscopy-guided ESI appeared to be a safe, minimally invasive option for managing pain from lumbar spinal stenosis (17). Ergin et al. indicated that fluoroscopic guidance for caudal epidural Tuohy needle placement without real-time imaging could result in inadvertent intravenous injection of the drug. In this study they found 4 of 10 cases that had intravenous leakage of drug when real-time fluoroscopic imaging was used. They recommended real-time imaging in addition to routine fluoroscopic guidance for caudal epidural procedures (18).

Cooper et al. (19) found fluoroscopic transforaminal ESIs to be effective nonsurgical treatment options for patients who suffered with degenerative lumbar stenosis and radiculopathy and should be performed, or at least considered prior to surgical intervention.

A cautionary study found a significant risk of serious neurological injury after cervical transforaminal ESIs. They wrote that, possibly via an embolic mechanism, secondary to an inadvertent intra-arterial injection of particulate corticosteroid, a distal infarct can occur. They also describe embolism to the distal basilar artery region which can cause midbrain, pons, cerebellum, thalamus, temporal and occipital lobe infarctions (20).

The answer to the question "What is the most effective treatment for acute low back pain?" asked in the *Journal of Family Practice* in February 2002 included the statement "There is no consistent evidence that epidural steroid injections are effective for acute low back pain (evidence grade: D)" (21).

Sciatica, or sciatic pain, is a common sequela of a HNP. Watts and Silagy (22) did a meta-analysis on the efficacy of ESIs in the treatment of sciatica and describe "quantitative evidence from meta-analysis of pooled data from randomized trials that epidural administration of corticosteroids is effective in the management of lumbosacral radicular pain." Then Carette et al. (23) did a RCT to evaluate the efficacy of up to three ESIs in the treatment of sciatic pain secondary to an HNP. They found that while ESIs with methylprednisolone could afford short-term decrements in leg pain and sensory changes in the lower extremities, they offered no significant functional benefit and did not reduce the need for surgery.

Southern et al. (24) found that after a follow-up of more than two years, the efficacy of fluoroscopically guided caudal ESIs in patients with chronic lumbar discogenic pain was poor. Furthermore, they noted that the patients who responded to injection had significantly lower initial, preinjection pain scores.

Twelve controlled trials found ESIs to be effective in six (25–30), and in six studies (31–36) ESIs were found to be no different than placebo or reference treatment. As these trials go back to the early 1970s, there are certainly better ways to perform these trials currently. Koes et al. (37) note that many, if not most, of these trials had significant methodological problems. They found that the best studies showed inconsistent results of ESIs and they concluded that the efficacy of ESIs had not been established. They felt that the benefits of ESIs, if any, appeared to be only of short duration.

There are studies favorable to interventional procedures. Nimgade et al. (38) found steroid injections for lateral epicondylosis are the most successful short-term intervention for pain relief. Active physical therapy was efficacious no matter what the time frame.

Delport et al. (39) treated patients with lumbar spinal stenosis with ESIs under fluoroscopy. Of 140 patients, 32% noted more than two months of pain relief; 39% reported less than two months of pain relief; and 29% noted no relief from the injections. Twenty percent had surgery. Of note, 53% noted better functioning, and 74% were at least somewhat satisfied with their treatment.

Rosen (40) found that 50% of patients with low back pain and sciatica with radicular symptoms who received ESIs received temporary relief. Long-term relief was seen in fewer than 25% of patients.

In one study, Butterman (41) found that ESIs were not as effective as discectomy in their ability to reduce symptoms and disability associated with HNPs in the lumbar region. He noted that ESIs did have a role: they were found to be effective for up to three years in almost 50% of patients who had not had improvement with six or more weeks of noninvasive care.

In a more ambitious study, looking at the place of minimally invasive procedures in the treatment of chronic low back pain (CLBP), Cahana et al. (42) noted the contradictory interventional literature. They found that there was moderate evidence (via small randomized, nonrandomized, single-group, or matched case–control studies) for medial branch neurotomy and limited evidence (nonexperimental one or more center studies) for intradiscal treatments in mechanical LBP. They found moderate evidence for the use of transforaminal ESIs, lumbar percutaneous adhesiolysis, and spinal endoscopy for lumbar radiculopathy. They found no "gold standard treatment" for CLBP.

It was noted that the conflicting information from various reviews of ESIs made it difficult for general practitioners to determine how or if they should be used. Hopayian and Mugford (43) indicated that the choice of methods used for systematic reviews may alter views about the medical evidence.

McLain et al. (5) noted that clinical studies have alternatively either supported or refuted the efficacy of ESIs in the treatment of patients with back and leg pain. They noted that steroid medications did benefit some patients with radicular pain, but the benefits were limited in duration, thereby making efficacy over time difficult to prove. They also indicated the need for good randomized, controlled trials to identify those patients most likely to benefit from ESIs and when and for how long.

A recent study found only moderate evidence for the use of transforaminal ESIs, along with lumbar percutaneous adhesiolysis and spinal endoscopy for pain resulting from lumbar radiculopathy (44).

DePalma and Slipman (45) using so-called evidence-informed information (see below) note that no well-designed studies of ESIs in CLBP have been designed to evaluate the efficacy of transforaminal ESIs in treating discogenic CLBP. The existing evidence appears to indicate that non-target-specific ESIs are effective for short-term improvement in nonspecific CLBP. Furthermore, one to three ESIs appear to be effective in reducing nonspecific CLBP in the short term.

Tong et al. (46) called into question the practice of giving ESIs to patients who were on SSDI/workers' compensation and/or had work requiring heavy lifting.

Slipman et al. (47) did an EBM analysis of the current literature and indicated that current studies gave only sparse evidence to support the use of interventional techniques in the treatment of lumbar zygapophysial joint-mediated low back pain. A more recent article found that no conservative treatment has been found to be effective for lumbar Z joint pain. Controlled trials indicated that intra-articular injections of steroids were no more effective than placebo treatment. Bogduk concluded that denervation of the lumbar Z joints remained the only available treatment (48).

Other data show similar findings. Nelemans et al. (49) showed, in their Cochrane Database EBM evaluation of RCTs of injection therapy for pain relief in patients with LBP, that convincing evidence for the effects of injection therapies for LBP is lacking and that there was a need for more and better designed trials.

Nelemans et al. (50) updated these data in 2007 specifically to evaluate the effectiveness of injection therapy in patients with low back pain lasting longer than one month. They reviewed 21 randomized trials. Only 11 studies compared active injections with placebo injections. The methodologic quality of many studies was considered low, with only three well-designed, explanatory trials (RCTs).

They concluded that convincing evidence was still lacking on the effects of injection therapies for low back pain.

Staal et al. (51), in a Cochrane review, state that there is insufficient evidence to support the use of injection therapy in subacute and chronic low back pain. They note that there may be a subpopulation that would benefit from this therapy.

In another Cochrane review, Peloso et al. (52) state that an epidural injection of a corticosteroid and local anesthetic seems to reduce pain and improve function for patients with chronic neck pain who also have associated arm symptoms, but there are not enough studies to indicate which drug is best to use.

The Therapeutics and Technology Assessment subcommittee of the American Academy of Neurology concluded that ESIs may result in some improvement in radicular lumbosacral pain between two and six weeks after the injection compared to control treatments (level C evidence), with the average magnitude of effect being small and possibly limited to a subgroup of patients. In general, ESIs for radicular lumbosacral pain do not affect average impairment of function or need for surgery, or provide long-term pain relieve beyond three months, and their routine use for these indications was not recommended. Finally, there was insufficient evidence to make any recommendation for the use of ESIs to treat radicular cervical pain (53).

Bogduk (34) found that while the literature endorses the use of ESIs, there are little compelling data on rationale and efficacy for the procedure. In a more recent paper, Bogduk (54) stated "The apparent efficacy of lumbar intra-articular steroids is no greater than that of a sham injection. There is no justification for the continued use of this intervention. Better outcomes can be achieved with deliberate placebo therapy."

Valet et al. (55) looked at the efficacy of ESIs in a RCT comparing prednisolone to saline administered to patients with sciatica. They found that the efficacy of saline could not be excluded, but ESIs provided no additional improvement.

Rozenberg et al. (56) did a review of 13 trials published between 1966 and 1997. They concluded that they could not determine if ESIs were effective in common LBP and sciatica.

A study by Lafuma et al. (57) looking at the cost-effectiveness of ESIs requiring in-hospital management for lumbosciatic syndrome found that adding an epidural injection as a first-line treatment to the rest and the use of nonsteroidal antiinflammatory medication resulted in additional costs and no gain in efficacy.

An editorial in the *British Medical Journal* (58) notes that evidence for the efficacy of ESIs for LBP is equivocal; they may be useful as adjunctive treatment in some patients with symptoms lasting longer than three months in the absence of indicators of "chronic pain," and in patients who may have radicular symptoms.

A review by the Institute for Clinical Systems Improvement looked at fluoroscopically guided transforaminal ESIs for lumbar radicular pain and found that they are generally safe, but there was insufficient evidence to comment on the efficacy of ESIs (59).

Zhou et al. (60) looked at quality assurance for interventional pain management procedures and noted that a good QA program was helpful. They did a survey of 566 patients and found that the majority had immediate pain relief after a procedure. No follow-up was done, however, to determine if the decrement in pain persisted, or for how long. A number of different interventional pain management procedures were involved.

In an effort to look at the costs of interventional procedures in the USA, Straus (34) noted that the costs of interventional treatment for spinal pain were minimally $13 billion in 1990, with costs growing 7% per year. Cost minimization analysis suggested that ESIs under fluoroscopy "may not be justified by the current literature."

The findings noted above are also found in the German literature where Hildebrandt (61) found that intra-articular injections of steroids offered no greater benefit than normal saline and that long-lasting success from this procedure was lacking.

Vad et al. (62) state that they did a randomized study to evaluate the efficacy of transforaminal ESIs. However, the study was not blinded or randomized—patients were "randomized by choice." The data, secondary to these significant methodological problems, are not objective.

Patients, in a retrospective study done by Lin et al. (48), who had failed conservative treatment for cervical pain and were otherwise surgical candidates were given a trial of cervical ESIs, which were found to be a reasonable choice for the nonoperative treatment of patients with symptomatic cervical disk herniations. Cervical ESIs are less studied than lumbar ESIs and have "less support" than lumbar and caudal ESIs (63).

A RCT looking at intradiscal steroid therapy for lumbar spinal discogenic pain found that intradiscal steroid injections did not improve clinical outcome in patients with discogenic back pain compared to placebo (64).

A systematic review of spinal cord stimulation identified 1 RCT, 1 cohort study, and 72 case studies. Taylor et al. (65) found the level of evidence for the efficacy of spinal cord stimulation in chronic back and leg pain was only "moderate."

Two studies of percutaneous vertebroplasty done in the same time period found, in one case, that the procedure was safe and useful (66), while the other noted that there were no data from controlled clinical trials or from studies with long-term follow-up and that the procedure was still investigational but may be appropriate for patients with no other treatment options (67).

Neurolytic blocks have long been used for the management of cancer pain. Its use for noncancer pain is increasing. It is noted that neurolysis should be used for noncancer pain only after a patient has failed an aggressive interdisciplinary pain management program (68).

Abram (69) notes that it is difficult to determine if interventional procedures are truly effective, and further, there are almost no data on whether or not they are cost effective. He makes a number of conclusions that bear further evaluation:

1. Some patients do obtain excellent and lasting pain relief with all interventional techniques, but the same can be found in placebo studies.
2. ESIs are widely used, but there are little good data regarding efficacy, and recruiting patients for a blinded, definitive outcome study would be very difficult.
3. There is minimal evidence, if any, suggesting that fluoroscopic translaminar, transforaminal, caudal or epiduroscopic ESIs are safer or more effective than

the older "blind" translaminar approach—no comparison studies have been done.

4. Steroid facet injections can give temporary and, on occasion, prolonged relief for some patients with axial back pain, but no evidence is noted that they are more effective or longer lasting than placebo.

5. Radiofrequency ablation of lumbar facet nerves is more effective than sham procedures and gives longer lasting relief than facet injections.

6. Intradiscal electrotherapy (IDET) studies have not shown good evidence for efficacy.

More recent data show that the IDET procedure provides only "modest" improvement but is less destructive, cheaper and safer than other invasive procedures. There is less functional improvement than possible improvement in pain. Patients can also report a worsening of pain from a variety of different factors after the procedure (70).

Another common interventional procedure is discography. Carragee (71) notes that the rate of low-pressure painful injections in subjects without chronic LBP is approximately 25% and correlates with both anatomic and psychosocial factors. False positives may be more apt to be seen in specific subgroups. It has also been noted that discography is not validated, and is painful in 30% to 80% of asymptomatic subjects, and at best care, may have a positive predictive value of only 50% to 60% for resolution of LBP after surgical removal of a suspected pain generator identified by discography (72).

Minimally invasive nuclear decompression using nucleoplasty can be used prior to fusion or arthroplasty, but the evidence does not support the current device for the treatment of back pain alone. Derby et al. (73) feel the procedure is better suited for patients with referred extremity pain and protrusions of less than 4 to 6 mm, minimal stenosis, and relatively good disk heights.

Haldeman and Dagenais (72) describe a relatively new concept. Those physicians who feel that EBM is important, ideally with associated multiple high-quality RCTs supporting, in this case, interventions, are possibly disappointed that none exist. They note that, from authors having great and long clinical experience, "evidence-informed," rather than evidence-based, recommendations can be given. They state that the major principle behind evidence-informed medical management is that an author should be aware of and use research evidence when it is available, but make personal recommendations based on clinical experience when it is not. Unfortunately, this concept appears to be used only for interventional pain medicine.

Boswell (74) described new practice guidelines written by the American Society of Interventional Pain Physicians (ASIPP), which were presented in 2005 (75). The conclusions of this publication are based on much the same published information, yet are very different. Note that these recommendations were developed from "all types of evidence." Furthermore, "if an evidence-based approach failed to provide adequate levels of evidence, consensus and expert opinions were utilized." This would unfortunately fail the EBM established tests for the highest reliability of evidence, or at the very least make them a low level IV or V evidence. There is no discussion of "evidence informed."

1. Transforaminal ESIs—moderate-level evidence was found for this procedure or selective nerve roots in preoperative evaluation of patients with negative imaging studies and clinical findings of nerve root irritation.

2. Evidence for interlaminar ESIs in managing lumbar radiculopathy was strong for short-term relief and limited for long-term relief. The evidence is presented as moderate for both short-term and long-term pain relief for cervical radiculopathy.
3. Evidence for transforaminal ESIs for lumbar nerve root pain was felt to be strong for short-term and moderate for long-term improvement. Moderate evidence for managing cervical nerve root pain was found. Evidence was limited in lumbar postlaminectomy syndrome and lumbar spinal stenosis. The effectiveness of transforaminal epidural steroid injections in axial low back pain, lumbar disc extrusions, and axial neck pain was indeterminate.
4. Evidence of lumbar and cervical medial branch blocks in decreasing chronic LBP and cervical pain was moderate.
5. Medial branch neurotomy via radiofrequency neurotomy was moderate to strong for short- and long-term relief of lumbar and cervical facet joint pain.
6. There was moderate evidence for efficacy of short-term and limited evidence for long-term improvement in managing LBP via intraarticular blocks, and evidence was negative for this procedure in managing neck pain.
7. Evidence for intra-articular sacroiliac joint injections was moderate for short-term relief (less than six weeks) and limited for long-term relief.
8. Evidence for spinal cord stimulation in failed back surgery patients as well as complex regional pain syndrome patients was strong for short-term relief (less than one year) and moderate for long-term relief.

In 2007 and 2008, the latest version of the ACOEM (American College of Occupational and Environmental Medicine) Occupational Medicine Practice Guidelines was written, which indicated some constraints might be considered on interventional treatment and sent to various groups for review, one being ASIPP, which took great umbrage at the guidelines (76).

CONCLUSIONS

It is interesting that so many different conclusions can be taken from essentially the same data. It would seem, therefore, that there is not yet enough evidence to give fully credible, unequivocal, EBM statements of efficacy.

Clinically speaking, the *adjunctive* use of interventional procedures has been found to be clinically useful when the procedures are done by a well-trained, interventional anesthesiologist. There are several issues here, however:

1. Adjunctive treatment should be the operational term.
2. Proper diagnosis should be established by a specialist in neurology, physiatry, or orthopedics prior to patients undergoing invasive treatments.
3. These procedures have possibly limited to moderate evaluative and analgesic appropriateness. Patients should be given ALL of the information—both the positive and negative aspects—as well as information on all alternative treatments prior to undergoing invasive procedures.
4. The insurance companies favor interventional pain medicine to the exclusion of interdisciplinary pain medicine treatment for chronic, noncancer pain patients. This has eliminated many outstanding programs, which have closed for lack of insurance reimbursement.

5. Finally, in today's cost-conscious medical environment, the minority of interventionalists who utilize the procedures as a form of lottery—performing as many procedures as possible on patients who are not showing responsiveness—need to stop. This is a waste of our valuable but limited medical resources.

REFERENCES

1. Ioannidis JPA, Cappelleri JC, Lau J. Issues in comparisons between meta-analyses and large trials. JAMA 1998; 279:1089–1093.
2. Boden SD, David DO, Dina TS, et al. Abnormal magnetic-resonance scans of the lumbar spine in asymptomatic subjects. A prospective investigation. J Bone Joint Surg Am 1990; 72(3):403–408.
3. Jensen MC, Brant-Zawadzki MN, et al. Magnetic resonance imaging of the lumbar spine in people without back pain. N Engl J Med 1994; 331(2):69–73.
4. Stadnik TW, Lee RR, Coen HL, et al. Annular tears and disk herniation: prevalence and contrast enhancement on MR images in the absence of low back pain or sciatica. Radiology 1998; 206(1):49–55.
5. Savage RA, Whitehouse GH, Roberts N. The relationship between the magnetic resonance imaging appearance of the lumbar spine and low back pain, age and occupation in males. Eur Spine J 1997; 6(2):106–114.
6. Sackett DL, Straus S, Richardson S, et al. Evidence-based Medicine: How to Practice and Teach EBM. 2nd ed. London: Churchill Livingston, 2000.
7. Friedly J, Chan L, Deyo R. Increases in lumbosacral injections in the medicare population: 1994–2001. Spine 2007; 32(16):1754–1760.
8. Boas RA. Nerve blocks in the diagnosis of low back pain. Neurosurg Clin N Am 1991; 2(4):807–816.
9. Medpac. Medicare Payment Advisory Commission Report to the Congress: Paying for Interventional Pain Services in the Ambulatory Settings. December 2001. www.medpac.gov/publications/contressional_reports/dec2001Pain Management.pdf.
10. Friedly J, Chan L, Deyo R. Geographic variation in epidural steroid injection use in medicare patients. J Bone Joint Surg Am 2008; 90(8):1730–1737.
11. HHS.CMS. 2001 Medicare physician/supplier procedure summary master file (formerly Part B Procedure File). June 30, 2002. Electronic file.
12. Merrill DG. Hoffman's glasses: evidence-based medicine and the search for quality in the literature of interventional pain medicine. Reg Anesth Pain Med 2003; 28(6): 547–560.
13. Moher D, Cook DJ, Jadad AR, et al. Assessing the quality of reports of randomized trials: implications for the conduct of meta-analyses. Health Technol Assess 1999; 3:1–100.
14. Moher D, Pham B, Jones A, et al. Does the quality of reports of randomized trials affect estimates of intervention efficacy reported in meta-analyses? Lancet 1998; 352: 609–613.
15. Cluff R, Abdel-Kader M, Cohen SP, et al. The technical aspects of epidural steroid injections: a national survey. Anesth Analg 2002; 95:403–408.
16. Smuck M, Fuller BJ, Chiodo A, et al. Accuracy of intermittent fluoroscopy to detect intravascular injection during transforaminal epidural injections. Spine 2008; 33(7):E205–E210.
17. Barre L, Lutz GE, Southern D, et al. Fluoroscopically guided caudal epidural steroid injections for lumbar spinal stenosis: a retrospective evaluation of long term efficacy. Pain Physician 2004; 7(2):187–193.
18. Ergin A, Yanarates O, Sizlan A, et al. Accuracy of caudal epidural injection: the importance of real-time imaging. Pain Pract 2005; 5(3):251–254.
19. Cooper G, Lutz GE, Boachie-Adjei O, et al. Effectiveness of transforaminal epidural steroid injections in patients with degenerative lumbar scoliotic stenosis and radiculopathy. Pain Physician 2004; 7(3):311–317.

20. Scanion GC, Moeller-Bertram T, Romanowsky SM, et al. Cervical transforaminal epidural steroid injections: more dangerous than we think? Spine 2007; 32(11):1249–1256.
21. Harwood MI. What is the most effective treatment for acute low back pain? J Fam Pract 2002; 51(2):www.jfponline.com/pages.asp?AID=1106.
22. Watts RW, Silagy CA. A meta-analysis on the efficacy of epidural corticosteroids in the treatment of sciatica. Anaesth Intensive Care 1995; 23(5):564–569.
23. Carette S, LeClaire R, Marcoux S, et al. Epidural corticosteroid injections for sciatica due to herniated nucleus pulposus. N Engl J Med 1997; 336:1634–1640.
24. Southern D, Lutz GE, Cooper G, et al. Are fluoroscopic caudal epidural steroid injections effective for managing chronic low back pain. Pain Physician 2003; 6(2):167–172.
25. Dilke TFW, Burry HC, Grahame R. Extradural corticosteroid injection in management of lumbar nerve root compression. Br Med J 1973; 2:635–637.
26. Breivik H, Helsa PE, Molnar I, et al. Treatment of chronic low back pain and sciatica: comparison of caudal epidural injections of bupivacaine and methylprenisolone with bupivacaine followed by saline. In: Bonica JJ, Albe-Fessard DG, eds. Advances in Pain Research and Therapy. Vol. 1. New York: Raven Press, 1976:927–932.
27. Yates DW. A comparison of the types of epidural injection commonly used in the treatment of low back pain and sciatica. Rheumatoid Rehabil 1978; 17:181–186.
28. Mathews JA, Mills SB, Jenkins VM, et al. Back pain and sciatica: controlled trials of manipulation, traction, sclerosant and epidural injections. Br J Rheumatol 1987; 26:416–423.
29. Ridley MG, Kingsley GH, Gibson T, et al. Outpatient lumbar epidural corticosteroid injection in the management of sciatica. Br J Rheumatol 1988; 27:295–299.
30. Bush K, Hillier S. A controlled study of caudal epidural injections of triamcinolone plus procaine for the management of intractable sciatica. Spine 1991; 16:572–575.
31. Beliveau P. A comparison between epidural anaesthesia with and without corticosteroid in the treatment of sciatica. Rheumatol Phys Med 1971; 11:40–43.
32. Snoek W, Weber H, Jorgensen B. Double blind evaluation of extradural methylprednisolone for herniated lumbar discs. Acta Orthop Scand 1977; 48:635–641.
33. Klenerman L, Greenwood R, Davenport HT,et al. Lumbar epidural injections in the treatment of sciatica. Br J Rheumatol 1984; 23:35–38.
34. Cuckler JM, Bernini PA, Wiesel SW, et al. The use of epidural steroids in the treatment of lumbar radicular pain: a prospective, randomized, double-blind study. J Bone Joint Surg Am 1985; 67:63–66.
35. Rocco AG, Frank E, Kaul AF, et al. Epidural steroids, epidural morphine and epidural morphine and epidural steroids combined with morphine in the treatment of post-laminectomy syndrome. Pain 1989; 36:297–303.
36. Serrao JM, Marks RL, Morley SJ, et al. Intrathecal midazolam for the treatment of chronic mechanical low back pain: a controlled comparison with epidural steroid in a pilot study. Pain 1992; 48:5–12.
37. Koes BW, Scholten RJ, Mens JMA,et al. Efficacy of epidural steroid injections for low-back pain and sciatica: a systematic review of randomized clinical trials. Pain 1995; 63:279–288.
38. Nimgade AS, Sullivan M, Goldman R. Physiotherapy, steroid injections or rest for lateral epicondylosis? What the evidence suggests. Pain Pract 2005; 5(3):203.
39. Delport EG, Cucuzzella AR, Marley JK, et al. Treatment of lumbar spinal stenosis with epidural steroid injections: a retrospective outcome study. Arch Phys Med Rehabil 2004; 85(3):479–484.
40. Rosen CD, Kahanovitz N, Bernstein R, et al. A retrospective analysis of the efficacy of epidural steroid injections. Clin Orthop Relat Res 1988; 228:270–272.
41. Butterman GR. Treatment of lumbar disc herniation: epidural steroid injection compared with discectomy. A prospective, randomized study. J Bone Joint Surg Am 2004; 86-A(4):670–679.
42. Cahana A, Mavrocordatos P, Geurts JW, et al. Do minimally invasive procedures have a place in the treatment of chronic low back pain? Expert Rev Neurother 2004; 4(3):479–490.

43. Hopayian K, Mugford M. Conflicting conclusions from two systematic reviews of epidural steroid injections for sciatica: which evidence should general practitioners heed? Br J Gen Pract 1999; 49(438):57–61.
44. Macrocordatos P, Cahana A. Minimally invasive procedures for the treatment of failed back surgery syndrome. Adv Tech Stand Neurosurg 2006; 31:221–252.
45. DePalma MJ, Slipman CW. Evidence-informed management of chronic low back pain with epidural steroid injections. Spine 2008; 8:45–55.
46. Tong HC, Williams JC, Haig AJ, et al. Predicting outcomes of transforaminal epidural injections for sciatica. Spine J 2003; 3(6):430–434.
47. Slipman CW, Bhat AL, Gilchrist RV, et al. A critical review of the evidence for the use of zygapophysial injections and radiofrequency denervation in the treatment of low back pain. Spine J 2003; 3(4):310–316.
48. Lin EL, Lieu V, Halevi L, et al. Cervical epidural steroid injections for symptomatic disc herniations. J Disord Tech 2006; 19(3):183–186.
49. Nelemans PJ, de Bie RA, de Bet HCW, et al. Injection therapy for subacute and chronic benign low back pain. Cochrane Database Syst Rev 2000; (2):CD001824.
50. Nelemans PJ, de Bie RA, de Vet HC, et al. WITHDRAWN: injection therapy for subacute and chronic benign low-back pain. Cochrane Database Syst Rev 2007; (3):CD001824.
51. Staal JB, de Bie R, de Vet HCW, et al. Injection therapy for subacute and chronic low-back pain. Cochrane Database Syst Rev 2008; (3). Art. no.: CD001824. DOI: 10.1002/14651858.CD001824.pub3.
52. Peloso P, Gross A, Haines T, et al. Cervical Overview Group. Medicinal and injection therapies for mechanical neck disorders. Cochrane Database Syst Rev 2007; (3). Art. no.: CD000319. DOI: 10.1002/14651858.CD000319.pub4.
53. Armon C, Argoff CE, Samuels J, et al. Assessment: use of epidural steroid injections to treat radicular lumbosacral pain: report of the Therapeutics and Technology Assessment Subcommittee of the American Academy of Neurology. Neurology 2007; 68(10):723–729.
54. Bogduk N. A narrative review of intra-articular corticosteroid injections for low back pain. Pain Med 2005; 6(4):287–296.
55. Valat JP, Giraudeau B, Rozenberg S, et al. Epidural corticosteroid injections for sciatica: a randomised, double blind, controlled clinical trial. Ann Rheum Dis 2003; 62(7): 639–643.
56. Rozenberg S, Dubourg G, Khalifa P, et al. Efficacy of epidural steroid in low back pain and sciatica. A critical appraisal by a French task force of randomized trials. Critical Analysis Group of the French Society for Rheumatology. Rev Rhum Engl Ed 1999; 66(2):79–85.
57. Lafuma A, Bouvenot G, Cohen C, et al. A pragmatic cost-effectiveness study of routine epidural corticosteroid injections for lumbosciatic syndrome requiring inhospital management. Rev Rhum Engl Ed 1997; 64(10):549–555.
58. Samanta A, Samanta J. Editorial: is epidural injection of steroids effective for low back pain? BMJ 2004; 328:1509–1510.
59. Institute for Clinical Systems Improvement. Fluoroscopically guided transforaminal epidural steroid injections for lumbar radicular pain. Bloomington, MN: Institute for Clinical Systems Improvement. August 2004.
60. Zhou Y, Furgang FA, Zhang Y. Quality assurance for interventional pain management procedures. Pain Physician 2006; 9:107–114.
61. Hildebrandt J. Relevance of nerve blocks in treating and diagnosis low back pain—is the quality decisive? Schmerz 2001; 15(6):474–483.
62. Vad VB, Bhat A, Lutz GE, et al. Transforaminal epidural steroid injections in lumbosacral radiculopathy: a prospective randomized study. Spine 2002; 27:11–15.
63. Hession WG, Stanczak JD, David KW, et al. Epidural steroid injections. Semin Roentgenol 2004; 39(1):7–23.
64. Khot A, Bowditch M, Powell J, et al. The use of intradiscal steroid therapy for lumbar spinal discogenic pain. Spine 2004; 29(8):833–837.

65. Taylor RS, Van Buyten JP, Buchser E. Spinal cord stimulation for chronic back and leg pain and failed back surgery syndrome: a systemic review and analysis of prognostic factors. Spine 2005; 30:152–160.
66. Levine SA, Perin LA, Hayes D, et al. An evidence based evaluation of percutaneous vertebroplasty. Manag Care 2000; 9(3):56–60, 63.
67. Grados F, Depriester C, Cayrolle G, et al. Long-term observations of vertebral osteoporotic fractures treated by percutaneous vertebroplasty. Rheumatology (Oxford) 2000; 39(12):1410–1414.
68. Jackson TP, Gaeta R. Neurolytic blocks revisited. Curr Pain Headache Rep 2008; 12(1):7–13.
69. Abram S. Efficacy of interventional therapies for low back and neck pain. In: Justins DM, ed. Pain 2005—An Updated Review: Refresher Course Syllabus. Seattle: IASP Press, 2005:123–129.
70. Derby R, Baker RM, Lee CH, et al. Evidence-informed management of chronic low back pain with intradiscal electrothermal therapy. Spine 2008; 8:80–95.
71. Carragee EJ, Alamin TF, Carragee JM. Low-pressure postive discography in subjects asymptomatic of significant low back pain illness. Spine 2006; 31(5):505–509.
72. Haldeman S, Dagenais S. What have we learned about the evidence-informed management of chronic low back pain? Editorial. Spine 2008; 8:266–277.
73. Derby R, Baker RM, Lee CH. Evidence-informed management of chronic low back pain with minimally invasive nuclear decompression. Spine 2008; 8:150–159.
74. Boswell MV. Evidence-based use of interventional techniques for chronic spinal pain. Lecture, American Academy of Pain Management, 16th Annual Clinical Meeting, San Diego, CA, September 24, 2005.
75. Boswell MV, Shah RV, Everett CR, et al. Interventional techniques in the management of chronic spinal pain: evidence-based practice guidelines. Pain Phys 2005; 8(1):1–47.
76. Machikanti L, Singh V, Derby R, et al. Pain Physician Review of Occupational Medicine Practice Guidelines for interventional pain management and potential implications. Pain Physician 2008; 11:271–289.

14

Acupuncture

Peter T. Dorsher

Mayo College of Medicine, Jacksonville, Florida, U.S.A.

INTRODUCTION

Acupuncture as an integral part of Traditional Chinese Medicine (TCM) has been in clinical use to treat human illnesses for at least 3000 years, and some archeological evidence dates acupuncture to be extant almost 5000 years (1). Though the principles of acupuncture were first described in the *Nei Jing* treatise about 200 BC (2), it is important to realize that other cultures in different eras have independently described similar principles for treating pain and human illness. Imhotep, physician to the Egyptian pharaohs ~2700 BC, is attributed to have described treatment principles similar to those of TCM (3); and Mayan curanderos circa 200–1000 AD described needling techniques ("jup" and "tok") using fish bones and rattlesnake fangs to treat pain and human illness at points that are often similar to those used in TCM (4). This suggests these healing traditions independently uncovered common underlying principles of human physiology that are present in health and disease.

Though a discussion of acupuncture in treating pain will be examined herein, it is important to note that only about 30% of all the world's literature regarding acupuncture examines its use in treating pain conditions (5). Interest in acupuncture, especially for its pain relieving properties, first began in the United States when James Reston, a NY times correspondent, reported excellent improvement in his postoperative pain with adjunctive acupuncture after undergoing an emergency appendectomy in China while covering Nixon's "ping-pong" diplomatic missions (6). Since then, basic science and clinical research into acupuncture's effects has produced an expanding body of evidence that demonstrates acupuncture's efficacy in treating a wide variety of conditions, including chronic pain.

Public interest in using acupuncture as part of their health care treatment has been increasing. In 1998, nearly 2 million Americans per year reported receiving acupuncture treatment, with a one-year prevalence of acupuncture use of 1%, which represents a 250% increase from 1990 estimates (7).

WHAT IS ACUPUNCTURE?

The term "acupuncture" was coined by Jesuit missionaries who observed this treatment during their travels to China in the 1600s and is derived from the Latin terms "acus" (needle) and "punctura" (to puncture). Acupuncture treatments stimulate rather precise anatomic locations (acupuncture points) by a variety of techniques (e.g., needle, laser, palpation) in order to produce clinical effects, including pain relief. The Chinese character for an acupuncture point can be roughly translated as "hole" and "position" (2). The acupoints are located by

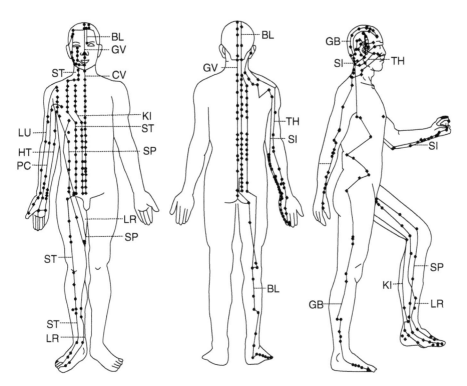

FIGURE 1 The 14 acupuncture principal meridians. *Abbreviations*: CV, conception vessel; GV, governing vessel; KI, kidney; BL, bladder; HT, heart; SI, small intestine; LR, liver; GB, gallbladder; PC, pericardium; TH, triple heater (energizer); LU, lung; LI, large intestine; SP, spleen; ST, stomach.

palpation for depressions between muscles, tendons, and/or bones; they are tender to palpation, especially when clinically involved in a pain condition. The 361 "classical" acupoints, which were described by ~200 AD, are the points found to be most frequently used and clinically important through centuries of acupuncture experience; but there are, theoretically, an infinite number of *ashi* ("that's it!") tender points that can be treated by acupuncture needling (2). Acupuncture points were initially grouped according to similar therapeutic properties, while the concept of channels (meridians) joining points with similar properties developed subsequently and was confirmed by the observed phenomenon of the spread of qi (energy, akin to referred pain spread from myofascial trigger points) along these pathways during treatments (2). Blood and qi are conceptualized to circulate in these channels. There are 14 principal meridians that the classical acupoints exist on: two midline channels and 12 others symmetrically arranged on each half of the body (Fig. 1).

PAIN TREATMENT IN ACUPUNCTURE
Pain in TCM can be approximated as "stuck" blood or qi (energy) in one or more of these meridians, and needles are placed to restore normal, unimpeded circulation of blood and qi in the affected channels. As an example, a temporal

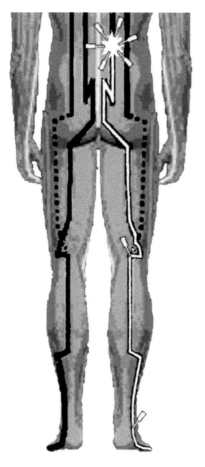

FIGURE 2 Acupuncture treatment for right S1 radiculopathy.

migraine headache is located in the distribution of the Gallbladder meridian. Needles would be placed in local tender points where the headache is present along the lateral aspect of the head, but also, points might be added near the lateral malleolus (GB-40) and/or in the first webspace of the foot (LR-3) to alleviate the headache. These distal ankle/foot points are conceptualized to help move the stuck blood and qi in the lateral head (causing the headache) downward in the Gallbladder channel away from the head region and restore normal circulation (producing relief of the migraine).

Another example would be treatment of an acute right S1 radiculopathy, as demonstrated in Figure 2. Note the bladder meridian, demonstrated in black, closely follows the distribution of the sciatic nerve through its lateral plantar branch to the 5th toe (S1 distribution). During an acupuncture treatment for the acute low back and leg pain symptoms from an S1 radiculopathy, the local painful area in the lumbar spine would be surrounded by acupuncture needles to help disperse the stagnant blood and/or qi there, and additional distal points at BL-40 behind the knee and BL-60 near the lateral malleolus could be selected to move the stagnant blood and/or qi from the lumbar spine. Note that patients with cystitis may also experience back pain in the low lumbar spine in the distribution of the bladder meridian, and that acupoints in that region of the back could be used to help treat the cystitis.

MYOFASCIAL PAIN SYNDROME DATA CONFIRM ACUPUNCTURE'S FINDINGS

The *Trigger Point Manual* (8,9) provides contemporary evidence of TCM's findings in treating pain. Though some myofascial pain theorists claim that trigger points (TrPs) in muscle can occur anywhere within a given muscle, many different researchers found similar locations for TrPs in muscles (8–11), which Travell and Simons' texts term "common" trigger point locations. These common TrP locations reflect the most clinically common and important trigger points found over the decades of their clinical experience, while classical acupoints similarly reflect the most clinically common and important acupuncture points found over many centuries (millennia) of acupuncture practice.

Recent data (12) demonstrate that over 93% of the ~255 common TrP locations described in the *Trigger Point Manual* are anatomically proximate to those of classical acupoints. Clinically, over 97% of these anatomically related trigger points and acupoints have similar pain uses described, and 94% have comparable somatovisceral effects. As examples, a sternocleidomastoid TrP associated with paroxysmal cough anatomically corresponds to acupoint ST-10, which is used to treat cough; and an upper trapezius TrP that is associated with tension headache and dizziness anatomically corresponds to acupoint GB-21, which is used to treat headache and vertigo. Finally, for anatomically corresponding TrPs and acupoints, the distributions of their myofascial referred pain and meridian distributions are similar in over 91% of instances. Two examples are presented in Figures 3 and 4. The marked anatomic, clinical (pain and somatovisceral), and physiologic (referred-pain to meridian) correspondences of the myofascial pain and acupuncture traditions in treating pain conditions strongly suggest that the *Trigger Point Manual* data is but a rediscovery of pain physiology principles outlined in the *Nei Jing* text 2000 years before!

EVIDENCE-BASED EVIDENCE OF ACUPUNCTURE'S EFFICACY FOR TREATING PAIN

In the past two decades, there have been a multitude of randomized, placebo-controlled clinical trials published that demonstrate the efficacy of acupuncture in treating pain conditions. In the German Acupuncture in Routine Care trials that examined over 3600 subjects receiving acupuncture for chronic neck pain (13), 56.5% of subjects who received acupuncture demonstrated significant improvements in their neck pain and disability scores compared to only 21.6% in the control group who received only usual care with medications and physical therapy ($p < 0.001$). Those receiving acupuncture had nearly a 30% reduction in pain scores *versus* only 5% reduction in controls; and the physical and psychological function of those receiving acupuncture, as measured by SF-36 scores, likewise, were clinically and statistically ($p < 0.001$) significantly improved compared to the control subjects (13). A 2007 Cochrane review of acupuncture in neck pain (14) concluded that for chronic mechanical neck disorders, the literature provides moderate evidence that acupuncture is more effective for pain

Scalene mTrP   Large Intestine Channel

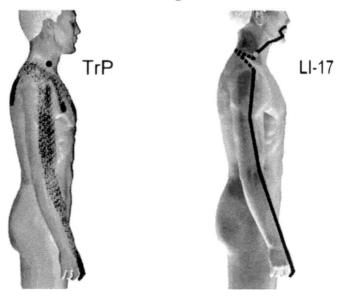

TrP   LI-17

FIGURE 3   Scalene TrP referred-pain compared to large intestine channel.

Gluteus Minimus mTrP   Gallbladder Channel

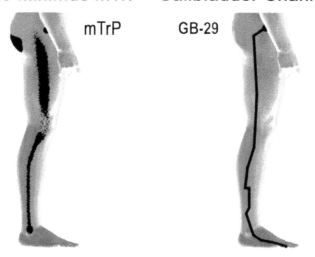

mTrP   GB-29

FIGURE 4   Gluteus minimus TrP referred-pain compared to Gallbladder channel.

relief than some types of sham controls, measured immediately posttreatment; that acupuncture is more effective than inactive, sham treatments measured immediately posttreatment and at short-term follow-up; and that there is limited evidence that acupuncture was more effective than massage at short-term follow-up. For chronic neck disorders with radicular symptoms, there is moderate evidence that acupuncture is more effective than a wait-list control at short-term follow-up; that acupuncture relieves pain better than some sham treatments, measured at the end of the treatment; that those receiving acupuncture report less pain at short-term follow-up than those on a waiting list; and that acupuncture is more effective than inactive treatments for relieving pain posttreatment, and this effect is maintained at short-term follow-up.

The GERAC (German Acupuncture Care) study of acupuncture for low back pain (15) was a randomized, multicenter, blinded, parallel-group trial that enrolled 1162 patients into three arms comparing true acupuncture, sham acupuncture, and conventional treatment (drugs, physical therapy, and exercise). Pain scales and back-specific and global functional scales were used to measure outcomes. Those subjects receiving acupuncture demonstrated clinically and statistically significant improvements in pain and back-related disability scores compared to those receiving conventional treatment (~55% responders in acupuncture groups *versus* only about 33% of conventional treatment group). A recent meta-analysis in 2005 of the acupuncture literature for treating low back pain (16) concluded that acupuncture is more effective than sham acupuncture (standardized mean difference, 0.54 [95% CI, 0.35–0.73]; seven trials) and no additional treatment (standardized mean difference, 0.69 [CI, 0.40–0.98]; eight trials) for providing short-term relief of chronic low back pain. This short-term relief seems to be sustained over the longer term, but its sustained effect is uncertain as longer term follow-up data are limited in quantity and quality.

Other large, placebo-controlled trials have demonstrated acupuncture's efficacy in treating knee osteoarthritis (17) and migraine headaches (18). The NIH Consensus Conference in 1977 concluded that there was evidence of acupuncture's efficacy in postoperative dental pain and that it may be useful in headache, menstrual cramps, back pain, and fibromyalgia (19). The WHO concluded that there is evidence that acupuncture may be helpful in treating a variety of pain conditions, including dental pain, tennis elbow, sciatica, low back pain, rheumatoid arthritis, headache, migraine, trigeminal neuralgia, intercostal neuralgia, and peripheral neuropathy (20).

A major challenge for acupuncture trials has been to find adequate placebo acupuncture interventions, since even minimal needling may produce physiologic responses. A variety of sham acupuncture needles have been designed that do not pierce the skin; but these devices are expensive and still stimulate cutaneous sensory fibers, which could still produce physiologic effects. Infrared lasers for stimulating acupoints have been developed that can penetrate up to 6 cm, which may permit blinding of both patients and operators to whether the laser is actually stimulating the studied acupoints.

Of note, low-frequency electroacupuncture (2–4 Hz) produces a slow onset, generalized analgesic response that persists after stimulation is stopped and is cumulative with repeated stimulation related to endogenous opioid release; this analgesic effect is blocked with naloxone (21).

CONCLUSIONS

Acupuncture has been in clinical use for at least 3000 years in China and elsewhere. Other civilizations in different eras including the ancient Egyptians and Mayans independently discovered similar treatment principles. The contemporary myofascial pain tradition also appears to have rediscovered similar clinical and physiologic findings as those of TCM. This suggests that there is a common underlying phenomenon (possibly neurophysiologic) that these different traditions are describing.

Basic science and clinical evidence has accumulated in the past 30 years that demonstrates acupuncture's efficacy in treating a variety of pain conditions including chronic mechanical neck and low back pain; and this analgesic effect, which can be reversed by naloxone, appears to be mediated by the endogenous opioid system.

Evidence will be forthcoming that these effects may result from stimulation of the peripheral nervous system that alters central nervous system and autonomic nervous system function. The acupuncture tradition may have uncovered, through its synthesis of thousands of years of clinical observations of human illnesses, a clinical mapping of the somatovisceral and viscerosomatic reflexes of the human body, which can be manipulated with acupuncture treatment to treat pain and illness. This may open new, safer treatments that use the body's endogenous control mechanisms to improve acute and chronic pain and disease states.

REFERENCES

1. Eckman P. In the Footsteps of the Yellow Emperor. San Francisco: Cypress Book Company, 1996:37–38.
2. O'Connor J, Bensky D. Acupuncture: A Comprehensive Text. Chicago: Eastland Press, 1981.
3. Campbell A, Cohen M. A short history. http://www.acupunctureaustralia.org/pages/ashorthistory.htm (website accessed 1/14/08).
4. Bowen-Jones A. The fascinating similarities between Chinese medicine and traditional Mayan healing. http://www.1421.tv/pages/evidence/content.asp?EvidenceID=398 (accessed 1/14/08).
5. Helms JM. Acupuncture Energetics: A Clinical Approach for Physicians. Berkeley: Medical Acupuncture Publishers, 1995.
6. Reston J. Now, let me tell you about my appendectomy in Peking. New York Times, July 26, 1971; 1:6.
7. Eisenberg DM, Davis RB, Ettner SL, et al. Trends in alternative medicine use in the United States, 1990–1997. JAMA 1998; 280:1569–1575.
8. Travell JG, Simons DG. Myofascial Pain and Dysfunction: The Trigger Point Manual. Vol. 1. Baltimore: Williams and Wilkins, 1983.
9. Travell JG, Simons DG. Myofascial Pain and Dysfunction: The Trigger Point Manual: The Lower Extremities. Vol. 2. Baltimore: Williams and Wilkins, 1992.
10. Birch S. Trigger point: acupuncture point correlations revisited. J Altern Complement Med 2003; 9:91–103.
11. Melzack R, Stillwell DM, Fox EJ. Trigger points and acupuncture points for pain: correlations and implications. Pain 1977; 3:3–23.
12. Dorsher PT, Fleckenstein J. Trigger points and classical acupuncture points: part 1: qualitative and quantitative anatomic correspondences. Dt Ztschr f Akup 2008; 51(2):15–24.
13. Witt CM, Jena S, Brinkhaus B, et al. Acupuncture for patients with chronic neck pain. Pain 2006; 125(1–2):98–106.

14. Trinh K, Graham N, Gross A, et al. Acupuncture for neck disorders. Spine; 32(2): 236–243.
15. Haake M, Muller HH, Schade-Brittinger C, et al. German acupuncture trials (GERAC) for chronic low back pain: a randomized, multicenter, blinded, parallel-group trial with 3 groups. Arch Int Med 2007; 167(17):1892–1898.
16. Manheimer E, White A, Berman B, et al. Meta-analysis: acupuncture for low back pain. Ann Int Med 2005; 142(8):651–663.
17. Berman BM, Lao L, Langenberg P, et al. Effectiveness of acupuncture as adjunctive therapy in osteoarthritis of the knee: a randomized, controlled trial. Ann Intern Med 2004; 141:901–910.
18. Linde K, Streng A, Jurgens S, et al. Acupuncture for patients with migraine: a randomized controlled trial. JAMA 2005; 293:2118–2125.
19. Acupuncture. NIH Consensus Statement. 1997; 15(5):1–34.
20. World Health Organization. Acupuncture: review and analysis of reports on controlled clinical trials. World Health Organization, Geneva, Switzerland, 2003.
21. Cheng RS, Pomeranz BH. Electroacupuncture analgesia is mediated by stereospecific opiate receptors and is reversed by antagonists of type I receptors. Life Sci 1979; 26:631–638.

Complementary and Alternative Medicine in the Management of Chronic Pain

Alan K. Halperin

Division of General Internal Medicine, Department of Medicine, University of Florida College of Medicine Jacksonville, Jacksonville, Florida, U.S.A.

Individuals suffering with chronic pain commonly seek out alternative and complementary practitioners and treatments. They are often overwhelmed and bewildered by the number and variety of different treatments and practitioners for chronic pain. Although there is an increasing body of published literature on the efficacy of complementary and alternative medicine (CAM), there are no established guidelines for aiding patients and physicians. This chapter first defines complementary and alternative medicine and reviews surveys of the prevalence and reason for their use in chronic pain and then reviews the scientific basis and published studies for the following commonly used modalities in chronic pain: acupuncture, massage, manipulation, herbs, movement, mind–body and other therapies. Finally, recommendations for the use of CAM services are suggested.

CAM DEFINITION

The National Center for Complementary and Alternative Medicine (NCCAM) defines complementary and alternative medicine (CAM) as a group of diverse medical and health care systems, practices, and procedures that are not presently considered to be part of conventional medicine (1). Complementary medicine uses its therapies in combination with conventional medicine whereas alternative medicine is used in place of conventional medicine. This definition is inadequate because it does not say what CAM is. Snyderman defines integrative medicine as follows: Integrative medicine is the term being used for a new movement that is being driven by the desires of consumers but that is now getting the attention of many academic health centers. Importantly, integrative medicine is not synonymous with CAM. It has a far larger meaning and mission in that it calls for restoration of the focus of medicine on health and healing and emphasizes the centrality of the patient–physician relationship. In addition to providing the best conventional care, integrative medicine focuses on preventive maintenance of health by paying attention to all relative components of lifestyle, including diet, exercise, stress management, and emotional well-being. It insists on patients being active participants in their health care as well as on physicians viewing patients as whole persons—minds, community members, and spiritual beings, as well as physical bodies. Finally, it asks physicians to serve as guides, role models, and mentors, as well as dispensers of therapeutic aids (2). Patients will be better served if their physicians are familiar with and value both conventional and CAM therapies and know how to integrate them.

There are five main domains of CAM and there is often overlap between them. (*i*) Whole medical systems: systems that have complete systems of theory and practice such as acupuncture. (*ii*) Mind–body medicine: variety of techniques that utilizes the mind's capacity to affect body functions and symptoms such as meditation, prayer, and mental healing. (*iii*) Biologically based practices: substances found in nature such as herbs and foods. (*iv*) Manipulative and body-based practices: manipulation by chiropractors or osteopathic physicians, yoga, and other movement therapies. (*v*) Energy medicine: the use of energy fields such as qi gong, Reiki, therapeutic touch and magnetic fields.

In 1993, Eisenberg published the landmark survey of CAM use in the United States (3). In this study, 34% of respondents reported the use of at least one CAM therapy within the last year. Expenditures totaled $13.7 billion, and 75% of expenditures were out of pocket. By 2002, the number of CAM uses had increased to 62% (4). Chronic pain, especially low back pain, is the most common condition for which patients seek CAM therapy. In a more recent survey of patients with neck or back pain, 37% had seen a conventional provider and 54% had used CAM within the last year (5). The most common CAM therapies included chiropractic, massage, and relaxation. These therapies were rated as very helpful by 61%, 65%, and 43%, respectively, whereas conventional providers were rated as very helpful by 27%. These statistics are consistent with increasing skepticism about the effectiveness and side effects of conventional pharmacologic (6,7) and interventional therapies (8,9).

CAM THERAPIES

Acupuncture

Traditional Acupuncture Theory
The discipline of acupuncture is highly complex. The reader is referred to acupuncture texts (10) for a more comprehensive description. All incorporate the concept of qi (chee). Qi, or life force, is responsible for growth and development and movement. Qi circulates through pathways, termed meridians. Along these meridians are over 361 acupuncture points that serve as energy centers. In addition to acupuncture points on the meridians, numerous acupuncture points exist in microsystems in the ear, hand, and scalp that correspond to body parts and systems. Two opposing forces exist in nature, yin and yang. These two forces regulate qi. When the body is in balance, there is a smooth flow of qi throughout the body. When there is blockage of the flow of qi, disease occurs, which can manifest as diseases, symptoms or emotions. The goal of the acupuncturist is to establish a diagnosis and determine the location of the blockage by performing a history and exam, especially of the pulse, tongue, and nails. Once the source of blockage is identified, stimulating acupuncture points by the insertion of needles restores the flow of qi and balance is restored to the body.

Modern Acupuncture Theory
Acupuncture originated in China at least 3000 years ago and has spread throughout Asia, Europe, and America. As a result, many different types of acupuncture have developed. Interest in the United States was stimulated by President Nixon's historic visit to China in 1972. During the visit, an American reporter,

James Reston, required an emergency appendectomy. In an article published in the *NewYork Times*, he described the use of acupuncture analgesia postoperatively. Since then, the practice of acupuncture has grown considerably in the United States. In 1997 the National Institute of Health issued a report detailing the efficacy of acupuncture in a variety of conditions such as back pain and nausea and vomiting related to chemotherapy. The NCCAM, the lead agency of the NIH in promoting research in CAM, has funded almost 50 studies related to acupuncture.

There has been much progress in understanding the biomedical explanations for acupuncture-induced analgesia (11). Several studies demonstrate increased endorphins and other endogenous opioids in the cerebral spinal fluid after acupuncture points were electrically simulated (EA) (12). The analgesic effects of acupuncture can be reversed in animals and humans by naloxone, an opioid antagonist (13). More recent studies show that low-frequency EA induces the release of encephalin and beta-endorphin and high-frequency stimulation releases dynorphin (14). In addition, low-frequency stimulation increased messenger RNA for the encephalin precursor protein and high-frequency stimulation increased RNA for dynorphin (15,16). fMRI studies demonstrate that different frequencies of electrical stimulation activate different parts of the brain. Low-frequency stimulation activates the contralateral primary and supplementary motor areas and ipsilateral superior temporal gyrus, whereas high-frequency stimulation activates the contra lateral inferior parietal lobules, anterior cingulated cortex, nucleus accumbens and pons (15). These studies suggest that acupuncture stimulates endogenous opioid production.

Other possible mechanisms include activation of the hypothalamic pituitary adrenocortical axis with resultant immune and sympathetic nervous system modulation (17) and inhibition of descending inhibitory control mechanisms. Advances in neural imaging using PET and fMRI have helped confirm the above observations. Acupuncture and pain share similar cortical pathways, but nervous system activities triggered by these two stimulations are opposite to each other (11).

Clinical Studies

Low Back Pain

Two meta-analyses (18,19) reported that acupuncture was effective for pain relief and improved function compared with no treatment. In addition, acupuncture, when added to conventional therapies, improved pain and function more than conventional therapies alone. Since then, two additional large high-quality studies have been reported. In one (20), 298 patients were randomized to acupuncture, minimal acupuncture (superficial needling), or wait list control. Both acupuncture groups had significant reduction in pain compared to wait list control. There were no differences in pain relief between the acupuncture and minimal acupuncture groups. A recent German study was the largest and most rigorous trial investigating the effect of acupuncture and low back pain (21). In this study, 1162 patients with low back pain were assigned to 10 true acupuncture sessions, sham acupuncture (superficial needling at non acupuncture points), or conventional therapy (drugs, physical therapy and exercise). The response rate six months after therapy (defined by improvement on several scales) was

48%, 44%, and 27%, respectively. Both acupuncture groups were significantly better than conventional therapy. There were no differences between true and sham acupuncture. The mechanism whereby sham acupuncture relieves pain is unknown. The observed differences could be attributed to placebo effect, differences in time contact with providers, or the nonspecific effects of needling in nonacupuncture points.

As a result of the study and other published studies, the German government decided to make acupuncture a covered benefit.

Neck Pain
A meta-analysis of 10 trials including 661 patients with chronic neck pain was recently reported (22). Patients who received acupuncture achieved better pain relief than sham treatments. Patients with radicular symptoms also improved. Since this publication, a large and rigorous German study has been published (23). In this study, 14,161 patients with chronic neck pain were randomized to receive acupuncture or a control group of no acupuncture. All subjects received routine medical care. Those who received acupuncture had significant improvement in pain compared with control. These effects were prolonged for six months.

Osteoarthritis
A meta-analysis recently reported on five well-designed, randomized clinical trials involving 1334 patients of acupuncture treatment for osteoarthritis of the knee (24). Acupuncture was superior to sham acupuncture for improving both pain and function. The largest study randomized 1007 patients with chronic osteoarthritis of the knee to standard care (NSAID and physiotherapy), acupuncture, or sham acupuncture (25). Success rates, defined as 36% improvement in the Western Ontario and McMaster Universities Osteoarthritis Index score (WOMAC) at 26 weeks, were 29% for standard care, 53.1% for acupuncture, and 51% for sham acupuncture. The acupuncture groups were superior to standard care, but there were no differences between true and sham acupuncture. The observed differences could be attributed to placebo effect, differences in time contact with providers, or the nonspecific effects of needling in nonacupuncture points.

Other Uses
In one randomized study of 100 patients with fibromyalgia, true acupuncture was no better than sham acupuncture in relieving pain (26). In another randomized study of 50 patients, acupuncture significantly improved the symptoms of fibromyalgia, such as pain, fatigue, and anxiety (27). Acupuncture use has also been reported in a variety of chronic pain conditions such as shoulder pain, epicondylitis, irritable bowel syndrome, chronic prostatitis, and others. However, there are not enough published reports to draw conclusions about their efficacy.

Massage
The term massage includes a variety of manual therapies. Common forms of massage include Swedish massage (superficial massage of muscles with lotion or oil), deep tissue massage, shiatsu (pressure over acupuncture points), thai massage (stretching in a sequence of postures), reflexology (pressure to points in feet

that are thought to correspond to body parts), rolfing (physical manipulation and movement to restore alignment), and craniosacral therapy (light touch to restore balance in the movement of cerebrospinal fluid). The mechanism by which massage improves pain is uncertain. Soft tissue massage, the most common form of massage therapy, is thought to act by modulating local blood flow and oxygenation in muscle. It also promotes mental relaxation, which may modulate immune system function and pain formation.

Clinical Studies
Three meta-analyses of massage for low back pain have been published (28–30). A total of nine studies were reviewed. All concluded that there is strong evidence that massage is effective for nonspecific low back pain. Both pain and function were improved. The beneficial effects of massage are enhanced when combined with exercise and education and when performed by an experienced therapist. No specific type of massage has been shown to be superior to others.

Manipulation
Manipulative therapies are one of the most commonly used CAM therapies. The neurophysiologic mechanisms whereby manipulation is effective in reducing pain have recently been reviewed (31). Biomechanical changes caused by spinal manipulation have physiological effects on the inflow of sensory information to the central nervous system. During spinal manipulation, there is from 0.71 to 1.62 mm axial displacement of vertebrae in the longitudinal plane. This movement suggests that mechanical processes may play a role in the biologic effects of spinal manipulation, affecting neural input, altering central processing, and affecting reflex somatomotor and somatovisceral output. Spinal manipulation affects many components of the peripheral and central nervous systems: proprioceptive afferents, dorsal roots, and dorsal root ganglia. Central sensitization may play a role in promoting pain, paraspinal muscle tone, altered vertebral movement, and other abnormal reflex responses. These neurophysiologic responses may all be altered by spinal manipulation.

Recently, there has been interest in medication-assisted manipulation or manipulation under anesthesia (MUA) (32). During MUA, anesthesiologists administer deep conscious sedation; then the manual therapist (chiropractor or osteopathic physician) performs a series of mobilization, stretching, and traction procedures to the spine and extremities; finally, a high-velocity, short amplitude thrust is applied to the spinous processes. Conscious sedation is thought to more effectively break up joint and soft tissue adhesions and increase ligament, tendon, muscle, and articular flexibility than can be accomplished in the awake state because of muscle guarding and pain.

Clinical Studies
Recent meta-analyses have reviewed the data on the efficacy of spinal manipulation (33). For chronic low back pain, the Cochrane Review showed that spinal manipulation was moderately superior to sham manipulation in relieving back pain. The difference averaged 10 to 19 points on the 100 point visual analog pain scale and 3.3 points on the RDQ function scale. There were no differences when compared to other therapies. Two additional studies have been reported since the meta-analyses. In one study of 681 patients, there were no differences in pain,

functional status or other outcomes between patients randomized to chiropractors *versus* medical management (34). In the largest study, 1334 patients with low back pain were studied (35). The patients were randomized into six groups: first to spinal manipulation delivered by the UK NHS, spinal manipulation in private premises, and "best care," and then to an exercise program. Both spinal manipulation and exercise alone achieved significant reduction of pain. However, the combination was superior to either alone.

Recently there has been increased interest in MUA, described above (36). No randomized clinical trials have been performed, but there have been several observational studies that support the procedure (36).

Biologically Based Studies

Several meta-analyses have reported on the efficacy of diet and herbs in relieving chronic pain (37,38). Harpagoside procumbens (devil's claw) has been studied in two dosage strengths, 50 mg and 100 mg. Over 500 patients have been studied. Compared with placebo, both dosage strengths clinically and significantly reduced pain. The Cochrane Review concluded that there is strong evidence that harpagoside reduced pain more than placebo in patients with acute episodes of nonspecific low back pain (37). It appears to have similar efficacy to rofecoxib 12.5 mg daily. Two trials including 261 patients have compared the analgesic effects of Salix alba (white willow bark) in doses of 120 mg daily and 240 mg daily. Salix alba's active ingredient is salicin, a derivative of salicylic acid, and is chemically related to aspirin. There is moderate evidence that it reduced pain more than placebo in the treatment of acute episodes of nonspecific low back pain and that it is similar in effectiveness to rofecoxib 12.5 mg daily. There is limited evidence that the cream is effective (37). There is not enough evidence to comment on the analgesic efficacy of other herbs or homeopathy.

Glucosamine and chondroitin sulfate alone and in combination have been studied in patients with osteoarthritis (39). Results have been contradictory. The largest study done in the US showed that glucosamine and chondroitin alone and in combination did not improve knee pain in osteoarthritis, compared with celecoxib (40). However, a subgroup analysis showed that the combination may be effective in patients with moderate-to-severe knee pain. There is also some evidence to suggest that the combination may have a positive structure-modifying effect and may, thus, slow the progression of osteoarthritis.

There is increasing interest in the role of diet as a pain modulator. There may be analgesic and antinociceptive properties of soybeans, sucrose, tart cherries, and other fruits and vegetables. No clinical studies have been performed.

Mind–Body Therapies

Mind–body medicine strategies such as meditation, guided imagery, yoga, biofeedback, hypnosis, tai chi, qi gong, and others are used by approximately 17% of the US population and prayer for healing is used by 45% (41). The concept that the mind, body, and spirit are integrally related is part of Traditional Chinese and Ayurvedic Medicine. This unity has persisted in Eastern healing traditions. In the West, beginning in the 16th Century, there has been an attempt to separate the body from spiritual and emotional dimensions, which has persisted to the present. Recently, however, there has been a resurgence of interest and research into the physiologic mechanisms whereby mind–body strategies influence health. All of the above strategies share common elements. With these techniques there is a reduction in sympathetic nervous system activity and stimulation of parasympathetic activity resulting in reduced blood pressure, respirations, heart rate, and stress hormones such as cortisol and norepinephrine. Since muscle tension appears to be mediated via the sympathetic nervous system, it is not surprising that these strategies have been useful in treating chronic pain. Mind–body therapies have a beneficial effect on immune system function and the release of numerous neuropeptides (such as serotonin and melatonin), which can affect mood and the perception of pain. Recent studies in brain imaging have revealed the interrelationship between body, mind and spirit in the perception of pain.

Yoga

Yoga originated in India over 2000 years ago. It has become very popular in the West. It involves aligning the body in postures (called asanas), breathing exercises, and meditation. Three recent trials have shown the promise of using yoga to treat chronic low back pain (42–44). The highest quality study (43) compared six weeks of yoga, exercise and self-care in 101 patients. Yoga was superior to exercise and self-care in improving back-related function. There were no differences in symptom botherness at 12 weeks, but yoga was superior at 26 weeks. Yoga appeared to be more effective in improving function and reducing pain, and the effects persisted for several months. The other studies have yielded conflicting results (42,44). Tai chi and qi gong are practices that originated in China and involve slow, controlled motions, and focused breathing. There are not enough studies to comment on their effectiveness.

Meditation

Meditation is a self-directed practice for relaxing the body and calming the mind. Most meditative techniques have come to the West from Eastern religious practices, particularly from India, China, and Japan, but meditation is a common practice of all cultures of the world. Although there are many types of meditation practices, the most common one in the West is mindfulness meditation. Introduced in 1979 by Kabat-Zinn, this type of meditation, termed mindfulness-based stress reduction (MBSR), is the awareness that emerges through paying attention on purpose, in the present moment and nonjudgmentally to the unfolding experience moment by moment (45). Numerous studies over the decades have shown beneficial effects on pain and anxiety, but comparison groups were not included in study design. In a recent pilot study in older adults with chronic back pain, 37 subjects were randomized to MBSR or wait list control (46). At the end of the 8-week study, the patients in the control group were crossed over to the MBSR program. In the MBSR group, pain acceptance scores, physical function scores, and activities engagement scores improved compared with controls. Pain scores, disability, and overall quality of life improved for the MBSR group, but did not achieve statistical significance. There is not enough evidence to comment on the efficacy of other mind–body medicine techniques such as progressive relaxation, biofeedback, guided imagery, and hypnosis. In some studies, many of these techniques have been combined.

A recent review of mind–body therapies concludes that multimodal therapies that combine stress management, training in coping skills, cognitive

behavioral training, and possibly, relaxation therapy are appropriate complementary therapies in the treatment of chronic low back pain (47).

Miscellaneous Therapies

Traction
A recent review of 10 randomized clinical trials of traction therapy concluded
that there was little evidence of efficacy (48). There have been two trials of intermittent vertebral decompression therapy. In this therapy, patients are attached to
a table with a pelvic harness and hold onto hand grips. The table separates with
a working pressure of 8.9–9.8 kg/cm^2 and the relaxation and distraction times
are set at 60 seconds each. One study compared vertebral axial decompression
with TENS (49). Success was defined as 50% improvement in pain on a VAS. The
treatment was successful in 68% of the vertebral axial decompression group and
0% in the TENS group. In a more recent study, 303 subjects with chronic LBP and
who failed at least two types of nonoperative interventions volunteered for an
observational study of vertebral axial decompression (50). The subjects received
24 treatments and there was no control group. There was a significant reduction
in pain and disability scores at discharge and at 30 days and 180 days postdis-
charge. This is a promising therapy that needs further investigation.

Prolotherapy
In prolotherapy, there are six weekly injections of 20–30 mL of a solution containing dextrose 12.5%, glycerin 12.5%, phenol 1%, and lidocaine 0.25% into multiple lumbosacral ligaments. The treatment was derived from sclerotherapy and is
thought to induce a localized inflammatory reaction with connective tissue proliferation. A review of published studies has yielded conflicting results (51).

Recommendations
Patients with chronic pain, practitioners of all types, and third party payers all
desire cost-effective interventions that result in improved pain and function.
Unfortunately, there is not enough support in the literature to make definitive
recommendations. For both conventional and CAM therapies, there is little evidence to support one treatment over others. Costs are out of control. Patients
often seek care from a potpourri of conventional and CAM providers including
primary care physicians, spine surgeons, neurologists, chiropractors, acupuncturists, massage therapists, physical therapists, psychologists, yoga therapists,
and others. It is confusing for patients with chronic pain and also providers
who attempt to stay current in effective therapies. The practitioner whom the
patient chooses will often determine the recommendations. Spine surgeons and
pain management specialists are likely to recommend more invasive approaches,
whereas chiropractors and acupuncturists and massage therapists will likely recommend more conservative approaches. Each has his/her expertise and also
financial incentives for recommending a certain approach. CAM therapists may
view surgeons and pain management specialists as too invasive. Physicians may
view chiropractors or acupuncturists as quacks. In this competitive marketplace,
all make their case for advocating a certain approach. How do patients know
who the experts are and which therapies are most likely to relieve pain, when
there is a lack of consensus on how best to manage chronic pain? There are no

simple answers, but the following recommendations seem reasonable: (*i*) Recommend noninvasive approaches first. The majority of those with chronic pain improve with time and do not require emergency surgery. CAM therapies are mostly noninvasive and have few side effects compared with most conventional therapies. (*ii*) Recommend therapies that require the patient to actively participate in their care. (*iii*) Recommend therapies that are beneficial for general health. For example, relaxation therapies, yoga, diet, and massage benefit overall well-being and can improve quality of life for those with and without pain. (*iv*) Recommend therapies that are consistent with the patient's beliefs. For example, those who do not believe in CAM approaches should be referred to conventional providers. Those who believe in CAM should be encouraged to consult CAM providers such as chiropractors, massage therapists, and acupuncturists. (*v*) Multiple approaches can be used simultaneously. Relaxation or meditation, yoga, massage, and acupuncture work synergistically. Together they may be better than individually. (*vi*) Physicians should become familiar with CAM therapies and providers to refer those who are interested. One way to become familiar is to experience various therapies.

REFERENCES

1. National Center for Complementary and Alternative Medicine. Available at http://nccam.nih.gov (accessed June, 2008).
2. Snyderman R, Weil AT. Integrative medicine bringing medicine back to its roots. Arch Intern Med 2002; 168:395–397.
3. Eisenberg DM, Kestrel RCA, Foster C, et al. Unconventional medicine in the United States: prevalence, costs and patterns of use. N Engl J Med 1993; 328:246–252.
4. Adv Data from Vital and Health Statistics. Complementary and alternative medicine use among adults: United States, No 343, 2004 pp (PHS) 2004–1250.
5. Wolsko PM, Eisenberg DM, Davis RB, et al. Patterns and perceptions of care for treatment of back and neck pain: results of a national survey. Spine 2003; 292–297.
6. Noble M, Tregear SJ, Treadwell JR, et al. Long-term opioid therapy for chronic non-cancer pain: a systematic review and meta-analysis of efficacy and safety. J Pain Symptom Manage 2008; 35:214–228.
7. Chou R, Huffman LH. Diagnosis and treatment of low back pain: A joint practice guideline from the American College of Physicians and American Pain Society. Ann Intern Med 2007; 147:505–514.
8. Boswell MV, Colson JD, Sehgal N, et al. A systematic review of therapeutic facet joint interventions in chronic spinal pain. Pain Physician 2007; 10:229–253.
9. Abdi S, Datta S, Trescot AM, et al. Epidural steroids in the management of chronic spinal pain: a systematic review. Pain Physician 2007; 10:185–212.
10. Helms JM. Acupuncture Energetics. Berkeley, CA: Medical Acupuncture Publishers, 1995.
11. Wang SM, Kain ZN, White P. Acupuncture analgesia: I. The scientific basis. Anesth Analg 2008; 106:602–610.
12. Clement-Jones V, McLoughlin L, Corer R, et al. Increased beta-endorphin but not met-enkephalin levels in human cerebrospinal fluid after acupuncture for recurrent pain. Lancet 1980; 2:946–949.
13. Han JS. Acupuncture: neuropeptide release produced by electrical stimulation of different frequencies. Neuroscience 2003; 26:17–22.
14. Han JS, Sun SL. Differential release of enkephalin and dynorphin by low and high frequency stimulation in the central nervous system. Acupunct Sci Int J 1990;1:19–27.
15. Guo HF, Tian JG, Wang X, et al. Brain substrates activated by electroacupuncture of different frequencies. Crain Res Mol Brain Res 1996; 43:157–166.

16. Zhang WT, Jin Z, Cui GH, et al. Relations between brain network activation and analgesic effect induced by low vs. high frequency electrical acupoint stimulation in different subjects: a functional magnetic resonance imaging study. Brain Res 2003; 982: 168–178.
17. Pan B, Castro-Lopes J, Coimbra A. Chemical sensory deafferentation abolishes hypothalamic pituitary activation induced by noxious stimulation or electroacupuncture but only decreases caused by immobilization stress. A c-fos study. Neuroscience 1997; 78:1059–1068.
18. Furlan AD, van Tulder MW, Cherkin DC, et al. Acupuncture and dry needling for low back pain. Cochrane Database Syst Rev 2005; 1:CD001351.
19. Manhelmer E, White A, Berman B, et al. Meta-analysis: acupuncture for low back pain. Ann Intern Med 2005; 142:651–663.
20. Brinkhaus B, Witt CM, Jena S, et al. Acupuncture in patients with chronic low back pain: a randomized controlled trial. Arch Intern Med 2006; 166:450457.
21. Haake M, Muller H, Schade-Brittinger C, et al. German Acupuncture Trials (GERAC) for chronic low back pain. Arch Intern Med 2007; 167:1892–1898.
22. Trinh KV, Graham N, Gross AR, et al. Cervical overview group. Acupuncture for neck disorders. Cochrane Database Syst Rev 2006; (3). Art. No.: CD004870.
23. Witt CM, Jena S, Brinkhaus B, et al. Acupuncture for patients with chronic neck pain. Pain 2006; 125:90–106.
24. White A, Foster NE, Cummings M, et al. Acupuncture treatment for chronic knee pain: a systematic review. Rheumatology 1007; 46:394–390.
25. Scharf HP, Mansmann U, Stretberger K, et al. Acupuncture and knee osteoarthritis: a three-armed randomized trial. Ann Intern Med 2006; 145:12–20.
26. Assefi NP, Sherman KJ, Jacobson C, et al. A randomized clinical trial of acupuncture compared with sham acupuncture in fibromyalgia. Ann Inern Med 2005; 143:10–19.
27. Martin DP, Sletten CD, Williams BA, et al. Improvement in fibromyalgia symptoms with acupuncture: results of a randomized controlled trial. Mayo Clin Proc 2006; 81:749–757.
28. Furlan AD, Imamura L, Irvin E. Massage for low back pain. Cochrane Database Syst Rev 2002; CD0019929.
29. Chou R, Huffman LH. Nonpharmacologic therapies for acute and chronic low back pain: a review of the evidence for an American Pain Society/American college of physicians clinical practice guideline. Ann Intern Med 2007; 147:492–502.
30. Imamura M, Furlan AD, Dryden T, et al. Evidence-informed management of chronic low back pain with massage. Spine J 2008; 8:121–133.
31. Pickar JG. Neurophysiologic effects of spinal manipulation. Spine J 2002; 2:357–371.
32. Dagenais S, Mayer J, Wooley JR, et al. Evidence-informed management of chronic low back pain with medicine assisted manipulation. Spine J 2008; 8:142–149.
33. Assendelft WJ, Morton SC, Yu EI, et al. Spinal manipulative therapy for low back pain. Ann Intern Med 2003; 138:871–881.
34. Hurwitz EL, Morganstern H, Harber P, et al. A randomized trial of medical care with and without physical therapy and chiropractic care with and without physical modalities for patients with low back pain: 6-month follow-up outcomes from the UCLA low back pain study. Spine 2002; 27:2193–2204.
35. UK BEAM Trial Team. United Kingdom back pain exercise and manipulation (UK Beam) randomized trial: effectiveness of physical treatments for back pain in primary care. BMJ 2004; 329:1377–1390.
36. Dagenais S, Mayer J, Wooley JR, et al. Evidence-informed management of chronic low back pain with medicine-assisted manipulation. Spine J 2008; 8:142–149.
37. Gagnier J, can Tulder MW, Berman B, et al. Herbal medicine for low back pain: a Cochrane Review. Spine 2007; 32:82–92.
38. Gagnier J. Evidence-informed management of chronic low back pain with herbal, vitamin, mineral and homeopathic supplements. Spine J 2008; 8:70–79.
39. Bruyere O, Reginster JY. Glucosamine and chondroitin sulfate as therapeutic agents for knee and hip osteoarthritis. Drugs Aging 2007; 24:73–580.

40. Clegg DO, Reda DJ, Harris CL. Glucosamine, chondroitin sulfate, and the two in combination for painful knee osteoarthritis. N Engl J Med 2006; 14:795–808.
41. National Center for Complementary and Alternative Medicine. Available at http://nccam.nih.gov (accessed June, 2008).
42. Galantino ML, Bzdewka TM, Eissler-Russo JL, et al. The impact of modified Hatha yoga on chronic low back pain: a pilot study. Altern Ther Health Med 2004; 10:56–59.
43. Sherman KJ, Cherkin DC, Erro J, et al. Comparing yoga, exercise, and a self-care book for chronic low back pain: a randomized controlled trial. Ann Intern Med 2005; 143:849–856.
44. Williams KA, Petronic J, Smith D, et al. Iyengar yoga therapy for chronic low back pain. Pain 2005; 115:107–117.
45. Kabat-Zinn J. Mindfulness-based interventions in context: past, present, and future. Clin Psychol: Sci Paract 2003; 10:144–156.
46. Marone NE, Greco CM, Weiner DK. Mindfulness meditation for treatment of chronic low back pain in older adults: a randomized controlled pilot study. Pain 2008; 134: 310–319.
47. Astin JA. Mind–body therapies for the management of pain. Clin J Pain 2004; 20: 27–32.
48. Gay RE, Brault J. Evidence-informed management of chronic low back pain with traction therapy. Spine J 2007; 8:234–242.
49. Sherry P, Kitchener P, Smart R. A prospective randomized controlled study of VAX-D and TENS for the treatment of chronic low back pain. Neurol Res 2001; 23:780–784.
50. Beattie PF, Nelson PT, Michener LA, et al. Outcomes after prone lumbar traction protocol for patients with activity-limiting low back pain: a prospective case series study. Arch Phys Med Rehabil 2007; 89:269–274.
51. Dagenais S, Mayer J, Halderman S, et al. Evidence-informed management of chronic low back pain with prolotherapy. Spine J 2008; 8:203–212.

16 Nonopiate Analgesics and Adjuvants

Gary W. Jay

Clinical Disease Area Expert-Pain, Pfizer, Inc., New London, Connecticut, U.S.A.

The purpose of this, and the next several chapters, is to give the reader basic clinical information regarding the medications mentioned elsewhere in this textbook.

There is no one way to use medications. It really depends on the patients with chronic noncancer pain and what they need. As will be noted below, there are some better methods of providing pain medication for the chronic noncancer pain patient, with specific reasons for both how and why. The use of adjunctive medication is also extremely important and will be discussed.

When a patient is initially seen, most physicians will follow the World Health Organization's three-step ladder (1), which divides pain into mild, moderate, and severe categories.

It is felt that mild pain should be treated with aspirin, acetaminophen (APAP), and nonsteroidal anti-inflammatory medications (NSAIDs), with or without the use of adjuvant medication.

For moderate pain, the World Health Organization indicates the use of mild narcotics (for the most part). These include codeine, hydrocodone, oxycodone, dihydrocodeine, and tramadol, with or without adjuvant medications.

Severe pain would mandate the use of the traditional opioids: morphine, hydromorphone, methadone, levorphanol, fentanyl, and oxycodone, with or without adjuvant medication.

Adjuvant medications include anticonvulsants, membrane stabilizers, N-methyl-D-aspartate (NMDA) antagonists, α_2 agonists, GABAnergic medications, and other agents including the antidepressants and neuroleptics. Opioids, antidepressants, and anticonvulsants will be discussed in the following chapters.

When used with opioids, NSAIDs may also be considered adjuvant medications. An important concept is multimodal (or balanced) analgesia, which is beneficial to both acute and chronic pain. This entails a rational combination of several analgesics, which have differing mechanisms of action to obtain improved efficacy and/or tolerability and safety when compared to similar or equianalgesic doses of a single drug (2).

For many years, NSAIDs have been used for treatment or management of mild to moderate pain, frequently in combination with APAP, which acts centrally and inhibits brain cyclooxygenase (COX) and nitric oxide synthase. New information has determined that APAP dosages of 4 g/day or more can induce hepatic abnormalities in normal healthy patients (3). NSAIDs can cause gastrointestinal symptoms and can potentially induce gastric bleeding. The selective COX-2 inhibitors were developed to deal with this problem, but they are now known to have potentially serious cardiovascular problems. New guidelines or statements from both the American (FDA) and European (EMEA) agencies indicate that when using NSAIDs, the smallest effective dose should be used for the shortest period of time (4). These reasons, among others, show the advantages of combining drugs at decreased dosages to give a better risk–benefit ratio for pain management. Weak opioids combined with APAP may be more beneficial, as more than one mechanism of action (MOA) are utilized (4, 5).

Studies have shown that combinations of NSAIDs and patient-controlled morphine analgesia offer advantages over morphine alone, another example of multimodal analgesia (6).

Multimodal analgesia is also used for outpatient surgery. These regimens should include nonopioid analgesics (i.e., local anesthetics, NSAIDs, COX inhibitors, APAP, ketamine, and α_2 agonists, for example) to supplement opioid analgesics. As this procedure may give good opioid-sparing effects, this may lead to a reduction in nausea, vomiting, constipation, urinary retention, sedation, and respiratory depression (7).

NONOPIOID ANALGESICS

The simple analgesics are easily chosen by the patient, if not the physician. They are inexpensive and easy to obtain. They include aspirin and APAP. Aspirin appears to work by inhibiting the synthesis of prostaglandin by blocking the action of COX, an enzyme that enables the conversion of arachidonic acid to prostaglandin to occur. Prostaglandins are synthesized from cellular membrane phospholipids after activation or injury, and sensitize pain receptors.

Aspirin, the prototypical NSAID, has anti-inflammatory and antipyretic properties, along with its pain-relieving properties. The recommended adult dose for treatment is 650 mg every six hours. Taking the aspirin with milk or food may decrease gastric irritation. Aspirin can also double bleeding time for four to seven days after taking 65 g. Peak blood levels are found after 45 minutes. The plasma half-life is two to three hours.

Acetaminophen (called Paracetamol in the United Kingdom)

This medication is used fairly universally for mild to moderate pain of all forms, including musculoskeletal pain, neuropathic pain, and even osteoarthritis (OA). An aniline derivative (coal tar analgesic), it is an antipyretic (with possible effects in the hypothalamic thermoregulatory center) and is very commonly used in combination drugs for pain and many other uses including combination cold (URI) preparations. It was first used clinically by von Mering in 1887 (8).

Acetaminophen, or N-acetyl-para-amino-phenol (APAP) appears to work centrally; its MOA appears far more complex than initially thought. Oral APAP has efficacy in the prevention of the development of hyperalgesia induced via direct activation of algetic spinal receptors (9). It is able to penetrate into the brain enabling both antipyresis and analgesic properties (10). The MOA of APAP appears to involve several systems:

- The eicosanoid system: APAP inhibits the COX enzyme and interferes with the conversion of arachidonic acid to prostaglandins (11, 12); COX-3 may be at least one site of APAP action (13).
- The serotonergic system: Up to fivefold increase in serotonin levels in multiple areas of the central nervous system (CNS) has been detected after APAP treatment (14). APAP analgesia is inhibited by tropisetron, an antiemetic and serotonin (5-HT) type 3 antagonist (15).

- The cannabinoid system: In the human CNS, paracetamol is metabolized to *P*-aminophenol which, via fatty acid amide hydrolase is transformed into *N*-arachidonoyl-phenolamine (AM404) (16). AM404 is a ligand at selective cannabinoid subtype 1 (CB1) receptors, as well as an agonist of transient receptor potential vanilloid type 1 receptors (TRPV1) and an inhibitor of fatty acid amide hydrolase, which would inhibit the reuptake and metabolism of anandamide, an endocannabinoid with analgesic properties (14, 16–19). The cannabinoids as well as endocannabinoids induce antinociceptive effects that are secondary mainly to CB1 receptors (20, 21).
- The opioid system: Cannabinoid-induced antinociception does appear to be associated with the release of opioid peptides into the brain (22). Opioid mu receptors, like the CB1 receptors found on many of the same neurons, are both associated with G proteins. The APAP metabolite AM404 may activate, at least in part, both the opioid and cannabinoid systems. The secondary interaction between CB1 and opiate receptors may then modulate other neurotransmitters including 5-HT, gamma-aminobutyric acid, both antinociceptive, as well as glutamate (21, 23, 24).

Naloxone (an opiate receptor antagonist) can prevent APAP's activity; APAP may be involved with the dynorphin system, as dynorphins interact with kappa receptors, and if they are blocked, the APAP-induced antinociceptive effects are reversed (25).

APAP is used for mild to moderate pain. It is considered first-line treatment for OA (26). It has few adverse effects except for hepatic toxicity, even leading to death, most typically found at dosages of 4 g/day or more, especially in patients with hepatic problems secondary to chronic alcohol abuse. Newer research finds the same problem (elevations in aminotransferase) in healthy adults taking 4 g of APAP a day for 14 days (3).

It is important to take a very specific history from patients regarding their APAP intake as they may neglect to tell you about APAP found in combination with other medications, which the patients may not even be aware of.

Its recommended dosage is 325 to 650 mg every four hours or 325 to 500 mg every three hours, with a maximum of 4 g (4000 mg) a day. The author tries to limit his patients' APAP to 2500 to 3000 mg a day, maximum. For moderate pain, 1 g may need to be given for optimal effectiveness, three times a day.

APAP is not extensively bound to proteins (only 10–25%). It has a high bioavailability (85–98%), a two-hour plasma half-life, and easily crosses the blood–brain barrier (BBB) with a peak concentration in the CSF in two to three hours.

Nonsteroidal Anti-inflammatory Drugs

NSAIDs are anti-inflammatory, analgesic, and antipyretic agents. They decrease prostaglandin production by inhibiting COX-1 and COX-2 enzymes. They are the drugs of choice for use in OA and rheumatoid arthritis for pain.

In June 2005, the FDA recommended a black box warning, which received final approval in January 2006 for CV events for all NSAIDs, prescription and over-the-counter forms. This black box warning noted NSAIDs could cause an increased risk of serious cardiovascular thrombotic events, myocardial infarction, and stroke, which could be fatal. This risk could increase with duration of use. Patients with cardiovascular disease or risk factors for cardiovascular disease may be at greater risk (27). This black box warning was in addition to the gastrointestinal black box warning regarding bleeding, ulcerations, and perforation of the stomach or intestines.

Renal events have also been reported with non-COX-2–specific NSAIDs as well as coxibs, including increased BUN, dysuria, urinary micturition frequency, hematuria, increased creatinine, renal insufficiency including renal failure, interstitial nephritis, albuminuria, urinary casts, cystitis, azotemia, nocturia, glomerular nephritis, polyuria, and more (28).

There are two type of NSAIDs: nonselective and selective (COX-2 inhibitors—only celecoxib remains in this group). All nonselective NSAIDs and coxibs are given at dosages that inhibit COX-2. This inhibition provides their antipyretic, anti-inflammatory, and analgesic effects. COX-2-selective drugs (celecoxib) might also be known as COX-1-sparing drugs, compared to nonselective NSAIDs (29).

Both nonselective and selective NSAIDs are considered second-line treatment for OA, as well as showing good efficacy for the pain of surgical procedures and other conditions that have an inflammatory component, such as dental surgery (30).

There are over 20 different NSAIDs in the United States in 10 different chemical classes:

1. Propionic acids (ibuprofen, naproxen, ketoprofen, ketorolac)
2. Indoleacetic acids (indomethacin, sulindac, etodolac)
3. Salicylic acids (nonacetylated)—(sodium salsalate, choline magnesium trisalicylate)—aspirin is acetylated
4. Phenylacetic acid (diclofenac)
5. Naphthylalkanone (Nabumetone)
6. Oxicam (Piroxicam)
7. Anthranilic acid (enolic)—(mefenamic acid, meclofenamate)
8. Pyrroleacetic acid (tolmetin)
9. Pyrazolone (phenylbutazone)
10. COX-2 inhibitors (celecoxib—rofecoxib and valdecoxib have been withdrawn from the market secondary to cardiovascular concerns)

The most frequently prescribed NSAIDs include the following:

*   Naproxen sodium (Anaprox), which reaches peak plasma levels in one to two hours, and has a mean half-life of 13 hours. It can be taken at 275 or 550 mg every six to eight hours, with a top dosage of 1375 mg/day.
*   Ibuprofen (Motrin) is prescribed in dosages of 600 and 800 mg per tablet. The suggested dosage for mild to moderate pain is 400 mg every four to six hours as needed.
*   Ketoprofen (Orudis) is a COX inhibitor but also stabilizes lysosomal membranes and possibly antagonizes the actions of bradykinin. Its peak plasma level is reached in one to two hours and has a two-hour plasma half-life. It is now over the counter (12.5-mg tablets) but is best used as 50- to 75-mg capsules. The recommended daily dosage is 150 to 300 mg a day in three or four

divided doses. GI side effects are generally mild. Care should be taken when given to a patient with impaired renal function.

- Ketorolac Tromethamine (Toradol) can be given orally or parentally for moderate to severe acute pain. Peak plasma levels occur after intramuscular injection in about 50 minutes. Its analgesic effect is considered to be roughly equivalent to a 10-mg dose of IM morphine. The typical injectable dose is 60 mg. Because of its potentially significant hepatic/renal side effects, the FDA has stated that Toradol should be given orally, after an IM injection of 60 mg, at 10 mg, every eight hours, for a maximum of five days.

The import of the different chemical classes is simple: not every NSAID will help every patient. If a patient does not receive relief from ibuprofen, the clinician should not try naproxen, which is in the same drug class, but another NSAID from another class should be utilized.

NSAIDs are extensively bound to serum albumin (95%). They are metabolized by the cytochrome P450 system (the CYP2C0 isoform) in the liver and excreted in the urine. Therefore, their use in patients with renal or hepatic dysfunction may be problematic. The half-lives of the NSAIDs vary greatly, ranging from an hour to longer than 55 hours.

NSAIDs may induce problems including constipation, confusion, headaches, and the aforementioned renal and hepatic toxicity, as well as GI ulcerations. They should be avoided in the elderly and those patients with congestive heart failure, coronary artery disease, hypertension, cirrhosis, and renal insufficiency. NSAIDs do have drug interactions, including ACE inhibitors, anticoagulants, beta-blockers, and loop diuretics.

The selective COX-2 inhibitor celecoxib has less risk of GI toxicity and has no reported effect on platelets/coagulation.

Risk factors for nonselective NSAID GI toxicity include combinations of NSAIDs; concomitant use of glucocorticoids and a past history of peptic ulcer disease, bleeding, or perforation. Again, their use in the older patient increases possible problems.

The idiosyncratic adverse effects of NSAIDs are also important to note and include the following:

- Rash
- Photosensitivity
- Tinnitus
- Aseptic meningitis
- Psychosis
- Cognitive dysfunction (especially in the elderly treated with indomethacin)
- Possible infertility
- Pulmonary infiltrates with eosinophilia
- Possible hypertension from naproxen and ibuprofen

Finally, long-term use of some NSAIDs appears to have accelerated cartilage damage in OA and some question the appropriateness of the use of NSAIDs in OA.

Some prescribing information:

- Ibuprofen (Motrin): Its half-life is 2 to 2.5 hours after multiple dosing. Typical adult dose is 1200 to 2400 mg/day.

- Naproxen: It is highly protein bound with a half-life of 12 to 15 hours. May use naproxen sodium 275- and 550-mg tablets twice a day.
- Ketoprofen (Orudis): It is 99% protein bound; its half-life is between 1.4 and 3.3 hours. It is available in 25, 50, and 75 mg and an extended-release 200-mg capsule. It can be taken three times a day.
- Oxaprozin (Daypro): Elimination half-life is between 50 and 60 hours after repeated doses—adult dose is 600 to 1200 mg/day. Patients can begin with a loading dose of 1800 mg.
- Etodolac (Lodine): The elimination half-life is six to seven hours. Maximum analgesia in one hour after oral dose. Doses range, in the adult, from 400 to 1200 mg/day.
- Indomethacin (Indocin): Elimination half-life is 2 to 11 hours. Adult dose is 75 to 150 mg/day.
- Diclofenac [Cataflam (potassium salt), Voltaren (enteric coated)]: It has a 75-minute half-life. The adult dose is 75 to 225 mg/day.
- Nabumetone (Relafen): A prodrug, metabolized to active metabolite with half-life of 24 hours. Adult dose is 1000 to 2000 mg/day.
- Ketorolac (Toradol): It is the only NSAID with parenteral usage; its half-life is four to six hours. Oral dosing is 10 mg three or four times a day. If given via IM or IV route, typically oral dosing is limited to four to five days.
- When using NSAIDs in the elderly, dosages should be decreased, in many cases, by 50%.
- Celecoxib (Celebrex): It has a half-life of 11 hours; adult dose is 100 to 400 mg a day.

Finally, it may be safe to give a COX-1 or COX-2 to patients with asthma and aspirin intolerance (31).

These medications are frequently sold in combination with other drugs such as caffeine, which exerts no specific analgesic effects, but may potentiate the analgesic effects of aspirin and APAP. There are aspirin–caffeine combination drugs (Anacin) and aspirin, APAP, and caffeine combinations (Excedrin Extra-Strength, Excedrin Migraine, and Vanquish). The recommended dosage is two tablets every six hours as needed.

MUSCLE RELAXANTS

Muscle relaxants are given for acute soft tissue spasm/pain by some clinicians. They are probably best utilized during the first one to three weeks post injury. They may be useful in patients with significant muscle spasm and pain. They are used appropriately after the development of muscle spasm after an injury such as a slip and fall, motor vehicle accident, work and athletic injuries, or over-stretching.

These medications work via the development of a therapeutic plasma level. Their exact MOA is unknown, but they do not directly affect striated muscle, the myoneural junction, or motor nerves. They produce relaxation by depressing the central pathways, possibly through their effects on higher CNS centers, which modifies the central perception of pain without effecting the peripheral pain reflexes or motor activity.

Carisoprodol (Soma) is a CNS depressant that metabolizes into a barbiturate, meprobamate, which makes it both addictive and particularly inappropriate to use for patients with pain from muscle spasm in addition to minor traumatic brain injury. It acts as a sedative and it is thought to depress polysynaptic transmission in interneuronal pools at the supraspinal level in the brain stem reticular formation. It is short lived, with peak plasma levels in one to two hours and a four to six hour half-life. Dosage is 350 mg every six to eight hours. It should not be mixed with other CNS depressants. It is also marketed in two other combined forms (with aspirin as Soma Compound) and with Codeine, for additional analgesic effects. It may be associated with postural hypotension, syncope, tachycardia, trembling, diplopia, blurred vision, and dyspnea, among other pharmacodynamic effects. Use caution in patients with hepatic and renal dysfunction.

Chlorzoxazone (Parafon Forte DSC) is a centrally acting muscle relaxant with fewer sedative properties. It is reported to inhibit the reflex arcs involved in producing and maintaining muscle spasm at the level of the spinal cord and subcortical areas of the brain. It reaches its peak plasma level in one to two hours, and duration of action is 6 to 12 hours. It is well tolerated, and side effects are uncommon. Dosage is 500 mg three times a day. Pharmacodynamic changes demonstrate a generally well-tolerated drug. Cautions include anaphylaxis.

Metaxalone (Skelaxin) is a centrally acting skeletal muscle relaxant which is chemically related to mephenoxalone, a mild tranquilizer. It is thought to induce muscle relaxation via CNS depression. Onset of action is about one hour, with peak blood levels in two hours, and duration of action is four to six hours. The recommended dose is 2400 to 3200 mg a day in divided doses (tablets are 400 mg each). It should be used carefully in patients with impaired liver function and should not be used at all in patients with significant renal or liver disease as well as a history of drug-induced anemias. Side effects include nausea, vomiting, GI upset, drowsiness, dizziness, headache, nervousness, and irritability as well as rash or pruritus. Jaundice and hemolytic anemia are rare. Use caution in patients with history of drug-induced anemias and with pre-existing liver damage. Serial liver function tests (LFTs) should be performed.

Methocarbamol (Robaxin) is a centrally acting skeletal muscle relaxant. It may inhibit nerve transmission in the internuncial neurons of the spinal cord. It has a 30- to 45-minute onset of action. Peak levels are found in about two hours, and its duration of action is four to six hours. It comes as 500- and 750-mg tablets. Tablets containing methocarbamol and aspirin (Robaxisal) are also available. The recommended dose of Robaxin is 750 mg three times a day. As with all of these medications, it should be taken for 7 to 10 days. It is well tolerated, with initial side effects which resolve over time, including lightheadedness, dizziness, vertigo, headache, rash, GI upset, nasal congestion, fever, blurred vision, urticaria, and mild muscular incoordination. In situations of severe, seemingly intractable muscle spasm, Robaxin may be given intravenously in doses of about 1 g every 8 to 12 hours.

Orphenadrine citrate (Norflex, Norgesic) is a centrally acting skeletal muscle relaxant with anticholinergic properties thought to work by blocking neuronal circuits, the hyperactivity of which may be implicated in hypertonia and spasm. It is available in injectable and oral formulations. The IM dose of Norflex is 2 mg, while the intravenous dosage is 60 mg in aqueous solution. The oral formulation (Norflex) is given in 100-mg tablets—one tablet every 12 hours. Norgesic is a combination form, including caffeine and aspirin and should be given one or two tablets every six to eight hours. Norgesic Forte, a stronger combination, is given one half to one tablet every six to eight hours. Because of its anticholinergic effects, it should be contraindicated in patients with glaucoma, prostatic enlargement, or bladder outlet obstruction. Its major side effects are also secondary to its anticholinergic properties and include tachycardia, palpitations, urinary retention, nausea, vomiting, dizziness, constipation, and drowsiness. It may also cause confusion, excitation, hallucinations, and syncope.

Many of these medications are given in combination with other drugs, including barbiturates (butalbital and meprobamate) and narcotics (codeine, oxycodone, propoxyphene, etc.) This is probably not a good idea, as the barbiturates and narcotics can easily help develop patient dependence.

A useful combination may include methocarbamol 750 mg three times a day for 10 days in patients with significant spasm, accompanied by ketoprofen, 75 mg, every six to eight hours as needed, with food as needed. For the acute posttraumatic soft tissue injury, one tablet of each taken together every six to eight hours for two to three doses works very well. These muscle relaxants are for acute cases of muscle spasm and pain. If there is no help within 10 days or so, they most probably won't work. In such cases, particularly in patients with painful muscle spasm lasting three weeks or longer, tizanidine would be the drug of choice.

Tizanidine has been used for painful conditions involving painful muscle spasm of three weeks' duration or longer, spasticity, myofascial pain, tension-type headache, acute low back pain, and fibromyalgia. This medication is very sedating, but it works well when given at h.s., rather than t.i.d. Peak effect is in one to two hours, with a duration of effect between three and six hours. Half-life is about 2.5 hours. It should be used with caution in patients with renal insufficiency. Adverse events may include hypertension, bradycardia, palpitations, prolonged QT interval, pruritus, and xerostomia. Dosages should be in the range of 12 to 16 mg given at night. Also, the generic forms of tizanidine are very frequently found to have side effects of hallucinations and vivid dreams, much more frequently than the nongeneric form (Zanaflex).

There are few high-quality, randomized controlled trials (RCTs) providing evidence of the effectiveness of muscle relaxants. It is felt that a combination of a skeletal muscle relaxant with an NSAID or with tramadol/APAP may be superior to single muscle relaxants (32).

OTHER ADJUNCTIVE MEDICATIONS

Other possible forms of adjunctive medications include NMDA receptor antagonists. There are no NMDA receptor antagonists approved for the treatment of pain; Memantine is approved for treatment of Alzheimer's disease. The NMDA receptor antagonists include ketamine, dextromethorphan, amantadine, magnesium, and methadone, an opiate which is considered to have a 10% NMDA receptor antagonism. These medications may, in the future, be very beneficial; particularly antagonists at the glycine-site NR2B sites, at which weak-binding channel blockers have shown an improved side effect profile in animal models of pain (33). Ketamine is used as an adjunctive therapy in the hospice setting when opioid therapy is not sufficient (34). Ketamine alone, or with midazolam, have long been used for sedating children undergoing minor operative procedures or painful procedures such as changing dressings for burn patients (35, 36).

Finally, subanesthetic dosages of ketamine used in analgesia appear to act largely as a dopamine D2 receptor agonist.

The α_2 agonists include clonidine and tizanidine. Clonidine is widely used, orally, transdermally, epidurally, and intrathecally, for the treatment of pain secondary to cancer, postoperative pain, neuropathies, postherpetic neuralgia, headaches, labor, and complex regional pain syndrome, restless leg syndrome, and orofacial pain.

Vistaril, an antihistamine, can also be used in combination with narcotics as an adjunctive medication to prolong and possibly amplify their effects.

Tramadol

Tramadol appears to be the most widely used analgesic for chronic noncancer pain of all types in the relatively (in parts) opiophobic European Union.

Tramadol is a centrally acting analgesic that is related structurally to codeine and morphine. It consists of two enantiomers, both of which are important in the drug's analgesic mechanisms. The (+)-tramadol and the metabolite (+)-O-desmethyl-tramadol (also called M1) are mu opioid receptor agonists. The (+)-tramadol also inhibits serotonin reuptake, while the (−)-tramadol enantiomers inhibit norepinephrine reuptake, enhancing inhibitory effects on spinal cord pain transmission (33).

Tramadol is rapidly absorbed after oral administration. It is rapidly distributed in the plasma, with about 20% plasma protein binding. It is metabolized by O- and N-demethylation and by conjugation forming glucuronides and sulfates. Tramadol and its metabolites are excreted mainly by the kidneys, with a mean elimination half-life of about six hours (33, 34). The O-demethylation of the drug to M1 is catalyzed by cytochrome P450 (CYP) 2D6 (35). The analgesic potency of tramadol is only 10% of that of morphine status post parenteral administration. Tramadol produces less constipation and problems with dependence than equianalgesic dosages of opioids (36). There are no respiratory or cardiovascular problems associated with the drug (37). M1 has a greater affinity to the mu receptor and is felt to be mainly responsible for tramadol opiate activity (36). It is felt that the dual activity (opioid and nonopioid) explains its effectiveness in pain that may not be responsive to opiates alone: neuropathic pain (38). Tramadol is felt to be one of the first-choice drugs for the treatment of neuropathic pain; it has been found to be effective in several placebo-controlled studies (39–45).

In a Cochrane evidence-based review, tramadol was found to be "an effective treatment for neuropathic pain" (46). The reviewers found five "eligible" RCTs, three comparing tramadol with placebo, one comparing tramadol with clomipramine, and one comparing tramadol with morphine. All three trials comparing tramadol to placebo were positive, with tramadol being superior to placebo. There was not enough evidence to develop a conclusion regarding tramadol versus morphine or clomipramine (47). It was determined that the NNT was 3.5 (NNT is the number needed to treat, to find one patient with a greater than 50% diminution of pain) (47).

Tramadol has been found to be useful in the treatment of fibromyalgia (48). It is also now thought to have antidepressant activity (49). For moderate to severe pain, start at 25 mg PO q.a.m., then increase by 25 mg/day every three days to 25 mg q.i.d., then increase by 50 mg/day every three days to 50 mg q.i.d.

Maximum dosage should not exceed 50 to 100 mg every four to six hours as needed. Typically, no more than 300 to 400 mg a day should be used. Large studies have found that tramadol abuse is statistically low, about 1 patient in 100,000 (49).

Antiarrhythmics

Antiarrhythmics block ectopic neuronal activity at central and peripheral sites (50). Lidocaine, mexiletine, and phenytoin—type I antiarrhythmics—stabilize neural membranes by sodium channel blockade. Lidocaine suppresses spontaneous impulse generation on injured nerve segments, dorsal root ganglia, and dorsal horn wide dynamic range neurons (51, 52). Lidocaine infusions have been used to predict the response of a given neuropathic pain disorder to antiarrhythmic therapy (53). Lidocaine may be effective at subanesthetic doses, and following nerve blocks analgesia may outlast conduction block for days or weeks (53–55). It has been reported that patients with peripheral nervous system (PNS) injury experience better pain relief than those with central pain syndromes (56). If a trial infusion of lidocaine is effective, a trial of oral mexiletine is worth considering.

Mexiletine and ketamine produced a moderate decrement of static but not dynamic allodynia associated with postherpetic neuralgia (57). Also, mexiletine was used to treat the peripheral neuropathy secondary to chemotherapy with taxol—a 50% improvement was seen (58).

Prior to starting mexiletine, a baseline electrocardiogram is recommended to determine if the patient has underlying ischemic heart disease. Dosages may be increased from 150 to 250 mg three times a day over several days. Taking the medication with food may minimize gastric side effects, which are common and a major reason for discontinuing the drug. Other side effects of mexiletine are nervous system effects such as tremor and diplopia. Once on a stable dose, a serum level should be obtained (the therapeutic range is between 0.5 and 2.0 mg/mL).

Topical Preparations of Local Anesthetics

Topical preparations of local anesthetics may be effective for neuropathic pain when there is localized allodynia or hypersensitivity. Topical blockade of small- and large-fiber nerve endings should reduce mechanical and thermal allodynia. A topical lidocaine patch (Lidoderm 5% lidocaine) has become available, which can be applied to painful areas in shingles (herpes zoster) and in more chronic forms of neuropathic pain such as diabetic neuropathy or the ischemic neuropathies created by prolonged peripheral vascular insufficiency. Up to three patches may be applied at one time to the painful area. The patches can be worn for up to 12 hours a day. However, the treating physician must ensure that the patient understands that chronic forms of neuropathic pain may require a longer therapeutic trial, for example, 30 days, before optimal symptomatic control can be determined. In patients with diabetic neuropathy, Rowbotham et al. (59) have found that the addition of topical lidocaine patches to exogenous GABAergic oral agents may provide further improvement of symptom control.

A topical cream, eutectic mixture of local anesthetic (EMLA cream), a mixture of lidocaine and prilocaine, may also be useful for cutaneous pain. The cream may be applied three or four times a day to the painful area.

Corticosteroids

Corticosteroids are clearly useful for neuropathic pain, particularly in stimulus-evoked pain such as lumbar radiculopathy. The anti-inflammatory effects of corticosteroids are well known, which may partly explain their efficacy for pain. When administered epidurally for treatment of discogenic radiculopathy, corticosteroids inhibit phospholipase A2 activity and suppress the perineural inflammatory response caused by leakage of disk material around the painful nerve root (60). However, corticosteroids also act as membrane stabilizers by suppressing ectopic neural discharges (61, 62). Therefore, some of the pain-relieving action of corticosteroids may be due to a lidocaine-like effect.

Depot forms of corticosteroids injected around injured nerves provide pain relief and reduce pain associated with entrapment syndromes. Corticosteroids are also effective if given orally or systemically. In cancer pain syndromes, steroids such as dexamethasone may be first-line therapy for neuropathic pain. The potential side effects of corticosteroids are well known and may be seen whether given orally, systemically, or epidurally.

As interventional treatment of pain becomes the most likely type of treatment a pain patient can receive, more steroids are being used than ever before, in spite of objective lack of level A or 1 evidence-based medicine. A number of $n = 1$ studies are published showing that "Corticosteroids cure pelvic pain" (63). Larger studies show that psychopathology/psychiatric comorbidity is associated with diminished pain relief after a medial branch nerve block with steroids (64), an issue that is most frequently ignored. Some RCTs are being done. In one, it was found that there were no differences in short-term outcomes found between local ultrasound guided corticosteroid injection and systemic corticosteroid injection in rotator cuff disease (65).

Finally, corticosteroid-induced psychosis was found in a patient following a cervical epidural, four medial branch blocks, four trigger point injections, and a tendon injection, all with corticosteroids, all performed in one treatment session. Seven days later, the patient developed psychotic episodes, with racing thoughts, anger, agitation, pressured hyperverbal speech, and paranoia. The symptoms resolved spontaneously within 7 to 10 days. This is possibly the first report of this known potential complication (66).

Baclofen

Baclofen is useful for trigeminal neuralgia and other types of neuropathic pain (67), particularly as an add-on drug. Baclofen is a GABA-B agonist and is presumed to hyperpolarize inhibitory neurons in the spinal cord (68), thereby reducing pain. This GABA effect appears to be similar to benzodiazepines, such as clonazepam. Side effects of baclofen can be significant and include sedation, confusion, nausea, vomiting, and weakness, especially in the elderly. A typical starting dose is 5 mg three times a day. Thereafter, the drug can be increased slowly to 20 mg four times a day. Abrupt cessation may precipitate withdrawal with hallucinations, anxiety, and tachycardia. The drug is excreted by the kidneys, and the dosage must be reduced in renal insufficiency.

Baclofen is more commonly being used intrathecally via an implanted pump for pain as well as spasticity. It is also being used for refractory cancer pain, neuropathic pain, and visceral pain (69–72).

Capsaicin

Capsaicin is a C fiber–specific neurotoxin and is one of the components of hot peppers that produces a burning sensation on contact with mucous membranes. Topical preparations are available over the counter and are widely used for chronic pain syndromes. Capsaicin is a vanilloid receptor (TRPV1) agonist and activates ion channels on C fibers that are thermotransducers of noxious heat (>43°C) (73). With repeated application in sufficient quantities, capsaicin can inactivate primary afferent nociceptors via desensitization. For patients with pain due to sensitized nociceptors, capsaicin may be effective, if they can tolerate the pain induced by the medication. The drug causes intense burning, which may abate with repeated applications and gradual inactivation of the nociceptors. However, in patients with tactile allodynia, which is probably mediated by large fibers, capsaicin may not be as effective. Capsaicin extracts are available commercially as topical preparations, containing 0.025% and 0.075% and should be applied to the painful area three to five times a day. The preparation may be better tolerated if it is used after application of a topical local anesthetic cream.

TRPVI (vanilloid) receptors have become a major research target for both agonists and antagonists, with multiple treatment indications including post-surgical pain, postherpetic neuralgia, diabetic neuropathic pain, OA, and others, including cancer (74). Further research has found evidence that TRPVI receptors on the central branches of dorsal root ganglion (DRG) neurons in the spinal cord may play an important role in pain modulation and nociceptive transmission (75). It has also been noted that capsaicin-induced calcium desensitizes the TRPVI channels and contributes to capsaicin-induced analgesia (76).

TRPV1 receptors, as neuronally expressed, are nonselective Ca(2+) preferring cation channels. Other than capsaicin, this channel is activated by different stimuli including heat, acid, certain arachidonic acid derivatives, and direct phosphorylation via protein kinase C (PKC—see below) (77).

Protein Kinase C (PKC) Inhibitors

Activation of PKC has been implicated in noted changes in pain perception. When activated by phorbol esters, PKC enhances thermal hyperalgesia in diabetic mice. Activated PKC also leads to enhancement of excitatory amino acids (EAAs) in dorsal horn neurons as well as trigeminal neurons. It is therefore possible that PKC may induce neuronal sensitization that produces hyperalgesia in diabetic neuropathy. Ruboxistaurin, a PKC inhibitor, may be a valid treatment for diabetic neuropathic pain (78–80).

TRPV1 and TRPV4 channels are coexpressed in certain DRG neurons and TRPV4 can be sensitized by PKC in the DRG neuronal cell bodies as well as in the central sensory and nonsensory nerve terminals. This PKC-induced sensitization may play a synergistic role in nociception (81).

REFERENCES

1. World Health Organization. Cancer Pain Relief with a Guide to Opioid Availability; World Health Organization; 1996.
2. Schug SA. Combination analgesia in 2005—a rational approach: focus on paracetamol-tramadol. Clin Rheumatol 2006; 25(suppl 1):S16–S21.

3. Watkins PB, Kaplowitz N, Slattery JT, et al. Aminotransferase elevations in healthy adults receiving 4 grams of acetaminophen daily: a randomized, controlled trial. JAMA 2006; 296(1):87–93.

4. Langford RM. Pain management today—what have we learned? Clin Rheumatol 2006; 25(suppl 7):2–8.

5. Schnitzer TJ. Update on guidelines for the treatment of chronic musculoskeletal pain. Clin Rheumatol 2006; 25(suppl 7):22–29.

6. Elia N, Lysakowski C, Tramer MR. Does multimodal analgesia with acetaminophen, nonsteroidal antiinflammatory drugs or selective cyclooxygenase-2 inhibitors and patient-controlled analgesia morphine offer advantages over morphine alone? Meta-analysis of randomized trials. Anesthesiology 2005; 103(6):1296–1304.

7. White PF. The changing role of non-opioid analgesic techniques in the management of postoperative pain. Anesth Analg 2005; 101(5 suppl):S5–S22.

8. von Mering J. Beitrage zur Kenntniss der Antipyretica. Ther Monatscyh 1983; 7:577–587.

9. Crawley B, Saito O, Malkmus S, et al. Acetaminophen prevents hyperalgesia in central pain cascade. Neurosci Lett 2008; 442:50–53.

10. Courad JP, Besse D, Delchambre C, et al. Acetaminophen distribution in the rat central nervous system. Life Sci 2001; 69:1455–1464.

11. Rowlinson SW, Kiefer JR, Prusakiewicz JJ, et al. A novel mechanism of cyclooxygenase-2 inhibition involving interactions with Ser-530 and Tyr-385. J Biol Chem 2003; 278:45763–45769.

12. Anderson BJ. Paracetamol (acetaminophen): mechanisms of action. Paediatr Anaesth 2008; 18:915–921.

13. Warner TD, Mitchell JA. Cyclooxygenase-3 (COX-3): filling in the gaps toward a COX continuum? Proc Natl Acad Sci U S A 2002; 99:13371–13373.

14. Smith HS. Potential analgesic mechanisms of acetaminophen. Pain Physician 2009; 12:269–280.

15. Picering G, Loriot MA, Libert F, et al. Analgesic effect of acetaminophen in humans: first evidence of a central serotonergic mechanism. Clin Pharm Ther 2006; 79(4):371–378.

16. Bertolini A, Ferrara A, Ottani A, et al. Paracetamol: new vistas of an old drug. CNS Drug Rev 2006; 12(3/4):250–275.

17. Sinning C, Bernhard W, Coste O, et al. New analgesics synthetically derived from the paracetamol metabolite N-(4-hydroxyphenyl)-(5Z,8Z,11Z,14Z)-icosatetra-5,8,11,14-enamide. J Med Chem 2008; 51(24):7800–7805.

18. Di Marzo V, Deutsch DG. Biochemistry of the endogenous ligands of cannabinoid receptors. Neurobiol Dis 1998; 5:386–404.

19. Hogestatt ED, Jonsson BA, Ermund A, et al. Conversion of acetaminophen to bioactive N-acylphenolamine AM404 via fatty acid amide hydrolase-dependent arachidonic acid conjugation in the nervous system. J Biol Chem 2005; 280:31405–31412.

20. Manzanares J, Julian MD, Carrascosa A. Role of the cannabinoid system in pain control and therapeutic implications for the management of acute and chronic pain episodes. Curr Neuropharmacol 2006; 4:239–257.

21. Rice ASC, Farquhar-Smith WP, Nagy I. Endocannabinoids and pain: spinal and peripheral analgesia in inflammation and neuropathy. Prostaglandins Leukot Essent Fatty Acids 2002; 66(2/3):243–256.

22. Palazzo E, de Novellis V, Petrosino S, et al. Neuropathic pain and the endocannabinoid system in the dorsal raphe: pharmacological treatment and interactions with serotonergic systems. Eur J Neurosci 2006; 24:2011–2020.

23. Schoffelmeer ANM, Hogenboom F, Wardeh G, et al. Interaction between CB1 and μ opioid receptors mediating inhibition of neurotransmitter release in rat nucleus accumbens core. Neuropharmacology 2006; 51:773–781.

24. Ruggieri V, Vitale G, Pini LA, et al. Differential involvement of opioidergic and serotonergic systems in the antinociceptive activity of N-arachidonoyl-phenolamine

(AM404) in the rat: comparison with paracetamol. Naunyn Schmiedebergs Arch Pharmacol 2008; 337:219–229.

25. Sandrini M, Romualdi P, Capobianco A. The effect of paracetamol on nociception and dynorphin A levels in the rat brain. Neuropeptides 2001; 35:110–116.

26. American College of Rheumatology Subcommittee on Osteoarthritis Guidelines. Recommendations for the medical management of osteoarthritis of the hip and knee: 2000 update. Arthritis Rheum 2000; 43:1905–1915.

27. World Health Organization (WHO) Pharmaceuticals Newsletter 2005; 3:8.

28. Barkin RL, Buvanendran A. Focus on the COX-1 and COX-2 agents: renal events of nonsteroidal and anti-inflammatory drugs-NSAIDs. Am J Ther 2004; 11:124–129.

29. Warner TD, Mitchell JA. COX-2 selectivity alone does not define the cardiovascular risks associated with non-steroidal anti-inflammatory drugs. Lancet 2008: 371(9608):270–273.

30. Barkin RL, Romano RJ. Nonopioid drugs for pain management. Patient Care 2004: 41–51.

31. Szczeklik A, Murray JJ; Celecoxib in Aspirin-Intolerant Asthma Study Group. Celecoxib in patients with asthma and aspirin intolerance. The Celecoxib in Aspirin-Intolerant Asthma Study Group. N Engl J Med 2001; 344(2):142.

32. Beebe FA, Barkin RL, Barkin S. A clinical and pharmacologic review of skeletal muscle relaxants for musculoskeletal conditions. Am J Ther 2005; 12:151–171.

33. Brown DG, Krupp JJ. *N*-methyl-D-aspartate Receptor (NMDA) antagonists as potential pain therapeutics. Curr Top Med Chem 2006; 6(8):749–770.

34. Legge J, Ball N, Elliott DP. The potential role of ketamine in hospice analgesia: a literature review. Consult Pharm 2006; 21(1):51–57.

35. Owens VF, Palmieri TL, Comroe CM, et al. Ketamine: a safe and effective agent for painful procedures in the pediatric burn patient. J Burn Care Res 2006; 27(2): 211–216.

36. Cheuk DK, Wong WH, Ma E, et al. Use of midazolam and ketamine as sedation for children undergoing minor operative procedures. Support Care Cancer 2005; 13(12):1001–1009.

37. Grond S, Sablotzki A. Clinical pharmacology of tramadol. Clin Pharmacokinet 2004; 43(13):879–923.

38. Desmeules JA. The tramadol option. Eur J Pain 2000; 4(suppl A):15–21.

39. Dworkin RH, Backonja M, Rowbotham MC, et al. Advances in neuropathic pain. Arch Neurol 2003; 60:1524–1534.

40. Stacey BR. Management of peripheral neuropathic pain. Am J Phys Med Rehabil 2005; 84(suppl 3):S4–S16.

41. Marchettini P, Teloni L, Formaglio Lacerenza M. Pain in diabetic neuropathy case study: whole patient management. Eur J Neurol 2004; (suppl 1):12–21.

42. Mullins CR, Wild TL. Pain management in a long-term care facility: compliance with JCAHO standards. J Pain Palliat Care Pharmacother 2003; 17(2):63–70.

43. Sindrup SH, Andersen G, Madsen C, et al. Tramadol relieves pain and allodynia in polineurpathy: a randomised, double-blind, controlled trial. Pain 1999; 83:85–90.

44. Waikakul S, Waikakul W. Penkitti P, et al. Comparison of analgesics for pain after brachial plexus injury: tramadol vs. paracetamol with codeine. Pain Clinic 1998; 11:119–124.

45. Harati Y, Gooch C, Sweenson M, et al. Double-blind randomized trial of tramadol for the treatment of the pain of diabetic neuropathy. Neurology 1998; 50:1842–1846.

46. Duhmke RM, Cornblath DD, Hollingshead JR. Tramadol for neuropathic pain. Cochrane Database Syst Rev 2004; 2:CD003726.

47. Cook RJ, Sackett DL. The number needed to treat: a clinically useful measure of treatment effect. BMJ 1995; 310:452–454.

48. Sumpton JE, Moulin DE. Fibromyalgia: presentation and management with a focus on pharmacological treatment. Pain Res Manage 2009; 13(6):477–483.

49. Reeves RR, Burke RS. Tramadol: basic pharmacology and emerging concepts. Drugs Today (Barc) 2008; 44(11):827–836.

50. Chabal C, Jacobson L, Mariano A, et al. The use of oral mexiletine for the treatment of pain after peripheral nerve injury. Anesthesiology 1992; 76:513–517.
51. Abram SE, Yaksh TL. Systemic lidocaine blocks nerve injury-induced hyperalgesia and nociceptor-driven spinal sensitization in the rat. Anesthesiology 1994; 80:383–391.
52. Swerdlow M. Anticonvulsant drugs and chronic pain. Clin Neuropharmacol 1984; 7:51–82.
53. Burchiel KJ, Chabal C. A role for systemic lidocaine challenge in the classification of neuropathic pains. Pain Forum 1995; 4:81–82.
54. Chaplan SR, Flemming BW, Shafer SL, et al. Prolonged alleviation of tactile allodynia by intravenous lidocaine in neuropathic rats. Anesthesiology 1995; 83:775–785.
55. Jaffe RA, Rowe MA. Subanesthetic concentrations of lidocaine selectively inhibit a nociceptive response in the isolated rat spinal cord. Pain 1995; 60:167–174.
56. Galer BS, Miller KV, Rowbotham MC. Response to intravenous lidocaine infusion differs based on clinical diagnosis and site of nervous system injury. Neurology 1993; 43:1233–1235.
57. Sasaki A, Serizawa K, Andoh T, et al. Pharmacological differences between static and dynamic allodynia in mice with herpetic or postherpetic pain. J Pharmacol Sci 2008; 108(3):266–273.
58. Yano T, Yamane H, Fukuoka R, et al. Evaluation of efficacy and safety of adjuvant analgesics for peripheral neuropathy induced by cancer chemotherapy in digestive cancer patients—a pilot study. Gan To Kagaku Ryoho 2009; 36(1):83–87.
59. Rowbotham MC, Davies PS, Verkernpinck C, et al. Lidocaine patch: double-blind, controlled study of a new treatment method for post-herpetic neuralgia. Pain 1996; 65:39–44.
60. Saal JS, Franson RC, Dobrow R, et al. High levels of inflammatory phospholipase A2 activity in lumbar disc herniations. Spine 1990; 15:674–678.
61. Castillo J, Curley J, Hotz J, et al. Glucocorticoids prolong rat sciatic nerve blockade in vivo from bupivacaine microspheres. Anesthesiology 1996; 85:1157–1166.
62. Devor M, Govrin-Lippmann R, Raber P. Corticosteroids suppress ectopic neural discharge originating in experimental neuromas. Pain 1985; 22:127–137.
63. Antolak SJ Jr, Antolak CM. Therapeutic pudendal nerve blocks using corticosteroids cure pelvic pain after failure of sacral neuromodulation. Pain Med 2009; 10(1):186–189.
64. Wasan AD, Jamison RN, Pham L, et al. Psychopathology predicts the outcome of medical branch blocks with corticosteroids for chronic axial low back or cervical pain: a prospective cohort study. BMC Musculoskelet Disord 2009; 10(1):22.
65. Ekeberg OM, Bautz-Holter E, Tveita EK, et al. Subacromial ultrasound guided or systemic steroid injection for rotator cuff disease: a randomized double blind study. BMJ 2009; 338:a3112.
66. Benyamin RM, Valleho R, Kramer J, et al. Corticosteroid induced psychosis in the pain management setting. Pain Physician 2008; 11(6):917–920.
67. Fromm GH, Terrence CF, Chattha AS. Baclofen in the treatment of trigeminal neuralgia: double-blind study and long-term follow-up. Ann Neurol 1984; 15:240–244.
68. Yaksh TL, Malmberg AB. Central pharmacology of nociceptive transmission. In: Wall PD, Melzack R, eds. Textbook of Pain. 3rd ed. Edinburgh, UK: Churchill Livingstone, 1994:165–200.
69. Newsome S, Frawley BJ, Argoff CE. Intrathecal analgesia for refractory cancer pain. Curr Pain Headache Rep 2008; 12(4):249–256.
70. Brennan PM, Whittle IR. Intrathecal baclofen therapy for neurological disorders: a sound knowledge base but many challenges remain. Br J Neurosurg 2008; 22(4):508–519.
71. Gronseth G, Cruccu G, Alksne J, et al. Practice parameter: the diagnostic evaluation and treatment of trigeminal neuralgia (an evidence based review): report of the Quality Standards Subcommittee of the American Academy of Neurology and the European Federation of Neurological Societies. Neurology 2008; 71(125):1183–1190.

72. Brusberg M, Ravnefjord A, Martinsson R, et al. The GABA(B) receptor agonist baclofen and the positive allosteric modulator CGP7930, inhibit visceral pain-related responses to colorectal distension in rats. Neuropharmacology 2009; 56(2):362–367.
73. Caternia MJ, Schumacher MA, Tominga M, et al. The capsaicin receptor: a heat-activated ion channel in the pain pathway. Nature 1997; 389:816–824.
74. Wong GY, Gavva NR. Therapeutic potential of vanilloid receptor TRPVI agonists and antagonists as analgesics: recent advances and setbacks. Brain Res Rev 2009; doi:10.1016/j.brainresrev.2008.12.006.
75. Spicarova D, Palecek J. The role of spinal cord vanilloid (TRPV1) receptors in pain modulation. Physiol Res 2008; 57(suppl 3):S69–S77.
76. Vyklicky L, Novakova-Tousova K, Benedikt J, et al. Calcium-dependent desensitization of vanilloid receptor TRPV1: a mechanism possibly involved in analgesia induced by topical application of capsaicin. Physiol Res 2008; 57(suppl 3):S59–S68.
77. Adcock JJ. TRPV1 receptors in sensitization of cough and pain reflexes. Pulm Pharmacol Ther 2009, doi:10.1016/j.pupt.2008.12.014.
78. Kamel J, Mizoguchi H, Narita M, et al. Therapeutic potential of PKC inhibitors in painful diabetic neuropathy. Exp Opin Invest Drugs 2001; 10(9):1653–1664.
79. Haslbeck M. New options in the treatment of various forms of diabetic neuropathy. MMW Fortschr Med 2004; 146(21):47–50.
80. Vinik AI, Bril V, Kempler P, et al. Treatment of symptomatic diabetic peripheral neuropathy with the protein kinase C beta-inhibitor ruboxistaurin mesylate during a 1-year, randomized, placebo controlled, double-blind clinical trial. Clin Ther 2005; 27(8):1164.
81. Cao DS, Yu SQ, Premkumar LS. Modulation of transient receptor potential vanilloid 4-mediated membrane currents and synaptic transmission by protein kinase C. Mol Pain 2009; 5:5.

17 Opioid Medications and Correct Medical Usage—An Update

Gary W. Jay

Clinical Disease Area Expert-Pain, Pfizer, Inc., New London, Connecticut, U.S.A.

The antinociceptive pain pathways have been described in detail in *Chronic Pain* (1). The descending pathways are opioid and monoaminergic based. The opioid analgesics appear to produce analgesia by inhibiting the ascending pain pathways (which carry nociceptive information to the brain), and activate the descending pain control pathways, which go from the CNS down the ventromedial medulla and down to the spinal cord dorsal horn. Opioids act in the periaqueductal gray (via μ receptors) to decrease GABAergic inhibition of the descending pathways.

The basic mode of opioid action is to inhibit the release of excitatory amino acids such as glutamate from peripheral nociceptors and postsynaptic neurons in the spinal cord dorsal horn.

After acute pain, algetic or pain-inducing chemicals are released from the nociceptors' terminals, including substance P, glutamate, calcitonin gene–related peptide (CGRP), neurokinins, and more. These chemicals will enable nociceptive information to reach the dorsal horn (via the substantia gelatinosa) and move rostrally via the ascending pain pathways. Locally, these algetic chemicals induce a neurogenic or sterile inflammation, the presence of which continues to feed nociceptive information centrally.

Glutamate will anneal to the *N*-methyl-D-aspartate (NMDA) receptor as well as the AMPA (alpha-amino-3-hydroxy-5-methyl-4-isoxazole propionic acid) receptor.

The AMPA receptor has a low threshold and quickly fluxes sodium and potassium through it. The NMDA receptor has a voltage-gated magnesium "plug." Typically, in acute pain this is not dislodged and the NMDA receptor provides only minimal stimulation.

As a consequence of the pathophysiology of chronic pain, the magnesium is forced out of the NMDA receptor (secondary to continuous stimulation, in part) and calcium fluxes through the receptor and into the cell, where it reacts with protein kinase C and nitric oxide synthase, which enables the formation of nitric oxide. The nitric oxide leaves the cell and reacts with guanyl synthase, which closes the sodium channel. This enables the development of pain that will not respond to opioids, as opioids can only work on the terminal if the sodium channel is open. A major goal is to prevent this from occurring by treating pain earlier rather than later.

Continued nociceptive stimulation will produce other phenomena, including "wind-up" secondary to continuous C-fiber stimulation to the dorsal horn which will enable the wide-dynamic range neurons, which are essentially "on–off" cells, to turn on and not go off, producing, with the help of the NMDA receptors, central sensitization with changes in perception inducing hyperalgesia, mechanical hypersensitivity, and allodynia. When this occurs, simple analgesics and even strong opioids may not be able to diminish the pain.

As noted, the NMDA receptors contribute significantly to these problems. They help effectuate wind-up; they stimulate apoptosis (along with increases of excitatory amino acids such as glutamate); and one can see the induction of cell death by "hyperstimulation" by the excitatory amino acids.

Neuronal plasticity occurs—new neuronal connections are made in the dorsal root ganglia (DRG) as well as the spinal cord dorsal horn. One example is the formation of new sympathetic neurons sprouting in the DRG. The sympathetic nervous system responds to pain only during pathological conditions. This enables greater hypersensitivity in the DRG and the corresponding areas of the dorsal horn.

CNS plasticity is the focus of a major research initiative.

When the sympathetic nerves sprout into the DRG's somatic nerves, this interaction makes the pain more difficult to treat.

Does all chronic noncancer pain (CNCP) involve sympathetic nervous system input? Probably yes, but to a lesser degree.

The use of opioids becomes important, as the majority of CNCP may not involve significant degrees of central sensitization. This is important in that the more significant the degree of central sensitization that exists, the less likely the opioids will be very effective in stopping the pain.

Opioids are used for moderate to severe pain. They are agonists of opioid receptors (μ, the most common; κ, dealing with spinal cord and supraspinal information and may contribute to nociception; and δ).

Genetic variations of the μ receptor exist. Patients respond differently to μ-opioid receptor agonists (2). When the μ receptor is genetically changed in mice, they may be insensitive to one opioid but remain sensitive to other opiates (3). This may also explain the phenomenon of incomplete opiate cross-tolerance in humans. The μ-opioid receptor gene is called *MOR1*, and genetic differences may explain differences in opiate effectiveness (4).

Evaluation of studies of long-term use of opioids on the quality of life of patients with CNCP identified both moderate/high-quality and low-quality evidence, indicating long-term treatment with opioids can lead to significant improvements in functional outcomes, including quality of life in patients with CNCP (5).

There are no randomized controlled trials of opiates that are longer than 12 weeks. There are, however, open-label trials lasting 6 to 24 months (6). Average pain relief was found to be 30% in 11 reviewed studies. The studies reviewed also found that the most common adverse events were constipation, nausea, and somnolence. Further, only 44% of 344 patients in the open-label trials remained on opiates between 7 and 24 months (6).

Other studies reviewed opiate use in neuropathic pain and general persistent noncancer pain in both very short (<24 hours) to intermediate-length studies (8–56 days). All these studies found opiates to be first-line drugs for pain treatment, as they separated well from placebo (7–10). When number needed to harm (NNH) was evaluated, the range for the common adverse events of nausea (3.6), constipation (4.6), drowsiness (5.3), vomiting (6.2), and dizziness (6.7) were determined (9).

Opioids are considered safe drugs in that they have been used for centuries and we know a fair bit about them. The most common adverse events include constipation, dizziness, nausea, vomiting, somnolence, and confusion. The serious adverse events include respiratory depression and death.

Addiction, a nonphysiological reaction, is also considered a serious adverse event.

Opioid medications have multiple routes of administration, including oral, IV, IM, SQ, sublingual, intranasal, inhaled, transdermal, vaginal, rectal, intrathecal, and epidural.

Opioids are either hydrophilic (propoxyphene, codeine, morphine, hydrocodone and oxycodone, hydromorphone and methadone) (which also has NMDA antagonistic properties) or lipophilic (fentanyl and sufentanil). The lipophilic drugs are more lipid soluble and have greater μ receptor affinity.

Another way of evaluating opiates is looking at them as weak or strong. Going along with the WHO three-step process, this may make more sense.

Weak Opiates:

- Codeine has a weak affinity to μ-opioid receptors; it is about 15% as potent as morphine (the opiate "gold standard"). It has a 2.5- to 3-hour half-life; major side effects include constipation and nausea; dosages greater than 65 mg every four to six hours are not appropriate. Most analgesic activity requires biotransformation to morphine by CYP2D6. Therefore, patients taking a CYP2D6 inhibitor may obviate the effectiveness of the drug.
- Hydrocodone (Vicodin, Vicoprofen, Lorcet, Lortab)—considered to be the most abused analgesic, per DAWN studies (Drug Abuse Warning Network); analgesic and antitussive; has active metabolites (hydromorphone, dihydrocodeine; renal dysfunction will be problematic; same half-life as codeine; typically found in combination with acetaminophen or an NSAID; use 1 to 2 q4–6 hours as needed. As with all PRN analgesics, limit use to 7 or 10 days. Its analgesic efficacy may depend on CYP2D6 activity. Available only as combination tablets with ibuprofen or acetaminophen or ASA. Watch for maximal acetaminophen intake >4 g/day.
- Oxycodone (Percodan, Percocet, Roxicet, Tylox)—elimination half-life of 3 to 3.5 hours; no active metabolites; effectiveness is 7.7 times the potency of codeine; typically found in combination with acetaminophen; has fewer side effects than morphine when given orally; no ceiling effect for analgesia; typically given 1 to 2 orally every four to six hours. The combination tablets have different strengths of oxycodone (2.5/325, 5/325, 7.5/325 and 500, 10/325 and 650), which should be monitored with appropriate dose escalation.
  - OxyContin, extended-release oxycodone, has many good characteristics: short half-life, long duration of action; no clinically active metabolites; easy titration, with a steady state found in 24 to 36 hours; no ceiling dose; minimal adverse effects; low first-pass effect; 60% to 87% bioavailability; no crushing/chewing. Comes in 10-, 20-, 40-, 60-, and 80-mg tablets. At least one review of studies on the use of controlled-release oxycodone has found it to be a good alternative in the treatment of CNCP (11). Unfortunately, this drug is subject to multiple misconceptions and has been given the appellation "hillbilly heroin" by the news. It was considered a major drug of diversion. Of interest is a recent note that OxyContin on the street is so

expensive that addicts are going back to heroin (11). It is second on the DAWN list of medications associated with overdoses.

- Meperidine (Demerol)—has 10% of the efficacy of morphine; has significant anticholinergic properties; has been associated with tachycardia, mydriasis; the half-life is three hours; its metabolite normeperidine (half-life of 15–30 minutes) is considered neurotoxic, with the ability to induce seizures and myoclonus. It is rarely used at this time.
- Propoxyphene (Darvon)—related to methadone; efficacy similar to that of codeine; half-life is 6 to 12 hours, but duration of effect is three to five hours; its demethylated metabolite norpropoxyphene has a very long half-life of 30 to 60 hours and can induce cardiotoxicity; it can induce seizures; it is also a weak competitive NMDA receptor antagonist. It should be used with care in the elderly if it should be used at all in this patient population. At the time this is being written, there is a movement for the FDA to withdraw this drug.
- Tramadol (Ultram) (also see chap. 23)—a synthetic analog of codeine, with oral potency equal to that of codeine; it inhibits norepinephrine and serotonin (5-HT$_3$) reuptake and has weak central opioid receptor activity (about 30%); half-life is 6.7 hours; peak plasma level in 2.3 hours; has active metabolite; analgesia from tramadol and its metabolite; typically used at 50 to 100 mg every six hours, maximum dose of 400 mg/day.
  ○ Possible seizure risk with concurrent tricyclic antidepressant, selective serotonin reuptake inhibitor (SSRI), monoamine oxidase inhibitor (MAOI), and opioid use
  ○ Serotonin syndrome has been reported with the combined use of tramadol and other serotonergic agents including tricyclic antidepressants, MAOIs, bupropion, SSRIs, buspirone, venlafaxine, etc.
  ○ Ultracet is tramadol (37 mg) in combination with acetaminophen. The combination of these two drugs has been found to have a possibly significant role in multimodal analgesia (12).
  ○ Tramadol can induce delirium in healthy elder patients (13).

Strong Opiates:

- Morphine—the prototypical opiate; half-life of two hours, but an analgesic effect lasting four to five hours; 50% of oral morphine reaches the central compartment within 30 minutes; it has active metabolites morphine-6-glucuronide (M6G) and morphine-3-glucuronide (M3G). M6G is found to be more potent than morphine when given intrathecally as well as less potent than morphine when comparing central effects; M3G has no affinity for the μ- and δ-opioid receptors and appears to have no analgesic potency; it can induce allodynia and hyperalgesia and, with higher dosages, myoclonus and seizures—this appears to induce antinociceptive activity. It can also bring on a syndrome similar to opioid withdrawal. Renal impairment will enhance the buildup of M3G and M6G. When given anally, M6G is found in much higher concentrations than M3G.
  ○ Has extended-release formulations: Kadian and MS-Contin, given every 8 to 12 hours, and Avinza, given once daily
  ○ MS-Contin—50% of oral dose reaches the central compartment within 1.5 hours and peaks at 2.5 to 4 hours; steady state is reached in 24 hours; no chewing/crushing

- ○ Kadian—peak level in 9 to 10 hours, lasts six to seven hours; typical use is q 12 hours; consider q.d. use in the elderly; no crushing or chewing
- ○ Avinza—once a day; no crushing or chewing; equal milligram doses over a 24-hour period with one Avinza and a six times a day immediate-release morphine (MSIR)
- Hydromorphone (Dilaudid)—an analog of morphine; given IV, 1.5 mg of hydromorphone is equivalent to 10 mg of morphine; duration of action is three to four hours; it is metabolized primarily to hydromorphone-3-glucuronide and accumulation of the hydromorphone-3-glucuronide, which is also not analgesically active, can induce neuroexcitatory side effects including allodynia, myoclonus, and seizures.
  - ○ Palladone, an extended-release formulation, was withdrawn secondary to overdosages when mixed with alcohol.
- Methadone—a synthetic μ-opioid agonist with approximately 10% NMDA antagonistic activity; considered equipotent to morphine when given parenterally; terminal elimination half-life is 50 to 120 hours; 90% protein bound; undergoes N-demethylation in liver and is excreted in urine; duration of analgesia is four hours; given chronically every six to eight hours; given in 5- and 10-mg tablets.
  - ○ Major problem is the half-life—clinically, one should wait at least five to seven days (longer is better) before adjusting methadone dose—if increased too soon, as steady state is not reached quickly, patient may develop significant sedation and/or overdosage—discordance between analgesic duration and half-life.
    - If patient develops respiratory depression, long half-life necessitates at least a 36- to 48-hour observation period; multiple dosages of opiate antagonist may be necessary.
  - ○ Cipro inhibits CYP1A2 and 3A4 (of the P450 system in the liver), thus increasing plasma levels of methadone.

The Federal Drug Administration (FDA) issued an alert/warning in November of 2006 regarding death, narcotic overdose, and serious cardiac arrhythmias secondary to methadone use. It noted that the duration of analgesic action (four to eight hours) was much shorter than its elimination half-life (8–59 hours) and suggested that physicians using the drug needed to be more knowledgeable about it.

Therapeutic levels of methadone were found to cause sudden death secondary to cardiac arrest. It is known that QTc prolongation and arrhythmogenesis can be induced by methadone (14–16). Methadone should not be a first-line opiate used for moderate to severe pain patients who are opiate naïve.

Methadone is well tolerated and effective in both cancer and noncancer chronic pain patients (17, 18).

- Fentanyl—oldest synthetic phenylpiperidine opioid agonist; 80 times more potent than morphine; it is very lipophilic; used IV for perioperative pain control; can be used epidurally or intrathecally. A buccal formulation has recently been approved.
  - ○ Duragesic transdermal therapeutic system—four dosages used for 72 hours per patch (25-, 50-, 75-, and 100-μg patches); reaches steady state within 12 to 24 hours; can have end-of-dose failure; after the generic

formulation of the patch, the Drug Enforcement Agency (DEA) gave notice of increased overdosage.

- o Actiq—given orally for transmucosal absorption; swallowed fentanyl has significant first-pass (hepatic and intestinal) metabolism; fentanyl does have good buccal mucosal absorption—what is not absorbed here is swallowed; high lipid solubility means rapid transit to CNS.
- o Fentora, an effervescent buccal tablet, has been used in the treatment of breakthrough pain. Dosages range from 100 to 800 μg.

A black box warning exists indicating that the use of fentanyl of any type is only for patients with cancer pain who are opioid tolerant; it is contraindicated in acute and postoperative pain. Actiq cannot be converted microgram per microgram. Actiq is still used for migraine in some emergency departments. It is dangerous to use any form of fentanyl on patients who are opiate naïve.

- Oxymorphone (Opana)—Dosages should be in the range of 5 to 20 mg q 4–6 hours, PRN. Peak action is in 30 minutes, with an average six-hour duration. Half-life is 7.2 to 9.4 hours. A relatively significant food effect on absorption exists.

USING NARCOTICS APPROPRIATELY

State and federal clinical practice guidelines do indicate that it is appropriate to ameliorate pain, and that the use of pain medications to do so is not illegal (19, 20). A set of "Frequently Asked Questions" was released by the DEA along with pain specialists from the University of Wisconsin in August 2004, the purpose of which was to indicate that physicians "cannot be arrested for properly prescribing narcotic pain killers that are the best treatment for millions of suffering patients" (21, 22). Unfortunately, the FAQ was withdrawn by the DEA and many statements retracted. This is discussed in greater detail below.

The Joint Commission for Accreditation of Health Care Organizations has determined that pain is the "Fifth Vital Sign" and mandated significant changes in hospital facilities to deal with this problem (23).

Undertreatment with opioid pain medication is becoming all too common for an estimated 40% to 70% of patients with chronic, intractable noncancer pain (24).

Medically, there are significant adverse effects of undertreatment of pain:

- Physical
  - o Increased pulse, blood pressure, and respiration
  - o Increased risk of cardiac event in patients so predisposed
  - o Increased risk of atelectasis, pneumonia
  - o Decreased tissue oxygenation, leading to muscle breakdown, poor healing, weakness
  - o Decreased activity and mobility leading to decreased recovery secondary to limited ambulation
  - o Increased risk of thromboembolic events
- Psychological
  - o Depression, anxiety disorders
  - o Sleep deprivation
  - o Anorexia
- Immunological

- Decreased immune response secondary to decreased nature killer cells
- Socioeconomic
  - Decreased productivity, loss of work
  - Increased use of health care resources
  - Familial breakdown

The treatment of the CNCP patient with only narcotics is problematic and most often leads to failure. The most appropriate treatment is within an inter-disciplinary pain management program (25–29). An important issue here is that part of the typical interdisciplinary program is the use and then weaning off of chronic opioid medications, as tolerated by the patient, and reflected by their continued and improved functionality.

Kalso et al. (6) note recommendations for the use of opioids in the CNCP patient. They indicate that the management of the patients' pain should be directed by the underlying cause of the pain. The prescribing physician should be aware of the patient's psychosocial status. Finally, they note that opioid treat-ment should not be considered a lifelong treatment.

The use of opioids in the CNCP patient does not have a routine, non-individualized answer. Clinically, many patients with CNCP with a very poor quality of life can improve their function with the use of time-release (around-the-clock, ATC) opioid pain medications. On the other hand, some patients may develop decreased functionality with chronic opioids. Therefore, *function* is the most important issue when dealing with pain patients and chronic opioid med-ications. If these patients are not showing an improved functionality on these medications, they may need to be stopped.

Most importantly, prior to the use of chronic opioid medications, the CNCP patients must have received all conservative and/or appropriate surgical treat-ment and failed it—meaning, their pain was not ameliorated and their function-ality continued to be poor or show further decline.

For patients who have had and failed all appropriate treatment, the use of chronic narcotics may certainly be appropriate on an individualized basis. There are several tenets that should be followed. First, these patients should receive long-acting opioids on an ATC basis to maintain an acceptable level of comfort. These medications provide a relatively flat dose–response curve, which engen-ders effective levels of analgesia without the peaks and valleys seen with short-acting pain medications, and therefore provide less risk for potential drug abuse.

There are four basic time-release medications:

- Duragesic patches (Janssen) (percutaneous Fentanyl)—used on the skin for, most typically, 72 hours at a time. This medication also enables the patient to stop taking pain pills multiple times a day, helping to extinguish a medication-related behavior. A generic patch with a different mechanism is now being used.
- Morphine sulfate—different time-release formulations: MS-Contin (Purdue Pharma Stamford, CT) and Kadian (King Pharmaceuticals, Bristol, TN); both formulations to be given, most typically every 12 hours; Avinza (King Phar-maceuticals), a once a day preparation. There are generic forms of MS-Contin.
- OxyContin (Purdue Pharma, Stamford, CT)—time-release oxycodone, typi-cally taken every 12 hours. It was this medication along with its nickname hillbilly heroin and multiple stories of drug abuse and drug diversion and

addiction that brought the current crises regarding the use of these medications to a head.

- Methadone (generic)—a very old medication, developed in the mid-20th century. This medication has a long half-life: it is not a "time-release" medication. It may be given every 8 to 12 hours. The difficulty in its use is twofold: poor understanding of its clinical attributes and use by many physicians and the fact that it is also used in specific government-approved heroin/opioid detoxification programs. Some pharmacies insist on having the words "for pain" on the prescription, or they would not fill it; another institutional problem for these patients—the stigma.

Many pharmacy formularies would not pay for the more expensive Oxy-Contin or Duragesic patches, leaving the morphine-derived time-release medications as well as methadone to be used. The problem here is natural selection. One of the breakdown products of morphine, M3G is pronociceptive and can induce significant side effects in the elderly as well as (less frequently) the young, including increased pain.

Even with a time-release medication, the CNCP patients on occasion need to be given a "breakthrough pain" medication, typically a short-acting, immediate-release opioid, which may be needed to lower nociceptive pain brought about by an acute exacerbation of pain secondary to any number of factors such as overactivity.

There are three types of breakthrough pain: incident or episodic—patients know what can cause the pain and take a pre-emptive, fast-acting pain medication. Next is idiopathic or spontaneous breakthrough pain, which comes on suddenly and not infrequently for no obvious reason. Lastly is end-of-dose failure, which is not as unusual as one would expect. Some patients will need to take MS-Contin or even OxyContin two or three times a day (q8h). Some patients use transdermal fentanyl patches, which are labeled to last 72 hours, but in some patients they may last only 48 hours. The physician can see the end-of-dose failure by the marked increase in breakthrough pain that occurs when the time-release medication has been metabolized and the blood level is dropping.

Breakthrough pain can be of moderate to severe intensity. It comes on quickly, typically in less than two to three minutes to maximal intensity. It can last, on average, 13 to 30 minutes, or longer, especially in cancer patients. For these reasons, the goal of treatment would be to use a pain medication with fast onset, such as transmucosal fentanyl.

The typical immediate-release medications used for breakthrough pain include the following:

- Ultram, Ultracet (Tramadol, with or without acetaminophen)—a medication which stimulates the μ-opioid receptors as well as affects serotonin and norepinephrine reuptake.
- Vicodin (Abbott Pharmaceutical, Abbott Park, IL)—hydrocodone and acetaminophen, given every four to six hours for breakthrough pain.
- Lorcet (Forest Pharmaceuticals, New York, NY), Lortab (UCB Pharma, Inc., Belgium), Norco (Watson Pharmaceuticals, Corona, CA)—hydrocodone and acetaminophen, to be used every four to six hours for breakthrough pain. Norco has the smallest dosages of acetaminophen, making the acetaminophen load lowest, and is therefore the least hepatotoxic, depending on the number utilized each day.

- Percocet (Endo Pharmaceuticals, Chadds Ford, PA)—oxycodone and acetaminophen, given every four to six hours for breakthrough pain.
- Roxicodone (Roxane Pharmaceuticals—a member of the Boehringer Ingelheim group of Pharmaceutical Companies (Ridgefield, CT)—oxycodone without acetaminophen, given every four to six hours for breakthrough pain.
- Actiq (Cephalon, Inc., Frazer, PA)—fentanyl oral transmucosal, an oralette or "lollypop" on a stick; allowed to dissolve in the mouth, with medication entering the system transmucosally; to be used every four to six hours for severe breakthrough pain. While labeled for breakthrough pain in cancer patients, it is now being used by many clinicians for moderate to severe breakthrough pain in the CNCP patients.

The use of immediate-release narcotics with acetaminophen and/or a nonsteroidal anti-inflammatory medication must be looked at carefully secondary to possible hepatotoxicity and nephrotoxicity.

In medical practice, physicians should use an extended-release (ATC) pain medication for the CNCP patient, with attention being focused on analgesia and improved function, as well as the number of breakthrough pain episodes. The extended-relief opioid typically enables an increased function, which may be responsible for the episodes of breakthrough pain that were not seen when the patient was bed/chair bound.

If the patient has more than three or four episodes of breakthrough pain, the ATC medications should be slowly increased, keeping an eye on continued improvement in function and the onset of drug-related problems such as sedation or poor cognitive function. If this occurs, the ATC medication should be decreased. Consideration of opioid rotation should be performed in such cases, as well as generally every four to six months as needed.

The use of breakthrough, instant/immediate-release pain medication for breakthrough pain should be limited to three to five times a typical day for a patient.

The science is important. There is no one perfect opioid that will work for all patients. Typical side effects, such as constipation, should be treated at the same time an opioid is started.

Individual responses to opioids may vary, possibly secondary to genetic factors, but this must be recognized. If one opioid does not give good analgesia with a small number of side effects, it should be changed. The use of an adjuvant to help with pain management and possibly allow a smaller dosage of opiate should always be considered.

When prescribing an opiate, always follow established principles and the guidelines and laws applicable from the state and the federal levels; follow both, but particularly whichever is most strict.

Pain management physicians must always document (while monitoring) the four A's: Analgesia; Activities of daily living; Adverse effects; and Aberrant drug-taking behaviors (30). By default, the pain management physician is responsible for identifying the rare drug abuser or drug diverter. When concerned, get a consult from an addictionologist and even cotreat with this clinician.

The use of chronic opioids alone should only be done after the patient has had, if needed, narcotic medication to help enable them to undergo appropriate rehabilitation. The initial use of chronic opioids is medically not indicated,

However, there is a very common caveat to this: a patient's insurance company may not pay for rehabilitation. Many will pay for interventional pain medicine, where a patient may receive a series of epidural steroid medications, for example, and be placed on pain medications simultaneously, but all will pay for pain medications (sometimes only specific pain medications, for extended and immediate release).

The new reality is that the pain management physician must provide care while preventing misuse and drug diversion. Physicians are being turned into police, creating a significant problem in the older established patient/physician relationship. Physicians feel that they cannot always/just cannot trust a pain patient who may divert a pain medication and get the physician into trouble. Patients are afraid, possibly with good reason, that even in the presence of real pain, their pain management needs may not be met.

DEFINITIONS

There are several definitions that must be kept in mind. They are presented with only a little variation, as the concepts and definitions are very important:

- *Physical dependence*: seen when the body has adapted to an opiate and there is a class-specific withdrawal syndrome that can be produced by the abrupt cessation, rapid dose reduction, and/or administration of an opiate antagonist. This is not addiction. It is associated with the following:
- *Tolerance*: a state of adaptation in which exposure to a drug can induce changes that cause the body to enable a diminution of one or more of the drug's effects over time, with all other conditions/aspects of disease being the same. If the physical disorder is getting worse, or progressing, it may cause a need for more medication. If a patient's functional activity is continuing to progress, he/she may need more medication to make up for the tolerance induced, and an increase in breakthrough pain secondary to activity.
- *Pseudoaddiction*: this is seen in pain patients who are seeking more pain medication, even doctor shopping to obtain these medications, secondary to the patient's real pain syndrome being undertreated. When the treatment enables the patient to achieve appropriate relief, all inappropriate behavior ends.
- *Addiction*: a primary, chronic, neurobiologic disease associated with genetic, psychosocial, and environmental factors which significantly influence its development and how it manifests. It is specifically characterized by behaviors that are typified by impaired control over drug use, compulsive use, craving the drug, and compulsive use in spite of self-induced harm.

A consensus document regarding these definitions was published in 2001 as a joint effort of the American Academy of Pain Medicine, The American Pain Society and the American Society of Addiction Medicine (31).

An important question is the risk of addiction and aberrant behavior. Portenoy and Savage (32) stated that addiction to opioids in the context of pain treatment is rare in those with no history of addictive behavior.

The Boston Collaborative Drug Surveillance Project looked at 11,882 inpatients who received an opioid while hospitalized; subsequently, only four cases of addiction could be identified (33).

Passik and Portenoy (34, 35) worked to develop a model of aberrant drug-taking behaviors. They felt that predictive behaviors included: selling prescription drugs; prescription forgery; stealing or borrowing another patient's drugs; injecting oral formulations; obtaining prescription drugs from nonmedical sources; concurrent abuse of related illicit drugs; multiple unsanctioned dose escalations; recurrent prescription losses. Behaviors felt to be less predictive included: aggressive complaining about a need for higher medication doses; drug hoarding during periods of reduced symptoms; requesting specific drugs; acquisition of similar drugs from other medical sources; unsanctioned medication dose escalation one to two times; unapproved use of the drug to treat another symptom; and reporting psychic effects not intended by the clinician.

TREATMENT PROCEDURES
CNCP patients should be seen monthly, at least for the first six months or more. If an escalation of the amount of breakthrough pain medication is seen, this may indicate a need to increase the time-release chronic narcotics.

In routine practice, the CNCP patients should be given a pain medication agreement, which indicates the possible side effects of narcotic usage (including sedation, nausea, vomiting, itching, loss of sexual function, and immunological problems, among others). Also, the patient must agree that only one physician will provide his/her narcotic pain medications, and the prescriptions will be taken to one (listed) pharmacy. Urine or blood tests may be performed at any time, and if an untoward substance (i.e., cocaine or narcotics not prescribed the pain specialist) is found in patients' urine or blood, or if their blood/urine level of the prescribed pain medication is very inappropriate, the physician may wean the patient off of their opioid medications and treat them without further use of narcotics or discharge them. Other reasons for tapering and ending opioid maintenance include evidence of opioid hoarding; obtaining pain medications from other prescribers; obtaining drugs from others (diversion); and uncontrolled dose escalation or other aberrant behaviors (frequent loss of one's medication—"my dog ate it"; reports of stolen medications without a proper police report; frequently calling in requesting medications earlier than should be indicated after being given a one-month drug prescription). A past history of substance abuse may be considered a relative contraindication for the use of chronic opioids. However, it is not felt that it is infeasible to treat a chronic pain patient with a history of drug abuse. These patients, as noted above, may need to be treated while they are being seen by an addictionologist.

In some practices, urine testing is felt to be an important part of managing a chronic pain patient safely. Appropriate urine testing can help the prescriber determine if the patient is taking the prescribed medication, if he/she is taking the correct dosages, and if there is any other untoward drug in his/her system. Some clinicians do this routinely; some do not do it at all. Some clinicians will have consenting patients observed, to be certain that the urine is theirs. Rare practices may frisk patients to be certain that they do not have a urine receptacle that they have used to transport "clean" urine. Both general class-specific urine testing should be done in combination with gas chromatography/mass spectrometry to find the identity of, or confirm the presence or absence of, a specific drug and/or its metabolites (36).

Another very useful tool is serial testing using drug-related questionnaires, such as the CAGE questionnaire (37), or the Pain Outcome Profile (POP+) developed by the American Academy of Pain Management (38).

The Web site www.legalsideofpain by former federal prosecutor Jennifer Bolen is an excellent resource for all physicians in pain management. Ms. Bolen has excellent examples of patient opioid medication agreements and informed consents for the use of opioids, as well as much more that is useful and should be mandatorily used, in one form or another by all pain management physicians (see chap. 25).

So-called "Universal Precautions" in pain medicine need to be remembered (39):

1. Diagnosis with appropriate differential
2. Psychological assessment
3. Informed consent for the use of opiates
4. Treatment agreements
5. Pain and function assessments
6. Trial of opiate therapy
7. Reassessment of pain and function
8. Regular assessment of the "4 A's"—Analgesia; Activities of daily living; Adverse events; Aberrant drug-taking behavior
9. Periodic review of diagnosis and comorbidities
10. Documentation (and lots of it!)

Chronic Opioid Use in Patients with CNCP

Two interesting studies from Canada note important facts which would most likely be replicated if done in the United States.

A report in 2001 by Moulin et al. (40) found that 340 Canadian pain patients with an average pain intensity of 6.3 (on a 1–10 scale) were taking medication for pain. Eighty percent complained of moderate to severe pain. Their average pain history was 10.7 years. Only 22% of these patients were taking opioid medications and two-thirds of these patients were only taking codeine preparations.

A more recent report (2003) found that a cohort of 154 Canadian pain patients had a mean pain score of 7.7 on a Likert scale (0–10), with a mean duration of pain being 4.7 years. Over 40% of these patients had not used opioids and about 25% had not used any other antineuropathic pain medication in spite of these high levels of pain (41).

A number of authors feel that while the use of opioids may be helpful to treat the CNCP patient, there are no specific guidelines and therefore a greater degree of hesitancy and fear exists (6,42–49). The "correct" way to use opiates as noted in these various studies is described above. The most basic points being: make certain the patient is examined and documentation is excellent; symptom control leading to improved function and quality of life is primary; chronic opioid therapy should be considered for both continuous nociceptive and neuropathic pain if all other appropriate therapies have been tried and failed, utilizing the proper time frame for the medications to work; know the psychosocial status of the patient; use ATC medications, with instant-release opioids for breakthrough pain; monitor treatment including re-examinations, functional assessments, and urine testing; the physician and the patient should have an appropriate opioid agreement which spells out the patient's rights and responsibilities.

Opioid therapy can be enhanced via the use of adjunctive medications (see chap. 23). These may include NMDA antagonists, clonidine, calcium channel blockers, alpha-2-adrenergic agonists, NSAIDs, gabapentinoids and neurokinin-1 (NK-1) receptor antagonists (50, 51).

The number of published opioid trials lasting longer than 6 to 12 weeks is very small. This leads to the concern regarding the safety of chronic narcotic usage. Reports show that there were 11 studies with 1025 patients that compared oral opioids with placebo and lasted for four days to eight weeks. Six trials had an open label follow-up of 6 to 24 months (7). The adverse events noted included constipation, nausea, and somnolence being the most common adverse events noted (at least one of the three) in 80% of patients. Also of interest is that only 44% of 388 patients placed in the open-label trails were still taking opioids after therapy for between 7 and 24 months, showing a relatively small group of patients continuing with long-term opioid treatment (7).

Another study looked at the impact of opioid use on CNCP patients. The authors found 11 studies which evaluated long-term opioid treatment for CNCP and also looked at quality of life and included 2877 patients. Six were randomized controlled trials and five were observational studies. The authors concluded that there was both moderate/high- and low-quality evidence indicating that long-term treatment with opiates can help CNCP patients develop an increased quality of life and significant improvements in function (5).

Maier et al. (52) looked at 121 patients with a three-year history of opioid use and found that the patients with long-term opioid use had significantly lower pain intensity and good improvements in quality of life, global assessments, and physical status. During the five years of this study, 33% had no change in opioid dosage, 16% had their dosages decreased, and 27% had a slight overall increase and 19% had significant dose increases (secondary to loss of opioid efficacy). It was concluded that there was a very low frequency of withdrawal in CNCP patients taking long-term opiates, and there was no evidence for tolerance development, especially if the treatment was performed in a pain center.

Several controlled studies of opioids in CNCP have shown pain relief of 30% to 50% with chronic dosing, but no development of significant tolerance, except for side effects such as nausea and sedation (53).

A more recent meta-analysis of the effectiveness and side effects of opioids when used for CNCP found that both weak and strong opioids outperformed placebo for both pain and function in all types of CNCP (54). The authors of this review also noted that better functional outcomes were found with other drugs which were, for pain relief, only outperformed by strong opioids (54). They also found that in spite of the typically short time for opioid trials, more than one-third of participants withdrew from the treatment (54).

The most common side effect/adverse event stemming from the use of opioids is constipation. Typically, when a patient is started on an opiate, a stimulant and stool-softening agent is stated at the same time. There are many patients who continue to have problems with significant constipation. A peripheral opioid receptor antagonist, methylnaltrexone, for the treatment of severe constipation has been found to be useful in managing opioid-induced constipation without significant adverse events including opiate withdrawal (55, 56). This drug, which is still in clinical development, can reverse morphine-induced gastrointestinal hypomotility (57–59).

It is also interesting to note that opioids have been ascribed anti-inflammatory properties (60).

Tolerance and Opioid-Induced Pain

Over time, continued opiate usage will induce "tolerance," a known effect, to the opioid analgesic effect (see above). It has been felt that most commonly, dose escalation is secondary to increasing pain, as a result of increasing nociception from ongoing disease processes. However, studies and additional clinical activity indicate that tolerance to different opioid effects can develop at different rates (selective tolerance); for example, one can rapidly develop tolerance to nausea and vomiting, sedation, and respiratory depression, but little if any tolerance to constipation and miosis (61). Patient dose variability (genetic polymorphism) can occur as differences in opioid receptor synthesis and differences in various opioid affinities of ligands causing a wide margin of dose variability in patients (61). It is felt that once tolerance to analgesic effects of a specific opiate has developed, simultaneous use of analgesics, which are mediated by different receptors, may help avoid further tolerance; this concept, known as multimodal analgesia, is growing more common and involves techniques such as opioid switching/rotation and the use of adjuvant medications.

Two possible mechanisms have also been postulated regarding the development of drug tolerance. First, a within-system mechanism, which involves opioid receptors downregulating at the highest affinity sites and uncoupling from G-proteins. The between-systems mechanism is proposed, with the opiate-activated opponent systems—the pain facility systems may be involved with the development of opioid tolerance (62). The first mechanism (within system) is the mechanism most often considered; other mechanisms indicate that chronic opiate treatment may also activate the pain facilitatory systems (NMDA receptors, nitric oxide production, and COX activation) during the development of opiate tolerance (62).

Data shows that opioids can increase pain through activation of the bulbospinal facilitation from the rostral ventromedial medulla (RVM); increased pain can decrease spinal opioid antinociceptive potency and finally blockade of pain restores the antinociceptive potency (63).

Tolerance can also be induced by a state of hyperalgesia that results from opioid exposure. The paradoxical or abnormal pain secondary to opiate therapy may also be secondary to neuroplastic changes in the brain and spinal cord, including the activation of the descending pain facilitation mechanism from the RVM. This may be developed, at least in part, by the increased activity of cholecystokinin (CCK) in the RVM. This may induce more pronociceptive events including the upregulation of spinal dynorphin levels and increased CGRP and substance P expression in the DRG. It then appears that opioids can initiate pain due to descending facilitation, upregulation of spinal dynorphin, and increased evoked release of excitatory neurotransmitters from primary afferents (64, 65). The neuroplastic changes secondary to chronic opioid utilization may be secondary to adaptive changes needed to promote increased pain transmission and induced tolerance (decreased antinociception) (66).

It has also been noted that chronic opioid use may be associated with the development of hyperalgesia (67). The use of chronic opiates does appear to induce the development of antinociceptive tolerance, which would necessitate increasing the doses of the opiate to maintain adequate analgesia. "Analgesic tolerance" has been associated with paradoxical pain in regions previously not affected by pain, as a result of sustained morphine utilization (67). Many neuropeptides and neurotransmitters (antagonists of algetic chemicals) have been able to block or reverse the antinociceptive tolerance (see below).

Chronic opioid use does upregulate substance P and calcitonin gene–related peptide, which in turn increases the release of algetic, or pain-inducing substances from primary afferent nerve fibers after stimulation. This is correlated with the onset of the abnormal pain states and the opioid antinociceptive tolerance (67).

The descending pain modulatory pathway from the brain stem RVM occurs via the dorsolateral funiculus (DLF) and maintains changes in the spinal cord secondary to abnormal pain states, paradoxical pain, and antinociceptive tolerance. Lesioning the DLF in animals prevented increased evoked algetic neuropeptide release and the development of antinociceptive tolerance and abnormal pain secondary to chronic opiate exposure (67).

Microinjecting lidocaine or a CCK antagonist into the RVM blocks both thermal and touch hypersensitivity and antinociceptive tolerance. It is concluded that chronic opioid exposure will enhance a descending pain facilitatory pathway from the RVM that is mediated by CCK, among other neuropeptides, and is essential for the maintenance of antinociceptive tolerance (67, 68). "Nociceptin," also called "orphanin FQ," or OFQ, is a ligand for the "opioid receptor–like 1" receptor. When injected into the RVM, OFQ suppresses firing of all types of neurons and blocks opioid-induced cell activation. In the medulla, OFQ can produce an antiopioid effect. It appears that depending upon in which region OFQ is placed, it may be able to produce either hyperalgesia or hypalgesia (69).

Chronic opioid administration induces increased expression of spinal dynorphin, which causes increased sensitivity to nonnoxious and noxious stimuli: a decrease in spinal antinociceptive properties (70, 71). Experimental use of a cannabinoid CB1 agonist to the spinal cord will also induce paradoxical/abnormal pain, inducing increased spinal dynorphin (71). Continuous morphine use induces neuroplasticity in primary afferents and the spinal cord and induces increased levels of CGRP and dynorphin (72). Dynorphin antiserum can block increased release of CGRP from rats given chronic morphine; so can lesions of the DLF (72).

NMDA receptor antagonists do decrease or prevent the development of tolerance to the antinociceptive effects of opioids (73, 74). It is thought that a range of NMDA receptor antagonists potentiate morphine-induced antinociception (73).

Another study found that the mechanism of tolerance to receptor-selective μ- and δ-opioids may be different compared to that associated with morphine tolerance (74). This would indicate that studies looking at paradoxical pain from chronic morphine utilization may not be generalizable to all opiates.

Specific neurons in the RVM include "off-cells," which are felt to inhibit nociceptive transmission, and "on-cells," which facilitate nociception. When these cells are tested with an NMDA antagonist, several things are noted: systemic morphine produces analgesia in part by involving an NMDA-mediated excitatory process to activate off-cells in the RVM. Secondly, activation of on-cells is mediated by a non-NMDA receptor, and this activation does not appear to be significant in regulating reflex responses to acute, noxious stimuli. Excitatory amino acid–induced excitation appears to work several ways in the RVM, activating off-cells and on-cells under different conditions (75).

Algetic or pain-inducing neuropeptides are involved in both the development of tolerance and paradoxical/abnormal pain. Sustained morphine use increases substance P and NK-1 receptor expression in the spinal cord dorsal horn. It also increases capsaicin-evoked substance P release and internalization of NK-1 receptors in the presence of noxious stimuli. It appears that NK-1 receptors have an important role in the expression of chronic morphine-induced hyperalgesia. It may also indicate that chronic opiate usage can induce changes that are similar to those found in inflammatory pain (76).

As noted earlier, CGRP has been found to be increased in the spinal cord dorsal horn during morphine tolerance. The opiate receptors appear to be involved in upregulation of CGRP and substance P following exposure to chronic opiates; protein kinase C appears to have a role in this upregulation (77). Prostaglandins are also upregulated (78). Both CGRP and substance P, which are colocalized and coreleased, are involved in the development of tolerance to spinal antinociceptive effects of μ- and δ-related agonists. CGRP antagonists may be helpful in the prevention and reversal of opioid tolerance (79–81).

CCK, which is enhanced in the RVM during chronic opiate exposure, may also decrease spinal morphine antinociception by causing a descending pain facilitatory mechanism to exacerbate spinal nociceptive activity. A CCK receptor antagonist may also be a useful tool in the prevention of paradoxical pain and analgesic tolerance (82).

Via the use of a 5-HT$_1$ A receptor agonist, it was determined that, as opioids produce bidirectional hypo- and proanalgesic activity, the 5-HT$_1$ A receptor activation counteracts the various aspects of opioid-induced pain. An interesting point is made by the authors of this study that opioid addiction may be self-therapy of opioid-induced pathological pain (83).

Another very important research target is CNS microglia. Spinal cord glia are important contributors to the creation of enhanced pain states secondary to the release of neuroexcitatory substances. Glia (microglia and astrocytes) also release neuroexcitatory substances in response to morphine, opposing its effects (84). After activation of microglial cells under neuropathic pain conditions induces proinflammatory cytokines including interleukin-1 beta, interleukin-6, tumor necrosis factor, complement components (C1q, C3, C4, C5, C5a), and multiple other substances that facilitate pain transmission (85).

Glia create and maintain enhanced pain states such as neuropathic pain and also compromise the efficacy of morphine and other opiates for pain control. Glia have essentially no role in pain under basal conditions, but pain is amplified when the glia become activated and induce the release of the proinflammatory products, those noted above and especially proinflammatory cytokines (86).

Glia are activated via multiple neuron-to-glia signals including neuronal chemokines, neurotransmitters, and substances released by damaged, dying, and dead neurons (86).

Glia become increasingly activated in response to repeated administration of opiates, which induces neuronal excitability via numerous mechanisms, including direct receptor-mediated actions, upregulation of excitatory amino acid receptor function, downregulation of GABA receptor function, as well as others (85, 86). These effects of glial activation amplify pain, decrease efficacy of opioid analgesia, contribute to the loss of opioid analgesia after repeated opioid administration (tolerance), and contribute to the development of opioid dependence (86, 87).

Toll-like receptors (TLR; a family of receptors that provide needed links between immune stimulants produced by microorganisms and the initiation of host defenses) are seemingly important players in this multifaceted problem. Activation of TLR4 induces the release of antimicrobial peptides, inflammatory cytokines, and chemokines, among other activities. TLR4-mediated glial activation is central to neuropathic pain, compromised acute opioid analgesia, and unwanted opioid side effects including tolerance, dependence, and reward. Selective antagonism of TLR4 has been shown to reverse neuropathic pain and potentiate opioid analgesia (88).

The p38 mitogen-activated protein kinases (p38 MAPK) are signaling molecules, part of a family of serine/threonine protein kinases, which play a role in cellular responses to external stress signals. Inhibitors of two members of the p38 family have anti-inflammatory effects via inhibiting the expression of inflammatory mediators (89). Activation of p38 MAPK in spinal microglia mediates morphine antinociceptive tolerance. Minocycline, a selective inhibitor of microglia activation, has been reported to attenuate peripheral inflammation-induced hyperalgesia by inhibiting p38 MAPK in the spinal microglia. These authors demonstrated that minocycline antagonizes morphine antinociceptive tolerance, possibly due to the inhibition of p38 activation in spinal microglia (90).

It was found that inhibiting neuronal nitric oxide synthase diminished morphine antinociceptive tolerance by reducing p38 MAPK activation in the spinal microglia (91). Another group provided evidence that p38 activation in spinal microglia played an important role in the development of tolerance to morphine analgesia (92).

Neuroglia
It has been found that glial activation contributes to a state of opioid analgesic tolerance, and the induced neuroglial communication is possibly responsible, at least in part, for the altered functional competence in δ-opioid receptor–mediated effects following morphine treatment; chronic morphine treatment has been found to involve the activation and hypertrophy of spinal glia cells (93).

Finally, a study notes that activity of endocannabinoids, mediated via CB1 receptors, contributes to both the development and maintenance of opioid tolerance by influencing the opioid-induced increase in spinal CGRP (94).

Sexual Dimorphism
More evidence is being found that indicates anatomical and neuropsychological differences exist between the nociceptive systems of males and females (95). Differences appear to exist between male and female perception of and response to pain (96). Women have been found to experience more severe and longer lasting pain than men (97).

Woman experience greater clinical pain, suffer greater pain-related distress, and show increased sensitivity to experimentally induced pain when compared to men. Some of the multifactorial issues helping to explain the sex differences include psychosocial factors (pain-related catastrophizing). Gonadal hormone levels in cycling women are also responsible for a substantial impact on pain perception and analgesic response. Women perceive more pain during their luteal phase, and estrogen antagonists provide long-term pain relief in certain situations (98).

Dyspnea exerts an inhibitory effect on pain; one study shows the inhibitory effect of dyspnea on pain sensation is less in females than in males, but the sex difference may not be explained by the female reproductive hormones alone (99). Another group looked at sexually dimorphic recruitment of spinal opioid analgesic pathways by the spinal application of morphine in rats, and found that in females, but not males, activation by intrathecal (IT) morphine of spinal κ-opioid receptors is a prerequisite for spinal morphine antinociception. Also, in females, but not males, IT application of antidynorphin antibodies substantially attenuates the antinociception produced by IT morphine. It was felt that the female-specific recruitment by IT morphine of a spinal dynorphin/κ-opioid receptor pathway results from organizational consequences of ovarian sex steroids and not the absence of testicular hormones (100).

Differences in analgesic responses to μ-opioid agonists have been seen, but the findings have varied. One study found women to have more a more robust response to morphine than men, in contrast to prior studies (101). Typically, the μ-opioid antinociceptive response is greater in male rats than in female rats (102). A recent study found sexual dimorphism in the opioid effects was related to the opioid receptors on which a particular opioid predominately acts (102).

Studies have found that the analgesic effect of kappa partial agonists (pentazocine, butorphanol, nalbuphine) is much greater in women than in men. This may be secondary to a naloxone-sensitive antinociceptive effect of these agonist/antagonists inducing decreased analgesia or increased pain (103, 104).

Other studies suggest that it is estrogen receptors in trigeminal neurons which modulate nociceptive responses via serotonin and other neuropeptides. It was thought that the variation in estrogen receptor signaling and neuropeptide plasticity in the trigeminal neurons may have an inducing effect on mensuration-related migraine (95).

Finally, inflammation and inflammatory disorders are thought to be sexually dimorphic, via neuroimmune mechanisms underlying sexual dimorphism in three possible aspects of the inflammatory process: plasma extravasation, neutrophil function, and inflammatory hyperalgesia (105).

Barriers to the Use of Opioids
There are patient and physician barriers to appropriate use of opioids: fears of addiction, medication dependence, and drug tolerance, with frequent lack of understanding of the differences between these issues.

Physicians are frequently afraid to prescribe opioids secondary to

- an inadequate understanding of pain management principles;
- inability to appropriately assess a patient's pain;
- fear/concern about regulation of controlled substances;
- fear that giving pain medication to one patient would make the physician a target of the DEA as well as other patients wanting/needing pain medications;
- fears of patient addiction and other problems leading to liability;
- concern about patients becoming tolerant to opioids, needing higher dosages, and needing them for extended periods of time (years);
- concern about side effects of opioids.

Patient barriers to appropriate opioid use include

- fear that pain means a disease is worse;
- concern that talking about pain would prevent a physician from dealing with a significant underlying disease;
- wanting to be a good patient and not alienate the physician by reporting pain;
- concerns about developing tolerance or addiction to pain medications;
- fear of showing "weakness";
- embarrassment to go to the pharmacy for these medications; further embarrassment that they may be construed a "drug addict," even though they have no aberrant drug-related behavior and a physiological reason for their pain.

Systemic/institutional barriers include

- restrictive regulation of controlled substances;
- poor access to treatment;
- poor access to pain management specialists;
- poor insurance.
  - The most appropriate treatment would not be reimbursed.
  - The most appropriate treatment is too costly for the patient.
  - Lack of rehabilitation benefits—"Bad Insurance."
    - Inability to obtain any rehabilitation or even just physical therapy or psychological care, as they are far more expensive than pain medications (an hour of physical therapy may bill at US $150 to $200, while a single generic Tylenol #4 tablet—one grain of codeine—costs only pennies).

Other barriers to pain relief:

- Pharmacies do not stock adequate and/or appropriate opioids.
- No continuity in patient care.

SUMMARY

The complexity of this subject is great, even though the medical aspects are fairly straightforward. It is the multitudes of other problems and barriers to appropriate pain management and opioid usage that make this problem so complex.

When one considers that the clinical definition of pain is simple—whatever the patient says it is—it is then up to the clinician to determine exactly what the patient means, utilizing a history, examination, and any necessary tests. Then appropriate treatment should be rendered. The utilization of chronic opioid analgesics is one very important treatment modality, which, when used appropriately, may help improve patients' function and ameliorate their pain.

In February 2009, the FDA issued a call for tightened regulations of extended-release oral medications, methadone, and patch opioid medications as well as for reducing diversion, overdoses, and inappropriate use of schedule II opioid medications (106). This may place more difficulty on physicians who utilize opioids in the treatment of CNCP patients and make continued treatment of these patients more onerous. While they are requesting more thorough risk management plans from the makers of these medications, the ramifications to the physician are not yet clear.

REFERENCES

1. Jay GW. Chronic Pain. New York: Informa Healthcare, 2007.
2. Pasternak GW. The pharmacology of mu analgesics: from patients to genes. Neuroscientist 2001; 7(3):220–231.
3. Rossi GC, Brown GP, Leventhal, et al. Novel receptor mechanisms for heroin and morphine-6 beta glucuronide analgesia. Neurosci Lett 1996; 216(1):1–4.
4. Pasternak GW. Molecular biology of opioid analgesia. J Pain Symptom Manage 2005; 29(5 suppl):S2–S9.
5. Devulder J, Richarz U, Nataraja S. Impact of long-term use of opioids on quality of life in patients with chronic, non-malignant pain. Curr Med Res Opin 2005; 21(10):1555–1568.
6. Kalso E, Allan L, Dellemijn PLI, et al. Recommendations for using opioids in chronic non-cancer pain. Eur J Pain 2003; 7(5):381–386.
7. Kalso E, Edwards JE, Moore RA, et al. Opioids in chronic non-cancer pain: a systemic review of efficacy and safety. Pain 2004; 112:372–380.
8. Watson CP, Watt-Watson JH, Chaipman ML. Chronic non-cancer pain and the long term utility of opioids. Pain Res Manage 2004; 9:19–24.
9. Eisenberg E, McNicol ED, Carr DB. Efficacy and safety of opioid agonists in the treatment of neuropathic pain of nonmalignant origin: systemic review and meta-analysis trials. JAMA 2005; 293:3043–3052.
10. Dworkin RH, Backonja M, Rowbotham MB, et al. Advances in neuropathic pain: diagnosis, mechanisms, and treatment recommendations. Arch Neurol 2003; 60:1524–1534.
11. Stiehl M. Controlled release oxycodone—a new option in the treatment of severe and very severe pain. Review of studies on neuropathic, physical activity-related and postoperative pain. NNW Fortschr Med 2004; 145(suppl 2):61–69.
12. Schug SA. Combination analgesia in 2005—a rational approach: focus on paracetamol–tramadol. Clin Rheumatol 2006; 25(suppl 1):S16–S21.
13. Kunig G, Datwyler S, Eschen A, et al. Unrecognized long-lasting tramadol-induced delirium in two elderly patients. Pharmacopsychiatry 2006; 39(5):194–199.
14. Chugh SS, Socoteanu C, Reinier K, et al. A community-based evaluation of sudden death associated with therapeutic levels of methadone. Am J Med 2008; 121(1):66–71.
15. Burgess FW, Pawasauskas J. Methadone analgesia: balancing the risks and benefits. Pain Medicine News Special Edition. December 2008:53–58.
16. Burgas FW, KRantz MJ, Barkin RL. Methadone: unintended mortality due to overdose and arrhythmia. Pain Medicine News. May/June 2007:1–6.
17. Fredheim OM, Kaasa S, Dale O, et al. Opioid switching from slow release morphine to oral methadone may improve pain control in chronic non-malignant pain: a nine-month follow-up study. Palliat Med 2006; 20(1):35–41.
18. Fredheim OM, Borchgrevink PC, Klepstad P, et al. Long term methadone for chronic pain: a pilot study of pharmacokinetic aspects. Eur J Pain 2007; 11(6):599–604.
19. Florida Administrative Code. Title 64, Department of Health, Board of Medicine, Chapter 64B8–9 Standards of Practice for Medical Doctors. 64B8–9.013 Standards for the Use of Controlled Substances for Treatment of Pain. Available at: http://www.medsch.wisc.edu/painpolicy/domestic/fllaw.htm. Accessed February 14, 2009.
20. Federation of State Medical Boards of the United States: Model policy for the use of controlled substances for the treatment of pain. May 2004. Available at: http://www.fsmb.org. Accessed February 14, 2009.
21. DEA issues new guidelines on pain drugs. Associated Press, August 11, 2004. Available at: http://www.msnbc.msn.com/id/5673456. Accessed February 14, 2009.
22. U.S. Department of Justice, Drug Enforcement Administration, with Pain & Policy Studies Group, University of Wisconsin. Frequently asked questions and answers for Health Care Professionals and Law Enforcement Personnel. Available at: http://www.deadiversion.usdoj.gov/. Accessed February 14, 2009.

23. Joint Commission on Accreditation of Healthcare Organizations. Pain Assessment and Management: An Organizational Approach. Oakbrook Terrace, Illinois: JCAHO, 2000:3.

24. Furrow BR. Pain management and provider liability: no more excuses. J Law Med Ethics 2001; 29(1):29–51.

25. Rosomoff HL, Rosomoff RS. Comprehensive multidisciplinary pain center approach to the treatment of low back pain. Neurosurg Clin N Am 1991; 2(4):877–890.

26. Cutler RB, Fishbain DA, Abdel-Moty E, et al. Does nonsurgical pain center treatment of chronic pain return patients to work? A review and meta-analysis of the literature. Spine 1994; 19:643–652.

27. Flor H, Fydrich T, Turk DC. Efficacy of multidisciplinary pain treatment centers: a meta-analytic review. Pain 1992; 49:22–30.

28. Chapman SL, Brena SF, Bradford LA. Treatment outcomes in a chronic pain rehabilitation program. Pain 1981; 11:255–268.

29. Turk DC, Loeser JD, Monarch ES. Chronic pain: purposes and costs of interdisciplinary pain rehabilitation programs. TEN 2002; 4(2):64–69.

30. www.fda.gov/ohrms/dockets/ac/02/slides/3820s2_05_passik.ppt. Accessed February 14, 2009.

31. Consensus document from the American Academy of Pain Medicine, The American Pain Society and the American Society of Addiction Medicine. Definitions related to the use of opioids for the treatment of pain. 2001.

32. Portenoy RK, Savage SR. Clinical realities and economic considerations: special therapeutic issues in intrathecal therapy—tolerance and addiction. J Pain Symptom Manage 1997; 14(3 suppl):S27–S35.

33. Porter J, Jick H. Addiction rare in patients treated with narcotics. N Engl J Med 1980; 302(2):123.

34. Passik SD, Portenoy RK, Ricketts PL. Substance abuse issues in cancer patients. Part 1: Prevalence and diagnosis. Oncology 1998; 12(4):517–521.

35. Passik SD, Portenoy RK, Ricketts PL. Substance abuse issues in cancer patients. Part 2: Evaluation and treatment. Oncology. 1998; 12(5):729–734.

36. Heit HA, Gourlay D. Urine drug testing in pain medicine. J Pain Symptom Manage 2004; 27(3):260–267.

37. Fiellin DA, Reid MC, O'Connor PG. Outpatient management of patients with alcohol problems. Ann Intern Med 2000; 133(10):815–827.

38. Federal Register 2004; 69(220):67170–67172.

39. Gourlay DL, Heit HA, Almahrezi A. Universal precautions in pain medicine: a rational approach to the treatment of chronic pain. Pain Med 2005; 6(2):107–112.

40. Moulin DE, Clark AJ, Speechley M, et al. Chronic pain in Canada. A patient survey. In: Proceedings of the 10th World Congress on Pain. San Diego, CA; 2002:93. Abstract.

41. Gilron I, Bailey JM. Trends in opioid use for chronic neuropathic pain: a survey of patients pursuing enrollment in clinical trials. Can J Anesth 2003; 50:42–47.

42. Nicholson B. Responsible prescribing of opioids for the management of chronic pain. Drugs 2003; 63(1):17–32.

43. Portenoy RK, Foley KM. Chronic use of opioid analgesics in non-malignant pain: report of 38 cases. Pain 1986; 25:171–186.

44. Portenoy RK. Opioid therapy for chronic nonmalignant pain: a review of critical issues. J Pain Symptom Manage 1996; 11(4):203–217.

45. Cowan DT, Allan L, Griffiths P. A pilot study into the problematic use of opioid analgesics in chronic non-cancer pain patients. Int J Nurs Stud 2002; 39(1):59–69.

46. Portenoy RK. Appropriate use of opioids for persistent non-cancer pain. Lancet 2004; 364(9436):739–740.

47. Breivik H. Opioids in chronic non-cancer pain, indications and controversies. Eur J Pain 2005; 9(2):127–130.

48. Reder RF. Opioid formulations: tailoring to the needs in chronic pain. Eur J Pain 2001; 5(suppl A):109–111.

49. Chou R, Clark E, Helfand M. Comparative efficacy and safety of long-acting oral opioids for chronic non-cancer pain: a systematic review. J Pain Symptom Manage 2003; 26(5):1026–1048.

50. Kalso E. Improving opioid effectiveness: from ideas to evidence. Eur J Pain 2005; 9(2):131–135.

51. Christo PJ, Grabow TS, Raja SN. Opioid effectiveness, addiction, and depression in chronic pain. Adv Psychosom Med 2004; 25:123–137.

52. Maier C, Schaub C, Willweber-Strumpf A, et al. Long-term efficiency of opioid medication in patients with chronic non-cancer-associated pain. Results of a survey 5 years after onset of medical treatment [abstract]. Schmerz 2005; 19(5):410–417.

53. Jovey JD, Ennis J, Gardner-Nix, et al. Use of opioid analgesics for the treatment of chronic noncancer pain—a consensus statement and guidelines from the Canadian Pain Society. Pain Res Manage 1998; 3:197–222.

54. Furlan AD, Sandoval JA, Mailis-Gagnon A, et al. Opioids for chronic noncancer pain: a meta-analysis of effectiveness and side effects. CMAJ 2006; 174(11):1589–1594.

55. Yuan CS, Foss JF, O'Connor M, et al. Methylnaltrexone for reversal of constipation due to chronic methadone use: a randomized controlled trial. JAMA 2000; 283(3):367–372.

56. Yuan CS, Foss JF. Oral methylnaltrexone for opioid-induced constipation. JAMA 2000; 284(11):1383–1384.

57. Yuan CS. Clinical status of methylnaltrexone, a new agent to prevent and manage opioid-induced side effects. J Support Oncol 2004; 2(2):111–117.

58. Greenwood-Van MB, Gardner CJ, Little PJ, et al. Preclinical studies of opioids and opioid antagonists on gastrointestinal function. Neurogastroenterol Motil 2004; 16(suppl 2):46–53.

59. Yuan CS, Doshan H, Charney MR, et al. Tolerability, gut effects, and pharmacokinetics of methylnaltrexone following repeated intravenous administration in humans. J Clin Pharm 2005; 45(5):538–546.

60. Walker JS. Anti-inflammatory effects of opioids. Adv Exp Med Biol 2003; 521:148–160.

61. Freye E, Latasch L. Development of opioid tolerance—molecular mechanisms and clinical consequences [abstract]. Anasthesiol Intensivmed Notfallmed Schmerzther 2003; 38(1):14–26.

62. Hsu MM, Wong CS. The roles of pain facilitatory systems in opioid tolerance. Acta Anaesthesiol Sin 2000; 38(3):155–166.

63. Vanderah TW, Suenaga NM, Ossipov MH, et al. Tonic descending facilitation from the rostral ventromedial medulla mediates opioid-induced abnormal pain and antinociceptive tolerance. J Neurosci 2001; 21(1):279–286.

64. Ossipov MH, Lai J, King T, et al. Underlying mechanisms of pronociceptive consequences of prolonged morphine exposure. Biopolymers 2005; 80(2/3):319–324.

65. Ossipov MH, Lai J, King T, et al. Antinociceptive and nociceptive actions of opioids. J Neurobiol 2004; 61(1):126–148.

66. Mao J, Price DD, Mayer DJ. Mechanisms of hyperalgesia and opiate tolerance: a current view of their possible interactions. Pain 1995; 62:259–274.

67. King T, Ossipov MH, Vanderah TW, et al. Is paradoxical pain induced by sustained opioid exposure an underlying mechanism of opioid antinociceptive tolerance? Neurosignals 2005; 14(4):194–205.

68. Ossipov MH, Lai J, Vanderah TW, et al. Induction of pain faciliatation by sustained opioid exposure: relationship to opioid antinociceptive tolerance. Life Sci 2003; 73(6):783–800.

69. Heinricher MM, McGaraughty S, Grandy DK. Circuitry underlying antiopioid actions of orphanin FQ in the rostral ventromedial medulla. J Neurophysiol 1997; 78(6):3351–3358.

70. Vanderah TW, Gardell LR, Burgess SE, et al. Dynorphin promotes abnormal pain and spinal opioid antinociceptive tolerance. J Neurosci 2000; 20(18):7074–7079.

71. Gardell LR, Burgess SE, Dogrul A, et al. Pronociceptive effects of spinal dynorphin promote cannabinoid-induced pain and antinociceptive tolerance. Pain 2002; 98(1/2):79–88.
72. Gardel LR, Wang R, Burgess SE, et al. Sustained morphine exposure induces a spinal dynorphin-dependent enhancement of excitatory transmitter release from primary afferent fibers. J Neurosci 2002; 22(15):6747–6755.
73. Fischer BD, Carrigan KA, Dykstra LA. Effects of N-methyl-D-aspartate receptor antagonists on acute morphine-induced and l-methadone-induced antinociception in mice. J Pain 2005; 6(7):425–433.
74. Bilsky EJ, Inturrisi CE, Sadee W, et al. Competitive and non-competitive NMDA antagonists block the development of antinociceptive tolerance to morphine, but not to selective mu or delta opioid agonists in mice. Pain 1996; 68(2/3):229–237.
75. Heinricher MM, Schouten JC, Jobst EE. Activation of brainstem N-methyl-D-aspartate receptors is required for the analgesic actions of morphine given systemically. Pain 2001; 92(1/2):129–138.
76. King T, Gardell LR, Wang R, et al. Role of NK-1 neurotransmission in opioid-induced hyperalgesia. Pain 2005; 116(3):276–288.
77. Belanger S, Ma W, Chabot JG, et al. Expression of calcitonin gene-related peptide, substance P and protein kinase C in cultured dorsal root ganglion neurons following chronic exposure to mu, delta and kappa opiates. Neuroscience 2002; 115(2):441–453.
78. Powel KJ, Quirion R, Jhamandas K. Inhibition of neurokinin-1-substance P receptor and protanoid activity prevents and reverses the development of morphine tolerance in vivo and the morphine-induced increase in CGRP expression in cultured dorsal root ganglion neurons. Eur J Neurosci 2003; 18(6):1572–1583.
79. Menard DP, van Rossum D, Kar S, et al. A calcitonin gene-related peptide receptor antagonist prevents the development of tolerance to spinal morphine analgesia. J Neurosci 1996; 16(7):2342–2351.
80. Powell KJ, Ma W, Sutak M, et al. Blockade and reversal of spinal morphine tolerance by peptide and non-peptide calcitonin gene-related peptide receptor antagonists. Br J Pharmacol 2000; 131(5):875–884.
81. Menard DP, van Rossum D, Kar S, et al. Alteration of calcitonin gene-related peptide and its receptor binding sites during the development of tolerance to mu and delta opioids. Can J Physiol Pharmacol 1995; 73(7):1089–1095.
82. Xie JY, Herman DS, Stiller CO, et al. Cholecystokinin in the rostral ventromedial medulla mediates opioid-induced hyperalgesia and antinociceptive tolerance. J Neurosci 2005; 25(2):409–416.
83. Colpaert FC, Deseure KR, Stinus L, et al. High-efficacy 5-HT1 A receptor activation counteracts opioid hyperallodynia and affective conditioning. J Pharmacol Exp Ther 2006; 316(2):892–899.
84. Watkins LR, Hutchinson MR, Johnson IN, et al. Glia: novel counter-regulators of opioid analgesia. Trends Neurosci 2005; 28(12):661–669.
85. Mika J. Modulation of microglia can attenuate neuropathic pain symptoms and enhance morphine effectiveness. Pharmacol Rep 2008; 60(3):297–307.
86. Watkins LR, Hutchinson MR, Ledeboer A, et al. Norman Cousins Lecture: Glia as the "bad guys": implications for improving clinical pain control and the clinical utility of opioids. Brain Behav Immun 2007; 21(2):131–146.
87. DeLeo JA, Tanga FY, Tawfik VL. Neuroimmune activation and neuroinflammation in chronic pain and opioid tolerance/hyperalgesia. Neuroscientist 2004; 10(1):40–52.
88. Hutchinson MR, Bland ST, Johnson KW, et al. Opioid-induced glial activation: mechanisms of activation and implications for opioid analgesia, dependence and reward. Scientific World Journal 2007; 7:98–111.
89. Kumar S, Boehm J, Lee JC. p38 MAP kinases: key signaling molecules as therapeutic targets for inflammatory disease. Nat Rev Drug Discov 2003; 2(9):717–726.
90. Cui Y, Liao XX, Liu W, et al. A novel role of minicycline: attenuating morphine antinociceptive tolerance by inhibition of p38 MAPK in the activated spinal microglia. Brain Behave Immun 2008; 22(1):114–123.

91. Liu W, Wang CH, Cui Y, et al. Inhibition of neuronal nitric oxide synthase antagonizes morphine antinociceptive tolerance by decreasing activation of p38 MAPK in the spinal microglia. Neurosci Lett 2006; 410(3):174–177.
92. Cui Y, Chen Y, Zhi JL, et al. Activation of p38 mitogen-activated protein kinase in spinal microglia mediates morphine antinociceptive tolerance. Brain Res 2006; 1069(1):235–243.
93. Holdridge SV, Armstrong SA, Taylor AM, et al. Behavioral and morphological evidence for the involvement of glial cell activation in delta opioid receptor function: implications for the development of opioid tolerance. Mol Pain 2007; 3:7.
94. Trang T, Sutak M, Jhamandas K. Involvement of cannabinoid (CB1)-receptors in the development and maintenance of opioid tolerance. Neuroscience 2007; 146(3):1275–1288.
95. Lipozencic J. The 1st world congress on gender-specific medicine men, women and medicine in a new view of the biology of sex/gender differences and aging. Acta Dermatovenerol Croat 2006; 14(2):132–134.
96. Schwarz JB. Gender differences in response to drugs: pain medications. J Gend Specif Med 1999; 2(5):28–30.
97. Sun LS. Gender differences in pain sensitivity and responses to analgesia. J Gend Specif Med 1998; 1(1):28–30.
98. Paller CJ, Campbell CM, Edwards RR, et al. Sex-based differences in pain perception and treatment. Pain Med. 2009; 10(2):289–299.
99. Nishino T, Isono S, Ishikawa T, et al. Sex differences in the effect of dyspnea on thermal pain threshold in young healthy subjects. Anesthesiology 2008; 109(6):1100–1106.
100. Liu NJ, von Gizycki H, Gintzler AR. Sexually dimorphic recruitment of spinal opioid analgesic pathways by the spinal application of morphine. J Pharmacol Exp Ther 2007; 322(2):654–660.
101. Fillingim RB, Ness TJ, Glover TL, et al. Morphine responses and experimental pain: sex differences in side effects and cardiovascular responses but not analgesia. J Pain 2005; 6(2):116–124.
102. Holtman JR Jr, Wala EP. Characterization of the antinociceptive effect of oxycodone in male and female rats. Pharmacol Biochem Behav 2006; 83(1):100–108.
103. Gear RW, Gordon NC, Miaskowski, et al. Sexual dimorphism in very low dose nalbuphine postoperative analgesia. Neurosci Lett 2003; 339(1):1–4.
104. Gear RW, Gordon NC, Miaskowski C, et al. Dose ratio is important in maximizing naloxone enhancement of nalbuphine analgesia in humans. Neurosci Lett 2003; 351(1):5–8.
105. Levine JD, Khasar SG, Green PG. Neurogenic inflammation and arthritis. Ann N Y Acad Sci 2006; 1069:155–167.
106. Pain management: FDA to tighten regulations of extended-release and patch meds. Drug War Chronicle 2009; (572). Available at http://www.stopthedrugwars.org. Accessed February 15, 2009.

18 Legal Issues in Pain Management

Jennifer Bolen

The Legal Side of Pain®, The J. Bolen Group, LLC, Knoxville, Tennessee, U.S.A.

Chronic opioid therapy (COT) is but one of many possible treatments to help people living with chronic pain conditions, and for some the only treatment. Because opioids are controlled substances, clinicians who prescribe them must be aware of the clinical and legal guidelines surrounding their use and strive to balance patient access to these medications with the obligation to prevent abuse and diversion. This chapter contains a basic discussion of federal and state laws governing the use of controlled medications for pain management. Clinicians should become familiar with these materials and use the brief question guide at the end of this chapter to open a dialogue with legal counsel concerning regulatory compliance and risk management needs for the medical practice. In addition to the question guide, clinicians will find a short resource list from which to compile a basic handbook on legal/regulatory materials.

BACKGROUND

On October 23, 2001, the U.S. Drug Enforcement Administration (DEA), together with 21 health care organizations issued a joint statement promoting pain relief and the prevention of abuse and diversion (1). The joint statement acknowledged that the undertreatment of pain is serious health problem in the United States, and encourages the aggressive treatment of pain (1). At the same time, and to encourage clinicians to guard against the nonmedical use of controlled medications, the joint statement recognized that the abuse and diversion of these medications is a real problem requiring clinicians to adopt reasonable measures as part of routine daily practice to undertake a benefit-to-risk analysis when considering these medications as part of a treatment plan.

Nearly eight years have passed since the issuance of the joint statement and the challenges for the pain clinician remain the same: addressing undertreated pain and preventing abuse and diversion. In May 2009, the nation's Director of National Drug Control Policy issued his report on the nonmedical use of prescription drugs, citing a serious threat to public health and safety because of the growing number of unintentional deaths involving prescription opioids (increasing 114% from 2001 to 2005) and treatment admissions (increasing 74% in a similar four-year period) (2).

Despite the strict requirements of federal and state Controlled Substances Acts and corresponding federal regulations, controlled prescribed medications (CPMs) are diverted from legitimate sources for illicit distribution and/or abuse (3). Typically, CPM diversion "involves individuals who doctor-shop and forge prescriptions, unscrupulous physicians who sell prescriptions to drug dealers or abusers, unscrupulous pharmacists who falsify records and subsequently sell the drugs, employees who steal from inventory, executives who falsify orders to cover illicit sales, individuals who commit burglaries or robberies of pharmacies, and individuals who purchase CPDs from rogue Internet pharmacies" (3). Another avenue of CPM diversion is "the sharing or purchasing of drugs between family and friends or individual theft from family and friends" (3).

In response to the growing problem of CPM diversion, the federal government has empowered the U.S. Food and Drug Administration (FDA) with authority to place additional requirements on pharmaceutical companies in connection with medications in the opioid class (4). The problem of nonmedical use of prescribed controlled substances is so bad that the DEA, FDA, and several professional pain organizations have labeled it a "public health crisis" (5). In early 2009, in an unprecedented attempt to better deal with the public health aspects of opioid abuse and diversion, the FDA began a series of meetings with industry members and other stakeholders in the pain community to address the nature and substance of one such control measure known as an Opioid REMS (Risk Evaluation and Mitigation Strategy). At the same time, the American Pain Society (APS) and the American Academy of Pain Medicine (AAPM) published clinical guidelines for the use of COT in the treatment of chronic noncancer pain (CNCP). These guidelines, published in the *Journal of Pain* (6), contain approximately 37 recommendations broken down into sections that closely parallel regulatory guidelines and rules on prescribing controlled medications to treat pain. The APS-AAPM guidelines present challenges to the pain clinician because many of the recommendations are based on weak evidence and clinicians may find themselves without the ability to fulfill these recommendations because of the structure of the current health care system—it does not always provide for risk management tools such as urine drug testing, specialist referrals, and combination therapies for the management of patients with CNCP.

Legal and medical professionals recognize that controlled medications are important to the treatment of pain and often may be the only treatment available for some patients. All stakeholders in the pain community share a responsibility for ensuring that prescription pain medications remain available to patients who need them and are subject to "safe use" and "safe handling" measures to prevent abuse and diversion. While there is no question that preventing prescription drug abuse and diversion is an important societal goal, the October 2001 Joint Statement makes clear that abuse prevention methods should not "hinder patients' ability to receive the care they need and deserve" (1). Pain clinicians should not fear prescribing controlled medications to their patients, so long as their prescribing is for a legitimate medical purpose and in the usual course of professional practice. Over time, the efforts of federal and state agencies, together with professional pain organizations, will bridge the gap between undertreating pain and inappropriate prescribing and achieve the balance described above. Risk management will always be a critical component of pain medicine, and the pain practitioner must develop a daily practice routine that balances the tasks of treating pain and minimizing risk.

INTEGRATION OF LAW AND MEDICINE
Law and medicine are closely integrated when treatment involves controlled medications. Pain clinicians should strive to understand federal and state legal standards relating to controlled substances, and to use these legal standards as the framework for regulatory compliance policies. It is equally important for

the pain clinician to evaluate current and relevant clinical guidelines, such as those issued in 2009 by APS-AAPM, and to follow them in good faith. The pain clinician's medical record documentation will play a crucial role in determining liability—administrative, civil, or criminal. The remainder of this chapter examines legal standards and parallel clinical guideline recommendations and offers the pain clinician suggestions on documentation and basic risk management protocols.

FEDERAL LEGAL/REGULATORY MATERIALS

Clinicians rarely receive formal training in legal and regulatory issues related to the prescribing of controlled substances. There are two basic levels of legal authorities for controlled substance prescribing: federal and state, with their own associated agencies. At the federal level (see Figure 1), there are three basic types of legal/regulatory materials: laws, regulations, and policy statements, the last of which includes the DEA's September 2006 *Final Policy Statement for the Dispensing of Controlled Substances for the Treatment of Pain* (the "Final Policy Statement") (7). Figure 1 contains a diagram of the three levels of federal legal materials and cites an example at each level.

The Controlled Substances Act of 1970

The federal Controlled Substances Act of 1970 (CSA) is the primary body of federal law governing the administration, dispensing, manufacturing, and prescribing of controlled medications. The CSA contains five (5) different "schedules" classifying the various substances under DEA's control. Federal law classifies each controlled substance into one of the five schedules based on

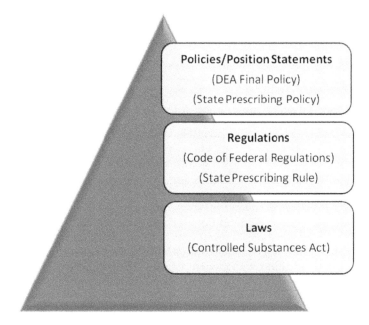

Policies/Position Statements

(DEA Final Policy)

(State Prescribing Policy)

Regulations

(Code of Federal Regulations)

(State Prescribing Rule)

Laws

(Controlled Substances Act)

FIGURE 1   Federal Legal/Regulatory Materials.

medicinal value, potential harmfulness, and the potential for abuse (8). Each state has its own controlled substance act, usually referred to as a Uniform Controlled Substances Act. States must use the federal CSA as the platform for their own CSAs, but a state may be more restrictive depending on its individual abuse and diversion problems. Thus, some states schedule medications that are not currently scheduled under federal law. Two examples include (*i*) tramadol and (*ii*) carisoprodol. As with the federal law, state CSAs prohibit the nonmedical use of controlled substances.

The Code of Federal Regulations

The Code of Federal Regulations explains individual aspects of the federal CSA. Title 21, Code of Federal Regulations, Part 1300, contains several sections directly relating to the prescribing of controlled substances. This section is limited to a discussion of three of the key federal regulations governing the prescribing of controlled substances. Pain clinicians should use online resources, such as the DEA Office of Diversion Control's website (9), to review relevant federal prescribing regulations. In addition, pain clinicians should review the DEA's *Practitioner's Manual* (10), published in September 2006.

21. CFR 1306.04—Purpose of Issue of Prescription

Section 1306.04 of Title 21, Code of Federal Regulations, sets forth the fundamental federal legal standard for a valid controlled substance prescription, regardless of the prescribed drug's schedule. A controlled substance prescription is effective or valid only if it is (*i*) issued for a legitimate medical purpose by an individual practitioner, who is (*ii*) acting in the usual course of his professional practice (11). While the prescribing clinician is primarily responsible for the "proper prescribing and dispensing of controlled substances," "a corresponding responsibility rests with the pharmacist who fills the prescription" (11). If the prescribing clinician or dispensing pharmacist knowingly prescribes or fills a controlled substance prescription outside the usual course of professional practice (or outside the usual course of legitimate and authorized research), then the individual practitioner may be "prosecuted" (12) under federal law. Section 1306.04 also *prohibits* prescribing clinicians from issuing a prescription order:

1. "to obtain controlled substances for supplying the individual practitioner for the purpose of general dispensing to patients" (13); and
2. "for the dispensing of narcotic drugs listed in any schedule for 'detoxification treatment' or 'maintenance treatment'" (14).

21. CFR 1306.05—Manner of Issuance of Prescriptions

Section 1306.05 of Title 21, Code of Federal Regulations, governs the technical aspects of issuing a controlled substance prescription. Section 1306.05(a) requires that "all prescriptions for controlled substances *shall be dated as of, and signed on, the day when issued*" (15). In addition, this section requires that the patient's full name and address be on the prescription and that the body of the prescription contain the "drug name, strength, dosage form, quantity prescribed, directions for use, and the name, address, and registration number of the practitioner" (16). Section 1306.05(a) also contains a requirement that Schedule II controlled substance prescriptions *must* be "written with ink or indelible pencil or typewriter and *shall* be manually signed by the practitioner." While a clinician's agent or secretary may prepare the body of the prescription, the prescribing clinician (DEA registrant) must be the one to sign the prescription form and will be held accountable by DEA if the prescription itself "does not conform in all essential respects to the law and regulations" (16). Once again, pharmacists have a "corresponding liability" if they dispense a controlled substance prescription that does not conform to the federal requirements. There are some important exceptions to the requirements of Section 1306.05(a), which apply to those individual practitioners who are exempt from registration, such as a hospitalist who uses the hospital's registration number (17). Section 1306.05(c) also contains directions for individual practitioners employed by one of the armed forces or the public health service.

21. CFR 1306.12—Refilling Prescriptions

Section 1306.12 prohibits the refilling of a prescription for a Schedule II controlled substance, subject to the "multiple prescriptions" exception created in 2007 by DEA pursuant to its rule-making authority. As of December 19, 2007, federal law permits an individual practitioner to issue "multiple prescriptions authorizing the patient to receive *a total of up to a 90-day supply of a Schedule II controlled substance,* **but only if the practitioner meets the following conditions**:

a. Each separate prescription is issued for a legitimate medical purpose by an individual practitioner acting in the usual course of professional practice;
b. The individual practitioner provides written instructions on each prescription (other than the first prescription, if the prescribing practitioner intends for that prescription to be filled immediately) indicating the earliest date on which a pharmacy may fill each prescription;
c. The individual practitioner <u>*concludes*</u> that providing the patient with multiple prescriptions in this manner does not create an undue risk of diversion or abuse;
d. The issuance of multiple prescriptions as described in this section is permissible under the applicable state laws; and
e. The individual practitioner complies fully with all other applicable requirements under the Act and these regulations as well as any additional requirements under state law" (18).

Of critical importance here is the fact that federal law *does not require* an individual practitioner to issue Schedule II prescriptions in this format, meaning that patients *do not have a legal right* to receive prescriptions in this format. Likewise, federal law *does not encourage* this practice, meaning the use of the multiple Schedule II prescriptions format is completely within the individual practitioner's discretion, and subject to the federal legal conditions set forth above, any additional state law conditions, and clinical guidelines and standards of care.

An equally important aspect of Section 1306.12 (the Final Rule) is the fact that DEA does not encourage individual practitioners to see their patients only once every 90 days when prescribing Schedule II controlled substances (19). Instead, DEA's position is that section 1306.12 requires individual practitioners to "determine on their own, based on sound medical judgment, and in accordance with established medical standards, whether it is appropriate to issue multiple prescriptions and how often to see their patients when doing so" (18). *This is a significant statement and one often disregarded by nonlawyer educators during lectures at pain conferences.* Quite simply, pain clinicians should remember that federal law *does not* encourage the "multiple Schedule II prescriptions" format. Thus, pain clinicians should carefully evaluate their use of this prescribing format and ensure that state law permits this practice and that each patient has been carefully evaluated—using a benefit-to-risk analysis—and document the rationale and safety measures for monitoring the patient during follow-up evaluations to prevent abuse and diversion.

DEA Policy Statements

Over almost a two-year period, beginning in November 2004 and ending in September 2006, DEA issued three policy statements relating to the use of controlled substances to treat pain (20). The *Interim Policy Statement* (November 2004) and the *Clarification Statement* (August 2005) both contain insight into DEA's position on prescribing of Schedule II controlled substances, and both ultimately give rise to the *Final Policy Statement* (September 2006) and the *Final Rule on Issuance of Multiple Prescriptions for Schedule II Controlled Substances* (November 2007) (discussed above). These three policy statements contain insight into DEA's position on registrant obligations. These statements are summarized below.

The DEA Interim Policy Statement—November 2004

In November 2004, following its October 2004, retraction of the FAQ and to explain its rationale or doing so, DEA published its Interim Policy Statement on Dispensing Controlled Substances to Treat Pain (the "Interim Policy Statement"). DEA said that "each of the [FAQ] factors—though not necessarily determinative—may indeed be indicative of diversion." Those factors, not viewed individually by the courts as indicative of criminal behavior (although prosecution on certain individual behaviors is possible), but in concomitant and recurrent patterns, included the following:

a. prescribing of an inordinately large quantity of controlled substances;
b. issuing large numbers of controlled substance prescriptions;
c. prescribing controlled substances without performing a physical examination;
d. the physician warned the patient to fill the controlled substance prescriptions at different drug stores;
e. the physician issued controlled substance prescriptions to a patient known to be delivering the drugs to others;
f. the physician prescribed controlled substances at intervals inconsistent with legitimate medical treatment;
g. the physician used street slang with patients rather than medical terminology to describe the controlled substances prescribed;
h. there was no logical relationship between the controlled substances prescribed and the treatment of the condition allegedly existing; and
i. the physician wrote more than one controlled substance prescription on occasions in order to spread them out.

These factors remain relevant today. However, it is important to note that DEA has stated that this does not mean that "the existence of any of [these] factors will automatically lead to the conclusion that the physician acted improperly" (21).

The DEA's Clarification Statement—August 2005

On August 26, 2005, DEA published a Clarification of Existing Requirements under the Controlled Substances Act for Prescribing Schedule II Controlled Substances, which DEA intended as a follow-up to its Interim Policy (November 2004) comments on prescriptions for Schedule II controlled substances. While not formally characterized as a "policy statement," this document provides insight into DEA's position on the use of Schedule II controlled substances to treat pain. "Schedule II controlled substances, by definition, have the highest potential for abuse, and are the most likely to cause dependence, of all the controlled substances that have an approved medical use" (22). "Physicians must use the utmost care in determining whether

a. their patients for whom they are prescribing schedule II controlled substances should be seen in person each time a prescription is issued; or
b. seeing the patient in person at somewhat less frequent intervals is consistent with sound medical practice and appropriate safeguards against diversion and misuse" (22).

"Physicians must also abide by any requirements imposed by their state medical boards with respect to proper prescribing practices and what constitutes a bona fide physician–patient relationship" (22). Subject to state laws which may prohibit prescribing in the absence of a face-to-face office visit, federal law permits physicians who regularly see each patient to issue a prescription for a Schedule II controlled substance for a legitimate medical purpose without seeing the patient in person, and may mail the prescription to the patient or pharmacy. DEA regulations state: "A prescription for a schedule II controlled substance may be transmitted by the practitioner or the practitioner's agent to a pharmacy via facsimile equipment, provided that the original written, signed prescription is presented to the pharmacist for review prior to the actual dispensing of the controlled substance, except as noted [elsewhere in this section of the regulations]" (23). Thus, as this provision of the regulations provides, faxing may be used to facilitate the filling of a Schedule II prescription, but only if the pharmacy receives the original written, signed prescription prior to dispensing the drug to the patient *and* only if state law permits it. Moreover, federal law *does not* set a specific limit on the number of days' worth of a Schedule II controlled substance that a physician may authorize per prescription. Some states, however, do impose specific limits on the amount of a Schedule II controlled substance that may be prescribed. Any limitations imposed by state law apply in addition to the corresponding requirements under federal law, so long as the state requirements do not conflict with or contravene federal requirements.

Remember, the essential federal legal standard is that a "prescription for a controlled substance be issued for a legitimate medical purpose in the usual course of professional practice." Both physicians and pharmacists "have a duty as DEA registrants to ensure that their prescribing and dispensing of controlled substances occur in a manner consistent with effective controls against diversion and misuse, taking into account the nature of the drug being prescribed." It took DEA a little more than a year after its Clarification Statement to publish a Final

Statement on Dispensing Controlled Substances to Treat Pain. Despite the large gap in time, DEA finally presented registrants with written materials containing regulatory boundaries on controlled substance prescribing.

DEA Final Policy Statement—September 2006

Federal case law makes clear: there is no "one size fits all" definition of legitimate medical purpose and usual course of professional practice. In administrative cases, the law is also clear: DEA evaluates each case on its own merits in view of the totality of the circumstances and individual facts tied to physician–patient relationships. DEA expects registrants to accept their responsibility and to put practices into place, as part of routine medical practice, to prevent abuse and diversion (24). According to a 2009 DEA administrative case involving the suspension and ultimate reinstatement of a physician's registration, DEA has the authority to suspend or revoke a registration if the registrant's behavior presents a threat to public health and safety (24). "A practitioner who ignores the warning signs that her patients are either personally abusing or diverting controlled substances commits 'acts inconsistent with the public interest,' 21 U.S.C. 824(a)(4), even if she is merely gullible or naive" (24).

The DEA Final Policy Statement contains the following critical language explaining DEA's position on DEA registrant responsibilities to prevent abuse and diversion when prescribing controlled medications to treat pain:

> *What are the general legal responsibilities of a physician to prevent diversion and abuse when prescribing controlled substances?*
>
> In each instance where a physician issues a prescription for a controlled substance, the physician must properly determine there is a legitimate medical purpose for the patient to be prescribed that controlled substance and the physician must be acting in the usual course of professional practice [internal citation omitted]. This is the basic legal requirement discussed above, which has been part of American law for decades. Moreover, as a condition of being a DEA registrant, a physician who prescribes controlled substances *has an obligation to take reasonable measures to prevent diversion* [internal citation omitted]. *The overwhelming majority of physicians in the United States who prescribe controlled substances do, in fact, exercise the appropriate degree of medical supervision—as part of their routine practice during office visits—to minimize the likelihood of diversion or abuse.* Again, each patient's situation is unique and the nature and degree of physician oversight should be tailored accordingly, based on the physician's sound medical judgment and consistent with established medical standards.
>
> *What additional precaution should be taken when a patient has a history of drug abuse?*
>
> As a DEA registrant, *a physician has a responsibility to exercise a much greater degree of oversight to prevent diversion and abuse in the case of a known or suspected addict than in the case of a patient for whom there are no indicators of drug abuse.* **Under no circumstances** may a physician dispense controlled substances with the knowledge they will be used for a nonmedical purpose or that they will be resold by the patient. Some physicians who treat patients having a history of drug abuse require each patient to sign a contract agreeing to certain terms designed to prevent diversion and abuse, *such as periodic urinalysis*. While such measures are not mandated by the CSA or DEA regulations, they can be very useful.
>
> *Can a physician be investigated solely on the basis of the number of tablets prescribed for an individual patient?*

The Supreme Court has long recognized that an administrative agency responsible for enforcing the law has broad investigative authority [internal citation omitted], and courts have recognized that prescribing an "inordinately large quantity of controlled substances" can be evidence of a violation of the CSA [internal citation omitted]. DEA therefore, as the agency responsible for administering the CSA, has the legal authority to investigate a suspicious prescription of any quantity. Nonetheless, the amount of dosage units per prescription will never be a basis for investigation for the overwhelming majority of physicians. As with every other profession, however, among the hundreds of thousands of physicians who practice medicine in this country in a manner that warrants no government scrutiny are a handful who engage in criminal behavior. In rare cases, it is possible that an aberrant physician could prescribe such an enormous quantity of controlled substances to a given patient that this alone will be a valid basis for investigation. For example, if a physician were to prescribe 1,600 (sixteen hundred) tablets per day of a schedule II opioid to a single patient, this would certainly warrant investigation as there is no conceivable medical basis for anyone to ingest that quantity of such a powerful narcotic in a single day. Again, however, such cases are extremely rare. The overwhelming majority of physicians who conclude that use of a particular controlled substance is medically appropriate for a given patient should prescribe the amount of that controlled substance which is consistent with their sound medical judgment and accepted medical standards without concern that doing so will subject them to DEA scrutiny (7).

Summary of Key Federal Legal Standards (Substantive Only)

By way of summary, the federal law sets forth the below-listed *substantive* legal standards that DEA registrants must follow when treatment involves controlled substances. For a more complete discussion of both substantive and technical requirements for controlled substance prescriptions, review the DEA Diversion website and the DEA's September 2006 *Practitioner's Manual*, which may also be found on the website.

1. Provides DEA authority to oversee the flow of controlled substances in the United States and gives DEA authority to register and oversee registrant activity through its administrative and enforcement arms.
2. Requires registrants to prescribe controlled substances for a legitimate medical purpose while acting in the usual course of professional practice.
3. Requires registrants to use reasonable measures, as part of routine daily medical practice, to prevent abuse and diversion.
4. Imposes a corresponding responsibility on pharmacists to ensure a legitimate medical purpose prior to dispensing a controlled substance prescription, and requires them to do so in the usual course of professional practice.
5. Provides for specific handling of controlled substances in Schedule II, and identifies certain exceptions to the federal rules requiring a written prescription for these medications, including a provision for faxing and emergency supply. Prohibits refills of Schedule II controlled substance prescriptions, unless the registrant is acting under the "multiple issuance" or "do not fill" rule of 21 CFR 1306.12 (described above). Registrants may not issue multiple prescriptions for Schedule II controlled substances unless state law authorizes them to do so.

6. Provides for specific handling of controlled substances in Schedule III, and includes a provision for oral prescribing and refills, subject to the legitimate medical purpose/usual course of professional practice rule.
7. Does not limit the quantity of any drug prescribed or dispensed, but does limit the number of refills permitted for each prescription for a Schedule III controlled substance.
8. With the exception of the Schedule II "multiple issuance" or "do not fill" rule, does not specify a quantity or duration to determine the clinician's ongoing use of a Schedule II controlled substance.
9. Does not establish a minimum or maximum dose for controlled substance prescriptions in Schedules II through V (some states DO set maximum doses for some controlled substances, so registrants should take care to review state law before prescribing).
10. Does not establish a "life" or period of validity for a Schedule II controlled substance prescription (some states DO set a "life" or period of validity, such as 7 days, 14 days, or 21 days, and registrants should take care to review state law before prescribing).
11. Does not limit the overall number of refills for Schedule III, IV, and V controlled substances, but does establish a rule of not more than five refills in six months (some states set more restrictions so registrants should check state law).
12. Permits the mailing of controlled substance prescriptions, subject to registrant discretion and policy suggestions.

State Legal/Regulatory Materials
State legal/regulatory materials in many ways parallel the federal framework, but there are differences in state policy–level material relating to the use of controlled medications to treat pain. While a state-by-state analysis of legal/regulatory materials is beyond the scope of this chapter, pain clinicians will find that the basic framework for state controlled substances acts, medical practice act regulations, and pain policy have many similarities and the same basic platform for critical elements. To date, all but three states (25) have regulations and/or policy or position statements specifically relating to prescribing controlled substances to treat pain.

There are three basic levels of state legal/regulatory materials:

1. *Laws*, such as a state's Uniform Controlled Substances Act; Medical, Nursing, and Pharmacy Practice Acts; and in some states an Intractable Pain Treatment Act;
2. *Regulations*, including professional licensing board rules outlining standards of professional conduct and often rules on prescribing controlled medications to treat pain; and
3. *Policy or Position Statements*, including state policies on the use of controlled medications to treat pain and the office-based treatment of opioid addiction.

Federation of State Medical Boards' Model Policy
Of critical relevance to many state licensing boards' position on prescribing controlled substances for the treatment of pain is the body of policy materials created by the Federation of State Medical Boards, located in Dallas, Texas (the FSMB).

The FSMB's mission is "to continuously improve the quality, safety, and integrity of health care through developing and promoting high standards for physician licensure and practice" (26). In 1997, and again in 2004, the FSMB published a *Model Policy for the Prescribing of Controlled Substances for the Treatment of Pain* (the *Model Policy*) (27). This document contains many helpful statements on the need for pain policy to achieve balance in patient care—access to pain management, including controlled medications, and measures to prevent abuse and diversion of those medications.

As with most state regulations and/or policy statements on prescribing controlled substances to treat pain, the FSMB's *Model Policy* contains seven (7) basic elements:

1. Patient Evaluation (History and Physical Examination);
2. Treatment Plan;
3. Informed Consent;
4. Treatment Agreements;
5. Periodic Review (Patient Follow-up Evaluation);
6. Consultations and Referrals; and
7. Medical Record and Regulatory Compliance.

Pain clinicians have an "ethical and professional responsibility" to assess patients' pain (27). When pain clinicians believe it is appropriate to prescribe controlled medications to treat pain, they must document their clinical rationale for doing so (the legitimate medical purpose requirement) and take those steps outlined in currently accepted standards of care or, in the absence of a directly applicable statement of such a standard, clinical guidelines, such as the APS-AAPM 2009 clinical guideline (usual course of professional practice requirement) (6). Failure to adhere to state rules and, without a documented reason, state policy or position statements may result in administrative and legal sanctions.

One of the easiest ways to signal the intent to comply with state legal/regulatory requirements on the use of controlled substances to treat pain is to incorporate key phrases from state prescribing rules and policies into the medical record. For example, if a state prescribing rule requires a risk–benefit analysis prior to prescribing a controlled substance, then the prescribing clinician should enter a note in the patient chart integrating or referring to the legal/regulatory language, as illustrated in Figure 2. This format is easily transferred into electronic medical record systems or templates.

"*The anticipated benefits for this patient's use of DRUG A are as follows:*

The potential risks related to the use of DRUG A are as follows:

I have discussed these matters with the patient in detail, and based on all of the information in my possession at this time, including statements made to me by the patient, I believe the benefits of using DRUG A outweigh the risks associated with use, and I am going to prescribe a trial of DRUG A to the patient as follows . . . ."

FIGURE 2 Example of patient chart note.

There is no legal requirement requiring clinicians to incorporate legal/regulatory language into the medical record, but pain clinicians should realize that licensing board investigators and law enforcement agents speak a different language when it comes to pain management and occasional references to the materials these individuals use on a daily basis may help prevent misunderstandings and, more importantly, provide the prescribing clinician with a reference point should there be a challenge to one's prescribing patterns. Once again, there is no magic formula for avoiding legal scrutiny. However, pain clinicians must do what they can to ensure evidence of good faith prescribing and patient care as part of routine medical practice. The remainder of this section contains a discussion of each of the key elements of the FSMB's *Model Policy*, providing a framework for state licensing board materials. Pain clinicians should also consult parallel recommendations contained in the APS-AAPM Clinical Guidelines on the Use of COT to Treat CNCP to ensure practice in compliance with generally accepted clinical standards of care (28).

Patient Evaluation and Risk Assessment

Both the *Model Policy* and the APS-AAPM COT guideline require pain clinicians to engage in a careful evaluation of the patient prior to prescribing COT. The evaluation process has many components, most of which are also referred to by state licensing boards in prescribing regulations and policies. Language in the APS-AAPM COT guideline and many state regulations and policy statements suggest that the evaluation and risk assessment process should take place *prior to prescribing controlled substances to the patient* (6). The difficulty with such a requirement is obvious: many patients present already using controlled substances to treat pain and the timing of many patient visits is such that patients are almost out of their medications, requiring a prescription to avoid the discomforts of acute withdrawal. Common sense tells us that pain clinicians must balance their role as health care providers with their legal and professional obligation to prevent abuse and diversion. Thus, early in any relationship between a pain clinician and a patient, prescribing should be done in a controlled and trial fashion to ensure pain management and minimize risk.

In the patient evaluation phase, legal/regulatory materials recommend that clinicians:

1. obtain information about the patient's past medical history;
2. evaluate a recent physical examination or perform a new, condition-specific physical examination and document the results in the medical record;
3. document the nature and intensity of the patient's pain, current and past treatments for pain, any underlying or coexisting diseases or conditions, the effect of pain on the patient's physical and psychological function; and
4. ascertain the patient's history of substance abuse (alcohol and drug) (29).

The APS-AAPM COT guideline (6) expands upon the "risk assessment" portion of patient evaluation, making the following very important recommendations that directly correlate with the legal/regulatory recommendations:

1.1 *Before initiating COT*, clinicians *should* conduct a history, physical examination, and appropriate testing, including an assessment of risk of substance abuse, misuse, or addiction (*strong recommendation, low-quality evidence*).

1.2 Clinicians *may* consider a trial of COT as an option if CNCP is moderate or severe, pain is having an adverse impact on function or quality of life, and potential therapeutic benefits outweigh or are likely to outweigh potential harms (*strong recommendation, low-quality evidence*).

1.3 A benefit-to-harm evaluation, including a history, physical examination, and appropriate diagnostic testing, *should* be performed and documented before and on an ongoing basis during COT (*strong recommendation, low-quality evidence*) (6).

"Proper patient selection is critical and requires a comprehensive benefit-to-harm evaluation that weighs the potential positive effects of opioids on pain and function against potential risks." "*Thorough risk assessment and stratification is appropriate in every case*" (30).

In 2009, risk assessment requires all pain management clinicians to be familiar with the various risk factors for opioid abuse and the methods for assessing risk and evaluating the potential for opioid-associated adverse effects. "A thorough history and physical examination, including an assessment of psychosocial factors and family history, is essential for adequate risk stratification. Implicit in the recommendation to conduct a comprehensive benefit-to-harm analysis is the recognition that an opioid trial may not be appropriate. Clinicians should obtain appropriate diagnostic tests to evaluate the underlying pain condition, and should consider whether the pain condition may be treated more effectively with nonopioid therapy rather than with COT" (6).

Newer risk assessment measures include screening tools that assess the potential risks associated with COT based on patient characteristics, such as environmental factors, experience with medications, experience with lawsuits, emotions and feelings, and several others (6). The APS-AAPM COT guideline states these tools "are likely to be helpful for risk stratification, though more validation and prospective outcome studies are needed to understand how their use predicts and affects clinical outcomes" (6). Unfortunately, however, the current health care system does not provide focused reimbursement methods for the use of these tools, making it just one more thing pain clinicians are told they "should" do prior to prescribing controlled substances. In addition, many clinicians have yet to review these tools (31) and decide whether and how to incorporate their use into the medical practice.

In summary, pain clinicians should consider the following measures in connection with patient evaluation:

1. verify the patient's self-report of medication usage with prior providers or through a state prescription drug monitoring program or pharmacy profile;
2. discuss medication options with the patient and determine whether patient has had a trial of nonopioids and document patient's response to same or reason why the trial was inappropriate or did not work;
3. review documentation from prior providers;
4. consider overall risk assessment issues and whether a urine drug test would support your prescribing rationale.

The pain clinician's rationale for the use of controlled substances is a critical documentation topic. Overall, the clinician should document their rationale for using controlled substances, medication quantity, the duration of use and, where applicable, medication combinations, and document one or more currently accepted clinical indications for the use of controlled substances. Doing so will go a long way to establishing a legitimate medical purpose.

Treatment Plan

After deciding whether to prescribe controlled substances to the patient, legal/regulatory materials require/suggest the use of a *written* treatment plan documenting the patient's diagnosis (or working diagnosis) and a summary of treatment goals and the time frame for reevaluating the patient's progress toward the same. The plan does not have to be elaborate, but it should clearly document the legitimate medical purpose for which controlled substances are prescribed and provide enough information to demonstrate that the clinician is acting within the usual course of professional practice. Most state licensing board rules/policies require some version of the following in connection with the treatment plan:

> The medical record should include (A) how the medication relates to the chief presenting complaint of chronic pain; (B) dosage and frequency of prescribed, (C) further testing and diagnostic evaluations to be ordered, (D) other treatments that are planned or considered, (E) periodic reviews planned, and (F) objectives that will be used to determine treatment success, such as pain relief and improved physical and psychosocial function (32).

Most states require clinicians to periodically review the treatment plan to ensure that the benefit-to-risk analysis remains the focus and to evaluate the necessary level of medical supervision to prevent abuse and diversion in the patient's individual case.

Informed Consent and Treatment Agreement

Informed consent and the agreement for treatment are critical components of most state rules/policies on prescribing controlled substances to treat pain. It is important to remember, however, that informed consent is a separate legal concept from a treatment agreement and one that is grounded in medical ethics. While it is possible to address informed consent and treatment agreement issues with the patient during a single visit, the better practice is to address these matters separately, using separate forms designed to reinforce the relevant subject matter with the patient. A full-blown discussion of the informed consent and treatment agreement is beyond the scope of this chapter.

Informed consent is the process by which the clinician fulfills the ethical responsibility to give the patient information from which he/she can make informed decisions about health care (33). It involves a process and a discussion with the patient about

1. the risks of the recommended treatment, including any medications prescribed;
2. the anticipated benefits of the recommended treatment;
3. any alternative or complimentary therapies; and
4. special issues related to the recommended treatment, such as treatment safety, driving, and decision-making (33).

Some states require a separate form documenting the informed consent process, while others permit the clinician to use a contemporaneous note describing it in the medical record. Be sure to check state licensing board requirements to ensure compliance. Also, a clinician's failure to provide the patient with adequate information may give rise to a claim of negligence. Check with legal counsel to ensure informed consent forms are current and written in conformance with state case law in mind. In summary, informed consent process and related documentation focuses on the patient's mindset and whether he/she has sufficient information to provide his/her consent to the recommended treatment. If the patient withholds information from a clinician about a material component of informed consent, such as withholding personal history of substance abuse, then any claim of negligence against the treating clinician may be mitigated by the patient's actions. These matters require careful legal analysis and are best left to the clinician's local legal counsel.

By contrast, a treatment agreement (often inappropriately referred to as a "narcotic contract") involves a form and a conversation between the patient and the clinician about the clinician's expectations of patient behaviors—what the patient must or must not do during the treatment period involving controlled substances. In fact, the treatment agreement is a unique tool arising out of state rules/policies on prescribing controlled substances to treat pain; informed consent is not and applies to any recommended medical treatment within the clinician–patient relationship. While both processes involve efforts designed to improve patient care and prevent abuse and diversion, the **informed consent** favors the patient's need for information *prior to making health care decisions* and the **treatment agreement** favors the clinician's need to set *behavioral boundaries* designed to protect the individual patient and the public's health and safety and to enforce them based on the individual patient's case.

The FSMB's *Model Policy* contains the following basic suggestions regarding the use of treatment agreements:

1. A written treatment agreement should be considered if the patient has a history of substance abuse (34).
2. The agreement should explain the purpose and terms of its use and should seek the patient's agreement to:
   a. use a single clinician for the prescribing of controlled substances;
   b. select a single pharmacy to use for filling controlled substance prescriptions (35);
   c. produce a blood/urine sample as requested for compliance and therapeutic testing; and
   d. bring with them to each office visit original medication bottles containing all remaining medication.
3. The agreement should clearly state the reasons for which controlled substance therapy or treatment overall may be discontinued (36).

It is vital that the pain clinician draft the treatment agreement using clear and simple language and even consider translating it into other languages to serve the entirety of the clinician's patient population. It is also important to remember that treatment agreements are part of the medical record and may be used in administrative hearings and court to address the clinician's prescribing habits. Often, treatment agreements and other practice forms are shown to hearing officers and jurors and provide an impression of the clinician's attention to detail and professionalism and tone toward patients. Thus, great care should be given to the drafting and review of treatment agreements and other office forms.

PERIODIC REVIEW AND RISK MONITORING

Periodic review involves patient follow-up care and medical supervision commensurate with the individual patient needs and the scope of the clinician's medical practice. Clinical standards of care require the clinician to evaluate the patient's progress (or lack thereof) toward the treatment plan goals and the patient's compliance with medication instructions—safe use and handling, etc. The timing of follow-up visits should be individualized to each patient, taking into consideration the patient's history, overall risk potential, and developing facts of patient care. Some state rules/policies require the clinician to see the patient at least every 12 weeks (37). Most states, however, do not suggest a specific follow-up period and leave the decision to the clinician, thereby requiring the clinician to exercise medical decision-making consistent with current standards of care and evolving patient needs. The language of the DEA's *Clarification Statement* (August 2005) and *Final Policy Statement* (September 2006), and its administrative opinion *in the matter of Jayam Krishna-Iyer* (January 2009), indicates growing regulatory emphasis on individualized treatment plans, follow-up periods, and patient risk monitoring. In many ways, periodic review emphasizes both sides of the balance issue—ensuring the patient's continued access to quality pain management, including where appropriate controlled medications, and routine measures as part of daily medical practice to prevent abuse and diversion. Pain clinicians may face regulatory scrutiny if patient follow-up does not include reasonable and regular means designed to prevent abuse and diversion, such as periodic urinalysis (38), medication counts (39) or attention to the amount of medication a patient has on hand and determining whether there is a need for the safe disposal of expired or unused medications, and other measures designed to address these concerns.

The APS-AAPM COT guideline provides the following recommendations in connection with patient monitoring:

> 5.1 Clinicians should reassess patients on COT periodically and as warranted by changing circumstances. Monitoring should include documentation of pain intensity and level of functioning, assessments of progress toward achieving therapeutic goals, presence of adverse events, and adherence to prescribed therapies (*strong recommendation, low-quality evidence*).
>
> 5.2 In patients on COT who are at high risk or who have engaged in aberrant drug-related behaviors, clinicians should periodically obtain urine drug screens or other information to confirm adherence to the COT plan of care (*strong recommendation, low-quality evidence*).
>
> 5.3 In patients on COT not at high risk and not known to have engaged in aberrant drug-related behaviors, clinicians should consider periodically obtaining urine drug screens or other information to confirm adherence to the COT plan of care (*weak recommendation, low-quality evidence*) (6).

According to a panel of experts who authored the APS-AAPM clinical guidelines on COT to treat CNCP:

> Clinicians should periodically reassess all patients on COT. Regular monitoring of patients once COT is initiated is critical because therapeutic risks and benefits do not remain static and can be affected by changes in

the underlying pain condition, presence of coexisting disease, or changes in psychological or social circumstances. Monitoring is essential to identify patients who are benefiting from COT, those who might benefit more with restructuring of treatment or receiving additional services such as treatment for addiction, and those whose benefits from treatment are outweighed by harms (6).

These guidelines state that the evidence is insufficient to guide precise recommendations on appropriate monitoring intervals. From a regulatory perspective, if this is the case with a patient, then the clinician should document this fact in the medical record.

Likewise, the APS-AAPM clinical guideline states:

Risk stratification is useful for guiding the approach to monitoring. In patients at low risk for adverse outcomes and on stable doses of opioids, monitoring at least once every three to six months may be sufficient. Patients who may need more frequent or intense monitoring, at least for a period of time after initiation of therapy or changes in opioid doses, include those with a prior history of an addictive disorder, those in an occupation demanding mental acuity, older adults, patients with an unstable or dysfunctional social environment, and those with comorbid psychiatric or medical conditions. For patients at very high risk for adverse outcomes, monitoring on a weekly basis may be a reasonable strategy (6).

It is important to note that the language of this clinical guideline may actually conflict with specific regulatory requirements in some states, such as Louisiana and New Jersey, both of which mandate that patients on chronic controlled substance therapy be seen at least every 12 weeks and, more frequently, depending on the patient's individual circumstances. Pain clinicians should document the interval for periodic review and supply a statement of the rationale for the period selected.

"There is general agreement that monitoring should routinely include assessment and documentation of pain severity and functional ability, progress toward achieving therapeutic goals, and presence of adverse effects" (6). Monitoring also include a complete and routine "clinical assessment for presence of aberrant drug-related behaviors, substance use, and psychological issues" (40).

Clinical and regulatory guidelines acknowledge that periodic urine drug screening can be a helpful tool to monitor patients using controlled medications (41). A detailed discussion of urine drug testing is beyond the scope of this chapter. However, several federal cases address the lack of urine drug testing and the failure to address the results of a urine drug test with the patient, indicating that the defendant-clinician's failure to use urine drug testing or the results of such toxicology tests as evidence of a lack of legitimate medical purpose and a provider acting outside the usual course of professional practice (42).

Overall, the pain clinician is responsible for determining whether the patient's response to controlled substance therapy is satisfactory and that ongoing use remains indicated. Many states suggest clinicians indicate a satisfactory response to controlled substance therapy by documenting facts associated with "the patient's decreased pain, increased level of function, or improved quality of life" (27). Many clinicians find themselves in hot water with licensing boards if they merely document the above-quoted phrase instead of making the effort to document facts demonstrating decreased pain, that is, the patient reports a decrease in pain from level 7 to level 4. Or, the patient reports "she is now working part time and doing house hold chores and engaging in social activities with her family—she states she went to the movies with her husband and children and sat through most of the movie without too much discomfort." In essence, clinicians should monitor the patient for "[o]bjective evidence of improved or diminished function ... and [consider] information from family members or other caregivers in determining the patient's response to treatment" (27). State legal/regulatory and clinical guidelines make very clear: "[i]f the patient's progress is unsatisfactory, the clinician should asses the appropriateness of continued use of the current treatment plan [especially one involving controlled substances] and consider the use of other therapeutic modalities" (27).

It is important to note that both clinical guidelines and legal/regulatory materials distinguish initial and ongoing treatment for "high-risk" patients. Pain clinicians should carefully review clinical and regulatory resources to ensure compliance. As questions arise, check with clinical colleagues and confirm practice policies with legal counsel.

CONSULTATIONS AND REFERRALS
The use of consultations and referrals is contemplated on an "as necessary" basis by both current clinical standards of care and state pain rules/policies. Some patients may need to see behavioral health specialists; others may need professionals qualified in addiction medicine or other specialty area. Unfortunately, the current health care system does not always support the use of necessary consultations and referrals, often making it difficult for both the clinician and the patient to address specific treatment concerns.

MEDICAL RECORDS
Pain clinicians are required to keep accurate and careful documentation of their interaction with patients and treatment recommendations. Like state regulations and policy statements, the *Model Policy* contains a list of medical records that pain clinicians should keep. Remember, state licensing boards and state laws may

---

The following list of Medical Records is quoted from the FSMB's Model Policy Statement on the Use of Controlled Substances for the Treatment of Pain (April 2004) (27). Similar lists appear in many state prescribing guidelines and regulations.
  "Medical Records—The physician should keep accurate and complete records to include

1. the medical history and physical examination,
2. diagnostic, therapeutic and laboratory results,
3. evaluations and consultations,
4. treatment objectives,
5. discussion of risks and benefits,
6. informed consent,
7. treatments,
8. medications (including date, type, dosage and quantity prescribed),
9. instructions and agreements and
10. periodic reviews.

  Records should remain current and be maintained in an accessible manner and readily available for review.

FIGURE 3 List of medical records.

TABLE 1 Key Legal/Regulatory Compliance Recommendations and Documentation Steps in the Treatment of Pain with Controlled Substances

Legal/Regulatory Component	Documentation Checklist
Patient Evaluation (History, Physical Examination, Risk Assessment)	*General patient history *Specific pain history *Past treatments for pain (including medication/procedures) and records from prior provider *Family and Patient history of chemical/substance abuse *Current report of pain (nature, intensity) *Condition-appropriate physical examination *Risk Assessment Questionnaire if Chronic Opioid Therapy is contemplated *Urine Drug Testing (point of care and laboratory confirmation), for illegal drugs and other controlled prescribed drugs *Electronic prescription drug monitoring program or patient pharmacy profile
Treatment Plan and Medication Trial	*Written treatment plan *Set goals for treatment and reasonable trial period *Discuss methods used to measure patient's progress and next steps outline *Set time for return visits using patient risk level (L, M, H) to guide decision making *Order additional testing (diagnostic and laboratory) *Use consultations and referrals as necessary *Take reasonable steps to prevent abuse and diversion via medication trial and safety steps
Informed Consent	*Informed consent is a process whereby the clinician discusses the (1) risks, including adverse effects, known side-effects, potential for addiction, (2) benefits, (3) alternatives to using controlled substances (if any), and (4) special issues, such as medication safety, driving, operating heavy machinery, making important decisions, caring for others, and carrying weapon. Clinicians should give patients a chance to ask questions. *Consider documenting informed consent SEPARATE from a Treatment Agreement. The two processes are not the same, and some state licensing boards make this point very clear. *The American Academy of Pain Medicine has a sample Informed Consent document on its website. Some states require a written, signed form; others allow a contemporaneous note in the patient's medical record. *Applies to both medications and treatments. Informed consent process is not unique to opioids, although the actual document usually is. *You should review your informed consent practices with your legal counsel.
Treatment Agreement	*Addresses practice boundaries and rules relating to obtaining, filling, and safe handling and usage of controlled substances. *Usually a written document discussing treatment accountability and drug boundary issues. *Should NOT be limited to opioids; Most state materials apply it to controlled substances rather than just opioids. *Should NOT be titled a Contract or a Narcotic Contract.

TABLE 1   (Continued)

Legal/Regulatory Component	Documentation Checklist
	*You should review this document with your legal counsel. *Most state licensing board rules/policies provide sample language for a treatment agreement; use this language and tailor it as appropriate to your practice. *The American Academy of Pain Medicine has a sample Treatment Agreement, but make sure you change the language to cover all controlled substances instead of leaving it as limited to opioids – especially for those who are in states that take this approach. *Remember, a Treatment Agreement is also a process and the pain clinician should address patient violations with balance in mind – access to pain care with obligation to prevent abuse and diversion. Failure to address aberrant patient behaviors may increase legal exposure.
Periodic Review	*Assess the patient periodically, based on the individual circumstances of each patient's case and according to the standard of care and state rules/guidelines. Some states require follow-up review at least every 12 weeks. Others require more frequent visits. *Standard of care may dictate more frequent visits due to the patient's risk level. *Remember to demonstrate reasonable measures to prevent abuse and diversion, such as periodic urine drug testing, medication counts, and referrals. *State rules/policies contain a checklist for follow-up care. *The APS-AAPM COT guideline contains additional suggestions.
Consultations and Referrals	*Use as necessary. *If patient's insurance does not cover, then document as much and advocate for coverage or alternatives. *Most state rules/policies suggest that consultations and referrals "are necessary" when a patient has a history of substance abuse and a pain condition necessitating controlled substances. Be sure to review these state materials.
Documentation	*Consult state rules/policies for a specific list of required documents.

require additional documentation, so pain clinicians should check with appropriate state agencies and their legal counsel to ensure compliance (Table 1). Medical record documentation often serves as a deciding factor in the outcome of legal challenges. While there can be no guarantee that having all of the items listed in Figure 3 will prevent a lawsuit, the better the pain clinician's documentation, the easier it is to explain the clinician's treatment rationale and the patient's consent to the same. In fact, solid documentation of the patient's informed consent to current and generally accepted treatments can mitigate risk and improve legal outcomes.

SUMMARY
The law is not designed to prevent the use of controlled substances to treat pain. Instead, federal and state legal/regulatory materials set boundaries within which

pain clinicians must operate to maintain their medical license and DEA registration. Familiarity with legal/regulatory boundaries enables pain clinicians to achieve balance in the treatment of chronic pain with controlled substances—treating pain while taking reasonable steps to prevent abuse and diversion. By integrating legal/regulatory principles with clinical guidelines through the creation and implementation of compliance and risk management policies, the pain clinician can minimize the potential for legal exposure. A good faith effort to comply with legal/regulatory directives and policies, together with clinical guidelines, may not stop a lawsuit but can certainly help determine its outcome and, most importantly, preserve patient access to quality medical care.

REFERENCES

1. Promoting Pain Relief and Preventing Abuse of Pain Medications: A Critical Balancing Act, A Joint Statement from 21 Health Organizations and the Drug Enforcement Administration, October 23, 2001. Available at: http://www.painpolicy.wisc.edu/dea01.htm.
2. National Prescription Drug Threat Assessment 2009, National Drug Intelligence Center, Drug Enforcement Administration. Available at: http://www.usdoj.gov/ndic/pubs33/33775/33775p.pdf. "Among the general population, nonmedical use of controlled prescription drugs was stable from 2003–2007, with 7 million Americans, aged 12 and older, reporting past month nonmedical use of prescription drugs. Pain relievers are the most widely diverted and abused, with one in five new drug abusers initiating with potent narcotics. Diversion and abuse of controlled prescription drugs cost public and private medical insurers an estimated $72.5 billion per year."
3. National Prescription Drug Threat Assessment 2009, National Drug Intelligence Center, Drug Enforcement Administration. Available at: http://www.usdoj.gov/ndic/pubs33/33775/33775p.pdf.<CE: Ref. 4, Duplicate Refs. 5 and 6.>
4. The Food and Drug Administration Amendments Act of 2007 (FDAAA), Public Law 110-85, 110th Congress. Available at: http://frwebgate.access.gpo.gov/cgi-bin/getdoc.cgi?dbname = 110_cong_public_laws&docid = f:publ085.110.
5. See, for example, Jayam Krishna-Iyer, MD. Suspension of Registration; Granting of Renewal Application Subject to Condition, 2009; 74(3):459–464 (DEA); and Chou R, et al. Clinical guidelines for the use of chronic opioid therapy in chronic noncancer pain. J Pain 2009; 10(2):113–130. Available at: www.sciencedirect.com.
6. Chou R, et al. Clinical guidelines for the use of chronic opioid therapy in chronic noncancer pain. J Pain 2009; 10(2):113–130. Available at: www.sciencedirect.com.
7. U.S. Drug Enforcement Administration, Final Policy Statement on Dispensing Controlled Substances for the Treatment of Pain. Federal Register 2006; 71(172):52716–52723. Available at: http://wais.access.gpo.gov (DOCID:fr fr06se06–139).
8. U.S. Drug Enforcement Administration, Codified Controlled Substances Act of 1970. Available at: http://www.deadiversion.usdoj.gov/21cfr/21usc/21ibusct.htm.
9. www.deadiversion.usdoj.gov.
10. U.S. Drug Enforcement Administration, Practitioner's Manual: An Informational Outline of the Controlled Substances Act 2006 Edition. Available at: http://www.deadiversion.usdoj.gov/pubs/manuals/pract/index.html. Clinicians should keep a copy of this manual in their office and review it periodically to ensure compliance with federal legal requirements for registration and prescribing.
11. 21 CFR 1306.04.
12. Here, prosecuted means both administrative and criminal actions. The ultimate direction of any investigation and prosecution is subject to a careful analysis of facts and legal authority of the regulatory agency, in this case the U.S. Department of Justice (DOJ) through DEA, who has authority to pursue administrative and criminal actions against registrants. When criminal actions are pursued, federal prosecutors

evaluate the investigative value of the case and decide whether to present the matter for prosecution. DEA often works with other law enforcement agencies on criminal cases involving prescribing clinicians and dispensing pharmacists. In administrative matters, DEA uses its own attorneys and its diversion investigators to initiate enforcement actions against DEA registrants. To learn more about these matters, use the DEA Diversion website at www.deadiversion.usdoj.gov.

13. 21 CFR 1306.04(b). The rationale for this rule is tied to the federal requirement of a separate registration for each dispensing location, because dispensing of controlled substances requires a great deal more paperwork and security that the act of prescribing. Pain clinicians should review the federal and state laws relating to dispensing controlled substances out of the medical practice and discuss these matters with legal counsel. While it may be that dispensing controlled substances provides an additional income stream to the clinician and the convenience of on-sight medications for patients, many clinicians find themselves unprepared to handle the significant increase of paperwork and DEA scrutiny.

14. 21 CFR 1306.04(c). Once again, narcotic treatment centers involve a separate registration and additional regulatory hurdles for clinicians who work in them. It is important to note, however, that the Drug Abuse Treatment Act of 2000 (DATA 2000) provides for special registration of qualified clinicians to prescribe controlled substances in Schedules III, IV, and V for the treatment of opioid addiction (commonly known as X-Registration for the prescribing of buprenorphine for detoxification within the privacy of the medical practice). To read more about these matters, consult the DEA Diversion website www.deadiversion.usdoj.gov.

15. "Issued" means the date the controlled substance prescription is released to the ultimate user, whether by hand delivery or posting via U.S. mail. *Citation*: Section 1306.05(a) makes clear "[a] practitioner may sign a prescription in the same manner as he would sign a check or legal document (e.g., J.H. Smith or John H. Smith)." In other words, pre- or postdating a controlled substance prescription is prohibited. *Important note*: While the act of pre- or postdating a prescription is prohibited under federal law, the act of providing fill date instructions, including a delayed fill date for a Schedule II controlled substance, *is not prohibited*. See the comments for 21 CFR 1306.12, concerning the issuance of multiple prescriptions for Schedule II controlled substances. Remember too that clinicians should consult individual state laws on multiple Schedule II prescriptions, because some states prohibit this prescribing format.

16. 21 CFR 1306.05(a).

17. 21 CFR 1306.05(b). Here, the individual practitioner must use the special registration number provided to the hospital and ensure that the following information is contained on the controlled substance prescription: the physician stamped, typed, or hand-printed on it, as well as the signature of the physician.

18. 21 CFR 1306.12 and U.S. Drug Enforcement Administration, Final Rule on Issuance of Multiple Prescriptions for Schedule II Controlled Substances, November 17, 2007 (effective December 17, 2007). Federal Register 2007; 72(222):64921–64930. Available at: http://wais.access.gpo.gov (DOCID:fr19no07–2).

19. U.S. Drug Enforcement Administration, Final Rule on Issuance of Multiple Prescriptions for Schedule II Controlled Substances, November 17, 2007 (effective December 17, 2007). Federal Register 2007; 72(222):64921–64930. Available at: http://wais.access.gpo.gov (DOCID:fr19no07–2).

20. Prior to the DEA's publication of its Final Policy Statement, DEA published two preliminary statements in the Federal Register: (1) U.S. Drug Enforcement Administration, Interim Policy Statement on Dispensing Controlled Substances for the Treatment of Pain. Federal Register 2004; 69(220):67170–67172. Available at: http://wais.access.gpo.gov (DOCID:fr16no04–82); and (2) the U.S. Drug Enforcement Administration, Clarification of Existing Requirements Under the Controlled Substances Act for Prescribing Schedule II Controlled Substances. Federal Register 2005; 70(165):50408–50409. Available at: http://wais.access.gpo.gov (DOCID:fr26au05–139).

21. U.S. Drug Enforcement Administration, Interim Policy Statement on Dispensing Controlled Substances for the Treatment of Pain. Federal Register 2004; 69(220):67170–67172. Available at: http://wais.access.gpo.gov (DOCID:fr16no04–82).

22. U.S. Drug Enforcement Administration, Clarification of Existing Requirements Under the Controlled Substances Act for Prescribing Schedule II Controlled Substances. Federal Register 2005; 70(165):50408–50409. Available at: http://wais.access.gpo.gov (DOCID:fr26au05–139).

23. 21 CFR 1306.11.

24. Jayam Krishna-Iyer, MD. Suspension of Registration; Granting of Renewal Application Subject to Condition, 2009; 74(3):459–464 (DEA).

25. To date, those three states include DE, IL, and IN. There is a great deal of pressure on these states to adopt some form of pain policy to ensure basic guidance to clinicians practicing in DE, IL, and IN.

26. www.fsmb.org (home page).

27. Federation of State Medical Boards, Model Policy for the Use of Controlled Substances for the Treatment of Pain (May 2004). Available at: http://www.fsmb.org/pdf/2004_grpol_Controlled_Substances.pdf.

28. The APS-AAPM document acknowledges that many of its recommendations are based on "weak evidence," because of the lack of data and evidence-based medicine studies on the treatment of chronic pain with opioids. Unfortunately, however, because these professional organizations published these clinical guidelines and structured them as "clinical recommendations," every attorney involved in any level of litigation (administrative, civil, or criminal) will work through hired medical experts and use the directives and specific language of the APS-AAPM guideline to measure the propriety of a defendant-clinician's prescribing habits. Thus, it is critical that pain clinicians attempt to follow these recommendations in good faith, and document reasons for varying from them—especially when the health care system inhibits or prevents compliance as is often the case with specific measures such as urine drug testing, behavioral medicine referrals, and even alternative means of treatment.

29. Federation of State Medical Boards, Model Policy for the Use of Controlled Substances for the Treatment of Pain (May 2004). Available at: http://www.fsmb.org/pdf/2004_grpol_Controlled_Substances.pdf; Texas Medical Board Rules [chap 170]. Available at: http://www.tmb.state.tx.us/rules/rules/ bdrules.php.

30. Chou R, et al. Clinical guidelines for the use of chronic opioid therapy in chronic non-cancer pain. J Pain 2009; 10(2):113–130. Available at: www.sciencedirect.com. According to the guideline, "[t]his approach is justified by estimates of aberrant drug-related behaviors (see Appendix B, Glossary), drug abuse, or misuse in patients with CNCP, which range from 0% to 50%, depending on the population evaluated and methods used to define and identify these outcomes [internal citation omitted]. Risk stratification pertaining to outcomes associated with the abuse liability of opioids—misuse, abuse, addiction and diversion—is a vital but relatively undeveloped skill for many clinicians [internal citation omitted]."

31. There are several tools, several of which are referenced by the APS-AAPM COT guideline: "Tools that appear to have good content, face, and construct validity include the Screener and Opioid Assessment for Patients with Pain (SOAPP) Version 1 (Appendix 3), the revised SOAPP (SOAPP-R), the Opioid Risk Tool (ORT) (Appendix 4), and the Diagnosis, Intractability, Risk, Efficacy (DIRE) instrument (Appendix 5). DIRE is clinician-administered and is designed to assess potential efficacy as well as harms. The SOAPP Version 1, SOAPP-R and ORT are patient self-report questionnaires that assess risk of aberrant drug-related behaviors." Chou R, et al. Clinical guidelines for the use of chronic opioid therapy in chronic noncancer pain. J Pain 2009; 10(2):113–130. Available at: www.sciencedirect.com.

32. State example comes from Texas Medical Board Rules, Texas Admin. Code, Title 22, Part 9, chap 170. Available at: http://www.tmb.state.tx.us/rules/rules/bdrules.php.

33. American Medical Association, Informed Consent. Available at: http://www.ama-assn.org/ama/pub/physician-resources/legal-topics/patient-physician-relationship-topics/informed-consent.shtml.

34. It is very important for pain clinicians to check state pain rules/policies for guidance on the use of treatment agreements. Many states recommend/suggest the use of treatment agreements if there is to be long-term prescribing of controlled substances. Thus, while the FSMB's Model Policy ties the use of a treatment agreement to the patient's known risk of substance abuse, many state rules/policies tie the use of a treatment agreement to all patients who are placed on long-term controlled substance therapy (not just opioid therapy). This distinction may be critical in any legal evaluation of the pain clinician's prescribing practices.

35. From a risk management perspective, pain clinicians should encourage patients to fill all of their prescriptions—controlled or not—at a single pharmacy to better enable the pharmacist to evaluate potential drug–drug interactions, provide additional patient education, and communicate possible drug conflicts to the pain clinician. While this may prove difficult in today's health care system largely due to the popularity or even required use of mail order pharmacies, the pain clinician may validly argue that such a control measure minimizes risk to not only the individual patient, but also to other stakeholders involved in patient's health care, including the health plan.

36. The American Academy of Pain Medicine publishes a sample treatment agreement on its website www.painmed.org. While this agreement is written for long-term opioid therapy, it can easily be tailored to meet the requirements of most state rules/policies by changing opioid therapy to controlled substance therapy. Pain clinicians should check with local legal counsel to ensure compliance with state licensing board expectations and current standards of care.

37. Louisiana and New Jersey are two states with such requirements. Readers should contact their medical board for more information.

38. Periodic urinalysis is cited as a term in a treatment agreement that is designed to prevent abuse and diversion, as stated in the DEA's Final Policy Statement (September 2006). In addition, periodic urinalysis (in one fashion or another) has been cited as an important risk management tool in several federal criminal case opinions (along with supporting trial transcripts). See, for example, US v. Williams, 445 F.3d 1302 (11th Cir. 2006); US v. Merrill, No. 06–14076 (11th Cir. 1/17/2008) (11th Cir. 2008).

39. Medication counts are often referred to as "pill counts" and are not always an accurate measure of a patient's compliance because it is relatively easy for a patient to save enough medication to remain consistent with expected medication usage. Some "patients" will go as far as borrowing or purchasing enough medication to meet count expectations. In many ways, counting medication may seem silly, but it can prove helpful especially when a patient is using a controlled substance for "breakthrough" pain management. Check with your state licensing board to determine its position on the value of medication counts in pain management.

40. The APS-AAPM clinical guidelines state: "Because patient self-report may be unreliable for determining amount of opioid use, functionality, or aberrant drug-related behaviors (internal citations omitted), pill counts, urine drug screening, family member or caregiver interviews, and use of prescription monitoring program data can be useful supplements. Although evidence is lacking on the accuracy and effects on clinical outcomes of formal screening instruments for identification of aberrant drug-related behaviors, use of tools with strong content, face, and construct validity, such as the PADT (Appendix 8 and 9) (internal citations omitted), is recommended as an efficient method of assessment and documentation."

41. Chou R, et al. Clinical guidelines for the use of chronic opioid therapy in chronic noncancer pain. J Pain 2009; 10(2):113–130. Available at: www.sciencedirect.com; U.S. Drug Enforcement Administration, Final Policy Statement on Dispensing Controlled Substances for the Treatment of Pain. Federal Register 2006; 71(172):52716–52723. Available at: http://wais.access.gpo.gov (DOCID:fr fr06se06–139).

42. US v. Williams, 445 F.3d 1302 (11th Cir. 2006); US v. Merrill, No. 06–14076 (11th Cir. 1/17/2008) (11th Cir. 2008).

19 Antidepressant Medications

Gary W. Jay

Clinical Disease Area Expert-Pain, Pfizer, Inc., New London, Connecticut, U.S.A.

The purpose of this chapter is to discuss the use of antidepressant medications (ADMs) in terms of their use for pain/analgesia.

TRICYCLIC ANTIDEPRESSANTS

Tricyclic antidepressants (TCAs) include amitriptyline, nortriptyline, desipramine, imipramine, and doxepin (which are used most frequently). Their starting dose is between 10 and 50 mg at night. It is best to start low and increase slowly. Dosages with effectiveness for pain are typically between 25 and 150 mg at night (q.h.s.). The most typical indications include neuropathic pain, fibromyalgia, and, in general, any type of chronic pain.

These medications work via a blockade of the reuptake of both serotonin and norepinephrine. They should be used with caution in the elderly and in patients with cardiovascular disorders, urinary hesitancy, or history of seizures. TCAs are contraindicated in patients with a history of recent myocardial infarction, narrow angle glaucoma, or within 14 days of the use of a monoamine oxidase inhibitor (MAOI).

TCAs should be used with caution with selective serotonin reuptake inhibitors (SSRIs) (as they increase the risk of serotonin syndrome), anticholinergic medications, antiarrhythmics, clonidine, lithium, and tramadol (which has the same reuptake inhibition). These medications should not be used in combination with drugs that prolong the QTc interval, as this may increase the risk for cardiac arrhythmia.

The major adverse effects of TCAs are secondary to cholinergic/muscarinic receptor blockade, histaminergic blockade (H1, H2), as well as blockade of the dopaminergic system. The anticholinergic side effects predominate and can include blurred vision, xerostomia, sinus tachycardia, constipation, urinary retention, confusion, and memory dysfunction. Histaminergic blockade can induce sedation, weight gain, dizziness, and hypotension. It also potentiates the effects of other CNS depressants. Alpha-1 adrenergic blockade can be associated with postural hypotension and dizziness. Blockade of dopaminergic receptors can induce extrapyramidal syndrome, dystonia, akinesia, neuroleptic malignant syndrome, tardive dyskinesia, and endocrine changes. Tachycardia and prolonged PR and QRS intervals with membrane stabilization can occur. The QT interval can become prolonged (1, 2).

An electrocardiogram is recommended if there is a history of cardiac disease. Electrocardiogram changes such as QRS widening, PR and QT prolongation, and T wave flattening can be induced by these agents as noted. TCAs may have quinidine-like actions, consistent with their sodium channel–blocking effects, particularly in patients with underlying ischemic cardiac disease or arrhythmias (3). Because abrupt discontinuation of antidepressants may precipitate withdrawal symptoms, such as insomnia, restlessness, and vivid dreams, a gradual taper over 5 to 10 days is recommended. Occasional blood levels as well as complete blood count (CBC) and hepatic studies are recommended to monitor for organ toxicity.

The TCA medication of choice is amitriptyline, a sedating TCA. Like all of the tricyclics, it works in the synapse to decrease reuptake of serotonin and, depending on the individual medication, norepinephrine. Amitriptyline, unlike the other TCAs, also works to repair the damage in stage 4 sleep architecture. It is the most sedating tricyclic. The typical dosage is between 10 and 50 mg at night. The author has found it rare to need more than 20 or 30 mg at night.

Doxepin is also a frequently used tricyclic. Anticholinergic side effects such as sedation are reduced (but not by much) when compared to amitriptyline. It does not work on the sleep architecture. It is used at the same dosage levels as amitriptyline.

Notice that the tricyclics are not used in their antidepressant dosages, anywhere from 100 to 350 mg a day. Even though the doses are low, their effectiveness in the treatment of pain is there.

Amitriptyline is indicated for use in neuropathic pain, while nortriptyline is more often used with fibromyalgia (4, 5). However, the increased sedation of amitriptyline may be useful in the treatment of fibromyalgia patients, although it is not FDA approved for this indication.

TCAs such as amitriptyline, desipramine, and imipramine, for example, block the induction of long-term potentiation by inhibiting actions on n-methyl-D-aspartate (NMDA) receptors (6).

TCAs have been used for years for the management of neuropathic pain syndromes, including diabetic peripheral neuropathy, postherpetic neuralgia, and migraine headache (6–8). However, pain relief is often modest and accompanied by side effects. Controlled studies indicate that approximately one-third of patients will obtain more than 50% pain relief, one-third will have minor adverse reactions, and 4% will discontinue the antidepressant because of major side effects (9). Fortunately, some patients obtain excellent pain relief.

Because comparisons between TCAs have not shown great differences in efficacy (8, 9), the choice of which antidepressant to use often depends on the side effect profile of a given drug. For example, when a patient is having difficulty in sleeping because of pain, a more sedating drug, such as amitriptyline, may be indicated. On the other hand, desipramine, which is less sedating, may be better tolerated in elderly patients.

TCAs have the lowest number needed to treat (NNT—the number of patients that need to be treated to achieve a 50% decrement in pain in one patient). The NNT for TCAs is 2.4 versus 6.7 for the SSRIs.

SELECTIVE SEROTONIN REUPTAKE INHIBITORS

The SSRIs include fluoxetine, paroxetine, and citalopram, escitalopram and sertraline, among others. These medications are not typically sedating, although for some patients they may be, and with the exclusion of those patients, they are energizing. They should be given in the morning. Fluoxetine and paroxetine should start at 10 to 20 mg a day and the dose can be increased to 60 to 80 mg. Sertraline should be given at 25 to 50 mg in the morning, up to 150 mg in divided doses. The doses should be divided, giving one when the patient gets up in the morning (around 7:00 AM) and one at noon. Patients should understand that taking these medications later than noon can, in many cases, give them problems sleeping.

The clinician can also safely combine 10 to 40 mg of fluoxetine or paroxetine, or 50 mg of sertraline given in the morning with a small dose of amitriptyline or doxepin (10–30 mg) at night. Inappropriate dosages of these two forms of medications can, rarely, induce the serotonin syndrome.

Compared with tricyclic agents, SSRIs for neuropathic pain have been relatively disappointing. In addition, they are more expensive than the older generic agents. Nonetheless, at relatively high doses (e.g., 60 mg), paroxetine is effective for diabetic neuropathy (10). Fluoxetine may also be useful in the treatment of rheumatic pain conditions, many of which have neuropathic components (11). SSRIs are better tolerated than TCAs and should be considered as first-line drugs in patients with concomitant depression. In this group, they may serve double duty.

SSRIs specifically blockade serotonin reuptake. They should be used cautiously in patients with a history of seizures. They should not be used in conjunction with MAOIs, as death has been reported (12).

There is an increased risk of the serotonin syndrome when SSRIs are combined with MAOIs, triptans, TCAs, bupropion, other SSRIs, buspirone, tramadol, and venlafaxine. Increased bleeding can be seen when used with warfarin (12).

The major side effects include nausea, diarrhea, anxiety, dyspepsia, diaphoresis, headache, insomnia, dizziness, tremor, nervousness, sedation, and sexual dysfunction.

SSRIs inhibit the CYP450 enzyme system and can cause delayed clearance of some medications, particularly those that use the CYP450 1A2 and 2D6 and 3A4 enzymes as metabolic substrates (1).

Norepinephrine–Serotonin Reuptake Inhibitors

These drugs include venlafaxine, duloxetine, and milnacipran. Venlafaxine can be started at 37.5 mg/day or b.i.d. and effective dosages are 150 to 300 mg/day. Duloxetine should be started at 20 mg b.i.d. and its effective dose is 60 mg/day. Milnacipran is used at dosages of 100 to 200 mg/day.

Venlafaxine is a novel phenylethylamine antidepressant that is chemically distinct from the older TCAs and the SSRIs. Although venlafaxine blocks serotonin and norepinephrine reuptake, its analgesic actions may be mediated by both an opioid mechanism and adrenergic effects (13). It appears to block serotonin reuptake at low dosages, and norepinephrine reuptake at high dosages, and dopamine at very high dosages (1). The drug may be at least as well tolerated as tricyclic agents and more effective for pain than standard doses of serotonin-selective drugs. Indeed, an initial report suggests that venlafaxine is effective for neuropathic pain (14). Venlafaxine should be started at one-half of a 37.5 mg tablet twice daily and titrated weekly to a maximum of 75 mg, taken twice a day. Nausea appears to be the most common side effect. An extended-release formulation of the drug was effective in relieving the pain associated with diabetic neuropathy. The NNT values for the higher dose of venlafaxine ER are comparable with those of the TCAs and gabapentin (15).

Venlafaxine has been used for the treatment of neuropathic pain (but is not FDA approved for this indication) (4).

It should be used with caution in hypertensive patients or patients with a history of seizures. It should be withdrawn slowly.

Venlafaxine has increased risk of serotonin syndrome when used with MAOIs, TCAs, SSRIs, tramadol, bupropion, and buspirone.

The most common adverse events include nausea, headache, nervousness, tremor, dry mouth somnolence, diaphoresis, constipation, and sexual dysfunction.

Duloxetine is a serotonergic and noradrenergic reuptake inhibitor with low affinity for other neurotransmitter systems. The most common adverse events are referable to the gastrointestinal and nervous systems. Duloxetine is primarily eliminated via the urine after significant hepatic metabolism via multiple oxidative pathways, methylation, and conjugation. The half-life is 12.1 hours. Duloxetine does cause inhibition of CYP 2D6. It should not be used in combination with nonselective MAOIs or CYP 1A2 inhibitors (16). It is effective for major depressive disorders as well as for the treatment of diabetic peripheral neuropathic pain (17–19).

Several double-blind, randomized, multicenter trails comparing duloxetine with placebo for the treatment of diabetic peripheral neuropathy have been done. In one, patients received duloxetine 60 mg daily, twice a day, or placebo. Duloxetine was superior to placebo in both dosages; discontinuations secondary to adverse events were more frequent in the duloxetine 60 mg/b.i.d. group (20).

In the second, a 12-week double-blind, placebo-controlled study in types 1 and 2 diabetics with peripheral diabetic neuropathy (PDN), both 60 and 120 mg/day dosages demonstrated statistically significant improvement in pain compared to placebo (21).

Duloxetine has also been found to be an effective and safe treatment for many symptoms associated with fibromyalgia in subjects with or without a major depressive disorder, particularly for women, who had the best outcomes, with significant improvement over most outcome measures (18, 22, 23).

Duloxetine is FDA approved for the treatment of neuropathic pain, fibromyalgia, and diabetic neuropathic pain.

Milnacipran, a new norepinephrine serotonin reuptake inhibitor, was approved in January 2009 for the treatment of fibromyalgia. This norepinephrine serotonin reuptake inhibitor preferentially blocks the reuptake of norepinephrine with higher potency than serotonin. Other than published studies, there is no clinical experience with this drug in the United States. The drug has been used in Europe, Asia, and Australia under the name Ixel. Milnacipran is said to block both serotonin and norepinephrine equally. Side effects include itching, sweating and chills, vertigo, headache, gastrointestinal complaints, orthostatic dizziness, depression, lethargy, hot flashes, and difficulty urinating. An exacerbation of hypertension can be seen at higher dosages (24, 25).

Norepinephrine–Dopamine Reuptake Inhibitor

Bupropion can be used as an antidepressant or for nicotine withdrawal. Dosages range, initially, from 75 to 150 mg/day to a maximum of 300 mg/day. It has been noted to help with neuropathic pain, but is not approved by the FDA for this indication (26).

The drug works by blockading the reuptake of norepinephrine and dopamine. It should not be used in patients with seizure disorders, anorexia, bulimia, or within 14 days of the use of MAOIs. Its toxicity is increased by levodopa and amantadine; there is an increased risk of seizure with agents that lower the seizure threshold. Common side effects include agitation, tremor, insomnia, nausea, headache, xerostomia, somnolence, hypertension, and tachycardia (12).

Atypical Antidepressants
Mirtazapine is an atypical ADM, described as a noradrenergic serotonin-specific antagonist. The drug facilitates enhanced noradrenergic and serotonergic output, which induces analgesia (1).

There are no reported problems with sexual dysfunction with this drug, and there is also a decrease in migraine headache as well as anxiety, agitation, depression, and insomnia (27–29).

BLACK BOX WARNING
Starting in 2004 the FDA requested a black box warning that children and adolescents taking antidepressants had an increased risk of suicide. In 2007, this warning was increased to include older patients and it reads, in part, "Antidepressants increased the risk compared to placebo of suicidal thinking and behavior (suicidality) in children, adolescents and young adults in short-term studies of major depressive disorder (MDD) and other psychiatric disorders." There did not appear to be a reported risk of suicide in adults over the age of 24.

This information should be kept in mind when prescribing antidepressants for pain or depression in the noted age groups, men and women up to the age of 24.

REFERENCES
1. Barkin RL, Barkin D. Pharmacologic management of acute and chronic pain: focus on drug interactions and patient-specific pharmacotherapeutic selection. South Med J 2001; 94(8):756–770.
2. Barkin RL, Fawcett J, Barkin S. Chronic pain management with a focus on the roll of newer antidepressants and centrally acting agents. In: Weiner RS, ed. Pain Management: A Practical Guide for Clinicians. 6th ed. New York, NY: CRC Press, 2002:415–434.
3. Glassman A, Roose S, Bigger J. The safety of tricyclic antidepressants in cardiac patients. Risk–benefit reconsidered. JAMA 1993; 269:2673–2677.
4. Sindrup SH, Otto M, Finnerup NB, et al. Antidepressants in the treatment of neuropathic pain. Basic Clin Pharmacol Toxicol 2005; 96(6):399–409.
5. Goldenberg DL, Burckhardt C, Crofford L. Management of fibromyalgia syndrome. JAMA 2004; 292(19):2388–2395.
6. Mico JA, Ardid D, Berrocoso E, et al. Antidepressants and pain. Trends Pharmacol Sci 2006; 27(7):348–354.
7. McQuay HJ, Tramer M, Nye BA, et al. A systematic review of antidepressants in neuropathic pain. Pain 1996; 68:217–227.
8. Max M. Antidepressants as analgesics. In: Fields HL, Liebskind JC, eds. Pharmacological Approaches to the Treatment of Chronic Pain: New Concepts and Critical Issues. Progress in Pain Research and Management. Vol 1. Seattle, WA: IASP Press, 1994:229–246.
9. Onghena P, van Houdenhove B. Antidepressant-induced analgesia in chronic nonmalignant pain: a meta-analysis of 39 placebo controlled studies. Pain 1992; 49:205–220.

10. Sobotka JL, Alexander B, Cook BL. A review of carbamazepine's hematologic reactions and monitoring recommendations. DICP 1990; 24:1214–1219.

11. Rani PU, Naidu MUR, Prasad VBN, et al. An evaluation of antidepressants in rheumatic pain conditions. Anesth Analg 1996; 83:371–375.

12. Lussier D, Beaulieu P, Fishbain D, et al. 2009 Overview of analgesic agents. Pain Medicine News Special Edition. December 2008:27–50.

13. Siegfried J. Long term results of electrical stimulation in the treatment of pain my means of implanted electrodes. In: Rizzi C, Visentin TA, eds. Pain Therapy. Amsterdam, The Netherlands: Elsevier, 1983:463–475.

14. Galer BS. Neuropathic pain of peripheral origin: advances in pharmacologic treatment. Neurology 1995; 45(suppl 9):S17–S25.

15. Rowbotham MC, Goli V, Kunz NR,et al. Venlafaxine extended release in the treatment of painful diabetic neuropathy: a double-blind, placebo controlled study. Pain 2004; 110(3):697–706.

16. Wernicke JF, Gahimer J, Yalcin I, et al. Safety and adverse event profile of duloxetine. Expert Opin Drug Saf 2005; 4(6):987–993.

17. Kirwin JL, Goren JL. Duloxetine: a dual serotonin–norepinephrine reuptake inhibitor for treatment of major depressive disorder. Pharmacotherapy 2005; 25(3):396–410.

18. Maizels M, McCarberg B. Antidepressants and antiepileptic drugs for chronic noncancer pain. Am Fam Physician 2005; 71(3):483–490.

19. Duloxetine (Cymbalta) for diabetic neuropathic pain. Med Lett Drugs Ther 2005; 47(1215/1216):67–68.

20. Raskin J, Pritchett YL, Wang F, et al. A double-blind, randomized multicenter trial comparing duloxetine with placebo in the management of diabetic peripheral neuropathic pain. Pain Med 2005; 6(5):346–356.

21. Goldstein DJ, Lu Y, Detke MJ, et al. Duloxetine vs. placebo in patients with painful diabetic neuropathy. Pain 2005; 116(1/2):109–118.

22. Arnold LM, Lu Y, Crofford LJ, et al. A double-blind, multicenter trial comparing duloxetine with placebo in the treatment of fibromyalgia patients with or without major depressive disorder. Arthritis Rheum 2004; 50(9):2974–2984.

23. Offenbaecher M, Ackenheil M. Current trends in neuropathic pain treatments with special reference to fibromyalgia. CNS Spectr 2005; 10(4):285–297.

24. Development of milnacipran for fibromyalgia hits a snag. Medscape Medical News. October 2005. Available at: medscape.com/viewarticle/538358. Accessed February 22, 2009.

25. Gendreau RM, Thorn MD, Gendreau JF, et al. Efficacy of milnacipran in patients with fibromyalgia. J Rheumatol 2005; 32:1975–1985.

26. Semenchuk MR, Sherman S, Davis B. Double-blind, randomized trial of bupropion SR for the treatment of neuropathic pain. Neurology 2001; 57(9):1583–1588.

27. Barkin RL, Chor PN, Braun BG, et al. A trilogy case review highlighting the clinical and pharmacologic applications of mirtazapine in reducing polypharmacy for anxiety, agitation, insomnia, depression and sexual dysfunction. J Clin Psychiatry 1999; 1:172–175.

28. Fawcett J, Barkin RL. Review of the results from clinical studies on the efficacy, safety and tolerability of mirtazapine for the treatment of patients with major depression. J Affect Disord 1998; 51:267–285.

29. Braverman B, O'Connor C, Barkin RL. Pharmacology, physiology and anesthetic management of antidepressants. In: Pharmacology and Physiology in Anesthesia. Philadelphia, PA: Lippincott Health Care Publications, 1993:1–15.

20 Anticonvulsant Medications

Gary W. Jay

Clinical Disease Area Expert-Pain, Pfizer, Inc., New London, Connecticut, U.S.A.

While the most common treatments for nociceptive pain include anti-inflammatory and opioid medications, anticonvulsant medications (ACMs) are first-line drugs for neuropathic pain. Both older (conventional) and newer ACMs may be used in patients with neuropathic pain, migraine, essential tremor, spasticity, restless legs syndrome, and several psychiatric disorders including bipolar disorder and schizophrenia (1, 2).

Food and Drug Administration (FDA)-approved ACMs and ADMs and a patch for neuropathic pain and fibromyalgia include the following:

- Carbamazepine: trigeminal neuralgia
- Duloxetine
  - peripheral diabetic neuropathy
  - fibromyalgia
- Gabapentin: postherpetic neuralgia
- Lidocaine Patch 5%: postherpetic neuralgia
- Pregabalin
  - peripheral diabetic neuropathy
  - postherpetic neuralgia
  - fibromyalgia
- Milnacipran: fibromyalgia

There is not a great deal of knowledge regarding the mechanism of action of most ACMs. Of note here are the multiple proposed mechanisms of action of multiple drugs, indicative of the uncertainty of the MOA (3).

- Sodium current blockade: carbamazepine, oxcarbazepine, lamotrigine, valproic acid, phenytoin, topiramate, zonisamide
- Calcium current blockade: gabapentin, pregabalin, carbamazepine, oxcarbazepine, zonisamide
- Increased GABA: topiramate, valproic acid, clonazepam, tiagabine
- Gabapentinoids: gabapentin, pregabalin—bind to the $\alpha_2\delta$ subunit of calcium channel; block calcium influx, prevent presynaptic release of neurotransmitters
- Reduced excitatory amino acids (i.e., glutamate): topiramate, lamotrigine, phenytoin, pregabalin, gabapentin
- Unknown: levetiracetam

When using ACMs, there are some clinical actions which may maximize their effectiveness, or appropriate patient use:

1. Always start low and go slow when titrating an ACM.
2. Understand the pharmacokinetics as well as the mechanistic differences between the ACMs.
3. In treatment-resistant patients (poor effectiveness), it is useful to combine two ACMs, if necessary, but be certain to use drugs with different modes of action.
4. All too frequently a patient will state that he or she has tried and failed an ACM, or many of them. Be certain to find out exactly what happened. Most commonly, a patient took a very low dose of an ACM for a very short period of time (less than that would be necessary to develop a steady state with clinical efficacy) and claimed lack of effectiveness, at which point, instead of insisting that the titration be continued appropriately, a different ACM is used, and the same problems persist. If an ACM is not titrated appropriately, the drug was really not used, as clinically there would not have been any effectiveness. Stopping a drug secondary to adverse effects is absolutely appropriate.
5. Push the ACM dosages until you see clinical effectiveness or you have to stop it secondary to side effects.
6. In many patients, maximal effectiveness (in the treatment of neuropathic pain) is found with ACMs given at 50% to 100% of their antiepileptic dosages. This does not hold true for the FDA-approved ACMs, which were approved at specific dosages for the treatment of neuropathic pain.

As a form of multimodal analgesia, oral gabapentin as well as pregabalin has been used perioperatively for adjunctive management of postoperative pain, as a supplement to opioids and other analgesics (4, 5).

The most commonly used ACMs and their typical doses include the following:

Name	Half-life (hr)	Dosing (mg/day)/regimen
Carbamazepine (Tegretol)	10–20	400–1200 mg/t.i.d.
Gabapentin (Neurontin)	5–9	1200–3600 mg/t.i.d.
Phenytoin (Dilantin)	12–36	300–600 mg/t.i.d. (q.h.s-nongeneric)
Oxcarbazepine (Trileptal)	8–10	300–1800 mg/b.i.d.
Topiramate (Topamax)	18–30	50–400 mg/b.i.d. or q.h.s
Lamotrigine (Lamictal)	15–30	50–300 mg/b.i.d.
Valproate (Depakote)	6–16	500–1500 mg/t.i.d.
Clonazepam (Klonopin)	18–50	0.5–6.0 mg/q.h.s.
Levetiracetam (Keppra)	6–8	1000–2000 mg/b.i.d.
Zonisamide (Zonegran)	25–60	100–400 mg/q.h.s
Tiagabine	5–10	12–44 mg/t.i.d.
Pregabalin (Lyrica)	5–6.5	75–300 mg/day

Anticonvulsants are useful for trigeminal neuralgia, postherpetic neuralgia, diabetic neuropathy, as well as central pain (6, 7). Although anticonvulsants have traditionally been thought of as most useful for lancinating pain, they may also relieve burning dysesthesias. Chemically, anticonvulsants are a diverse group of drugs, are typically highly protein bound, and undergo extensive hepatic metabolism.

Carbamazepine has a long history of use for neuropathic pain, particularly trigeminal neuralgia. Carbamazepine is chemically related to the tricyclic antidepressant imipramine, has a slow and erratic absorption, and may produce numerous side effects, including sedation, nausea, vomiting, and hepatic enzyme induction. In 10% of patients, transient leukopenia and thrombocytopenia may occur, and in 2% of patients hematologic changes can be persistent, requiring stopping the drug (8–10). Aplastic anemia is the most severe complication associated with carbamazepine, which may occur in 1:200,000 patients. Although requirements for hematologic monitoring remain debatable, a complete blood cell count, hepatic enzymes, blood urea nitrogen (BUN), and creatinine are recommended at baseline; and these are checked again at 2, 4, and 6 weeks, and every 6 months thereafter. Carbamazepine levels should be drawn every 6 months and after changing the dose to monitor for toxic levels and verify that the drug is within the therapeutic range (4–12 mg/cc). Patients with low pretreatment white blood cell counts are at increased risk of developing leukopenia (WBC < 3000/mm^3). Because toxicity is entirely unpredictable, it is important to instruct patients to recognize clinical signs and symptoms of hematologic toxicity, such as infections, fatigue, ecchymosis, and abnormal bleeding, and to notify the physician if they develop. Check hepatic enzymes and CBC routinely to rule out (possibly aplastic) anemia and hepatic dysfunction. Also, check the patient's ECG, if one has not been done recently; do one to look for arrhythmias and evaluate the QT interval. To improve compliance, carbamazepine should be started at a low dose (e.g., 50 mg twice daily) and increased over several weeks to a therapeutic level (200–300 mg typically three times a day).

Oxcarbazepine is an analog of carbamazepine, but typically is not associated with blood dyscrasias, nor hepatic insult.

Phenytoin also has well-known sodium channel-blocking effects and is useful for neuropathic pain (11). However, it is less effective than carbamazepine for trigeminal neuralgia (12). We have also noted that neuropathic pain caused by structural lesions causing nerve or root compression can paradoxically increase when phenytoin is administered. Phenytoin has a slow and variable oral absorption, some of which is dependent upon GI motility and transit time. Toxicity includes CNS effects and cardiac conduction abnormalities. Side effects are common and include hirsutism, gastrointestinal and hematologic effects, and gingival hyperplasia (13). Allergies to phenytoin are common, and may involve skin, liver, and bone marrow. Phenytoin doses in the range of 100 mg twice or three times a day may be helpful for neuropathic pain; therapeutic blood levels are in the range of 10 to 20 mg/ml. There are numerous potential drug interactions, including induction of cytochrome P450 enzymes, which may accelerate the metabolism of other drugs. Because of side effects and toxicity, phenytoin is not a first-line drug for neuropathic pain.

Valproic acid appears to interact with sodium channels but may also increase GABA metabolism. The principal nonantiepileptic, FDA-approved, use of valproic acid is for the prophylaxis of migraine headache (14). Potential toxicity includes hepatic injury and thrombocytopenia, particularly in children on multiple antiepileptic medications, although valproic acid is generally considered safe for adults.

Divalproex sodium is better tolerated than valproic acid. The recommended starting dose is 250 mg twice daily, although some patients may benefit from doses up to 1000 mg/day. As a prophylactic drug, valproic acid can reduce the frequency of migraine attacks by about 50% (14). Although there is little published information on the efficacy of valproic acid for neuropathic pain syndromes, based on its mechanism of action it may be useful alone or in combination with other adjuvant drugs. The drug may be associated with weight gain, pancreatitis, and hepatic injury as well as hair loss. A "fetal valproate syndrome" exists, so it should not be used in pregnant women.

Clonazepam may be useful for radiculopathic pain and neuropathic pain of a lancinating character. Clonazepam enhances dorsal horn inhibition by a GABAergic mechanism. The drug has a long half-life (18–50 hours), which reduces the risk of inducing an abstinence syndrome on abrupt withdrawal. The major side effects of clonazepam include sedation and cognitive dysfunction, especially in the elderly. Although the risk of organ toxicity is minimal, some clinicians recommend periodic complete blood count (CBC) and liver function tests for monitoring. Starting doses of 0.5 to 1.0 mg at bedtime are appropriate to reduce the incidence of daytime sedation.

Topiramate was found to be identical to placebo in three placebo controlled trials for painful diabetic neuropathy, while a fourth, independent placebo-controlled trial used different methods to assess topiramate efficacy and tolerability. It was found that in this one study, topiramate monotherapy reduced pain and body weight more effectively than placebo (15). The drug may be associated with weight loss and cognitive dysfunction. Topiramate was approved for migraine prophylaxis by the FDA in 2004.

Gabapentin is a popular anticonvulsant for neuropathic pain. Gabapentin was approved for use in the United States in 1993, as an adjunctive treatment of adults with partial epilepsy. Almost immediately after its release, physicians began to use gabapentin for various neuropathic pain disorders, such as diabetic peripheral neuropathy and postherpetic neuralgia. The structural similarity of gabapentin to GABA suggested that the drug might be useful for neuropathic pain. Although tricyclic antidepressants have been proven clinically effective for neuropathic pain for years, they often fail to provide adequate pain relief or cause unacceptable side effects. Therefore, when gabapentin became available, its benign side effect profile quickly made it very popular among physicians. Although initial enthusiasm for the drug was based largely on word of mouth, anecdotal published reports, discussions at clinical meetings and animal studies have substantiated the efficacy of gabapentin in various types of neuropathic pain. Over time, a growing consensus concerning the usefulness of gabapentin has emerged supported by well-controlled clinical trials.

It is clear that gabapentin is not a direct GABA agonist, although indirect effects on GABA metabolism or action may occur. A leading hypothesis suggested that gabapentin interacts with a novel receptor on a voltage-activated calcium channel (16). Research has shown that it interacts with the $\alpha2\delta$ subunit on the voltage-gated calcium channel (17). The inhibition of voltage-gated sodium channel activity (such as that occurs with classical anticonvulsants, e.g., phenytoin and carbamazepine) and amino acid transport, which alters neurotransmitter synthesis, may also occur. Although gabapentin is not an NMDA antagonist, there is evidence that gabapentin interacts with the glycine site on the NMDA receptor (18).

Ligation of rat spinal nerves L5 and L6 (the Chung model) produces characteristic pain behaviors, including allodynia, which are typical of neuropathic pain. Chapman et al. (19) demonstrated that gabapentin reduces pain in the Chung model. Gabapentin appears to act primarily in the CNS, in contrast to amitriptyline, which seems to act centrally and peripherally (20). Gabapentin also is effective in reducing pain behavior in phase 2 of the formalin test, a model of central sensitization and neuropathic pain (21). Gabapentin reduces spinally mediated hyperalgesia seen after sustained nociceptive afferent input caused by peripheral tissue injury. Gabapentin also enhances spinal morphine analgesia in the rat tail-flick test, a laboratory model of nociceptive pain (21).

Gabapentin is effective in reducing painful dysesthesias and improving quality-of-life scores in patients with painful diabetic peripheral neuropathy (23). Of patients randomized to receive gabapentin, 56% achieved a daily dosage of 3600 mg divided into three doses per day. The average magnitude of the analgesic response was modest, with a 24% reduction in intensity at the completion of the study compared with controls. Side effects were common. Dizziness and somnolence occurred in about 25% of patients, and confusion occurred in 8% of patients.

Morello et al. (24) compared gabapentin with amitriptyline for diabetic neuropathy and found both equally effective. However, the number needed to treat (NNT) for the tricyclic antidepressants is 2.5 and 4.2 for gabapentin (25–27).

Postherpetic neuralgia (PHN) is another difficult neuropathic syndrome. PHN affects approximately 10% to 15% of patients who develop herpes zoster, and is a particularly painful syndrome associated with lancinating pain and burning dysesthesias. The incidence of PHN is age related, with up to 50% of patients older than 60 years developing persistent pain after a bout of herpes zoster. Pain relief usually requires pharmacological therapy. Unfortunately, most medications are not very effective. For example, only about one-half of patients obtain adequate relief with antidepressants.

Rowbotham et al. (28) evaluated the efficacy of gabapentin for the treatment of PHN. Of patients taking gabapentin, 65% achieved a daily dosage of 3600 mg. Although the average magnitude of pain reduction with gabapentin was modest, with approximately a 30% reduction in pain compared with controls, statistically pain reduction was highly significant. In addition, gabapentin improved sleep parameters and quality-of-life scores. Adverse effects that occurred more commonly in the gabapentin group included somnolence (27%), dizziness (24%), ataxia, peripheral edema, and infection (7–10%). Based on the data of Rowbotham and colleagues, it was reasonable to consider gabapentin as first-line therapy for postherpetic neuralgia.

The FDA approved gabapentin for use in postherpetic neuralgia in 2002.

Gabapentin probably is at least as effective as antidepressants, with fewer contraindications. Gabapentin may be used as monotherapy or add-on/adjunctive treatment. Other possible adverse reactions include confusion, dizziness, and possible weight gain.

Gabapentin is generally well tolerated, even in the geriatric population, and has a safer side effect profile than tricyclic antidepressants. In the PHN study, the majority of patients were titrated to 3600 mg/day, and the median patient age was 73 years. The kidneys excrete gabapentin, and the dosage must be reduced for patients with renal insufficiency (29).

Pregabalin is also a GABA analog, with a similar structure and function to gabapentin. A new class of anticonvulsants was named the "Gabapentinoids" of which these two drugs are the first known for inclusion. Pregabalin (Lyrica) is indicated/approved for the treatment of neuropathic pain associated with both diabetic peripheral neuropathy and postherpetic neuralgia, adjunctive treatment of partial seizures, as well as fibromyalgia (see chap. 12) (30).

Pregabalin has negligible hepatic metabolism; it is not protein bound and has a plasma half-life of about six hours. Most of the oral dose (95%) is found unchanged in the urine. Peak plasma levels are found in about one hour post oral doses; oral bioavailability is greater than 90% (31).

The time to peak concentration is 1.5 hours, while a food effect increased this to 3 hours. A steady state is reached in one to two days. Pregabalin does not bind to plasma proteins. Mean half-life is 6.3 hours. It should be used in lesser dosages in patients with renal insufficiency, as it is metabolized renally (31, 32).

The most common adverse events seen in >10% of patients include dizziness, somnolence, peripheral edema, infection, and dry mouth (31, 32).

Pregabalin binds to the $\alpha 2\delta$ subunit protein of the voltage-gated calcium channels, like gabapentin, and reduces the release of excitatory neurotransmitters (e.g., glutamate, norepinephrine, serotonin, dopamine, and substance P) (33, 34).

Several randomized clinical trials show pregabalin to be superior to placebo in the treatment of neuropathic pain (PHN and DPN) at doses of 300 to 600 mg/day. Sleep was improved. Common adverse events included dizziness, peripheral edema, weight gain, and somnolence (35).

Randomized controlled studies of pregabalin in painful diabetic peripheral neuropathy were also done and showed the drug to be superior to placebo in doses of 300 to 600 mg/day. Improvements in sleep were also seen (36–38).

While many countries in the European Union have approved pregabalin, it was also evaluated for use in Canada for the treatment of peripheral neuropathic pain. The past treatment was reviewed. It was noted that the number of subjects with >50% reduction in pain increased when pregabalin was compared to placebo. Withdrawal due to adverse events was more frequent with pregabalin than placebo. The authors concluded that while pregabalin appeared effective in the treatment of peripheral neuropathic pain, no evidence was found that it offered advantages over the treatments currently being used in Canada (39).

Pregabalin was the first drug approved for use in fibromyalgia, based on two RCTs of approximately 1800 patients (40). The initial two studies considered of a 14-week study, with some patients showing reductions in pain during the first week. Approximately 70% of patients on a total daily dose of 300 mg/day of pregabalin, and 78% of those on a total daily dose of 450 mg/day experienced improvement on the patient global impression of change scale compared to 48% of those on placebo. The 600 mg/day dose was no more effective than the lower doses, and there was evidence of dose-related side effects (40).

The second trial, a six-month randomized withdrawal study, found that at the end of the double-blind phase, 61% of placebo patients had loss of therapeutic response to pregabalin, *versus* 90 (32%) of the pregabalin group, demonstrating the durability of effect for relieving FMS pain (41).

Other clinical cautions for other ADMs include the following:

- Lamotrigine—can be associated with Stevens–Johnson syndrome/toxic epidermal necrolysis; visual blurring with long-term use.
- Levetiracetam—caution if used with carbamazepine; may have typical GI and CNS side effects (nausea, ataxia, headache, dizziness, and sedation).
- Zonisamide—contraindicated in patients with sulfonamide hypersensitivity, can be associated with renal calculi.

SUICIDALITY AND ACMs

In July of 2008, the FDA had an advisory board which recommended against a black box warning regarding an increased risk of suicidal thoughts and behaviors. In December of 2008, the FDA announced that it would require makers of ACMs to add a warning to their drug labels, but not a black box warning, regarding this problem.

The FDA based their actions on the agency's meta-analysis of 199 clinical trials, with 43,000 subjects, of 11 ACMs being taken for multiple indications, which showed that patients taking antiepileptics had almost twice the suicidal behavior or thoughts when compared to a placebo group (0.37% vs. 0.22%) (42).

The Advisory Board did not dispute the FDA's findings.

The FDA stated that "all patients who are currently taking or starting on any antiepileptic drug for any indication should be monitored for notable changes in behavior that could indicate the emergence or worsening of suicidal thoughts or behavior or depression" (43).

REFERENCES

1. White PF. The changing role of non-opioid analgesic techniques in the management of postoperative pain. Anesth Analg 2005; 101(5 Suppl):S5–S22.
2. Mico JA, Ardid D, Berrocoso E, et al. Antidepressants and pain. Trends Pharmacol Sci 2006; 27(7):348–354.
3. Lussier D, Beaulieu P, Huskey A, et al. 2009 Overview of Analgesic Agents. Pain Medicine News Special Edition, December 2008:27–50.
4. Hurley RW, Cohen SP, Williams KA, et al. The analgesic effects of perioperative gabapentin on postoperative pain: a meta-analysis. Reg Anesth Pain Med 2006; 31(3):237–247.
5. Agarwal A, Gautam S, Gupta D, et al. Evaluation of a single preoperative dose of pregabalin for attenuation of postoperative pain after laparoscopic cholecystectomy. Br J Aneasth 2008; 101(5):700–704.
6. Swerdlow M. Anticonvulsants in the therapy of neuralgic pain. Pain Clin 1986; 1:9–19.
7. Hegarty A, Portenoy RK. Pharmacotherapy of neuropathic pain. Semin Neurol 1994; 14:213–224.
8. Hart RG, Easton JD. Carbamazepine and hematological monitoring. Ann Neurol 1982; 11:309–312.
9. Sotgiu ML, Lacerenza M, Marchettini P. Effect of systemic lidocaine on dorsal horn neuron hyperactivity following chronic peripheral nerve injury in rats. Somatosens Mot Res 1992; 9:227–233.

10. Vanderah TW, Gardell LR, Burgess SH, et al. Dynorphin promotes abnormal pain and spinal opioid antinociceptive tolerance. J Neurosci 2000; 20:7074–7079.

11. McCleane GJ. Intravenous infusion of phenytoin relieves neuropathic pain: a randomized double-blinded, placebo controlled, crossover study. Anesth Analg 1999; 89:985.

12. Blom S. Trigeminal neuralgia: its treatment with a new anticonvulsant drug G-32883. Lancet 1962; 1:839–840.

13. Brodie MJ, Dichter MA. Antiepileptic drugs. N Engl J Med 1996; 334:168–175.

14. Matthew NT, Saper JR, Silberstein SD, et al. Migraine prophylaxis with divalproex. Arch Neurol 1995; 52:281–286.

15. Raskin P, Donofrio PD, Rosenthal NR, et al. Topiramate vs. placebo in painful diabetic neuropathy: analgesic and metabolic effects. Neurology 2004; 63:865–873.

16. Chaplan SR. Neuropathic pain: role of voltage-dependent calcium channels. Reg Anesth Pain Med 2000; 25:283–285.

17. Gee NS, Brown JP, Dissanayake VU, et al. The novel anticonvulsant drug, gabapentin (Neurontin) binds to the alpha2delta subunit of a calcium channel. J Biol Chem 1996; 271:5768–5776.

18. Jun JH, Yaksh TL. The effect of intrathecal gabapentin and 3-isobutyl gamma-aminobutyric acid on the hyperalgesia observed after thermal injury in the rat. Anesth Analg 1998; 86:348–354.

19. Chapman V, Suzuki R, Chamarette HLC,et al. Effects of systemic carbamazepine and gabapentin on spinal neuronal responses in spinal nerve ligated rats. Pain 1998; 75:261–272.

20. Abdi S, Lee DH, Chung JM. The anti-allodynic effects of amitriptyline, gabapentin, and lidocaine in a rat model of neuropathic pain. Anesth Analg 1998; 87:1360–1366.

21. Shimoyama M, Shimoyama N, Inturrisi CE, et al. Gabapentin enhances the antinociceptive effects of spinal morphine in the rat tail-flick test. Pain 1997; 72:375–382.

22. Sindrup SH, Gram LF, Brosen K, et al. The selective serotonin reuptake inhibitor paroxetine is effective in the treatment of diabetic neuropathy symptoms. Pain 1990; 42:135–144.

23. Backonja MM, Beydoun A, Edwards KR, et al. Gabapentin for the symptomatic treatment of painful neuropathy in patients with diabetes mellitus. A randomized controlled trial. JAMA 1998; 280:1831–1836.

24. Morello CM, Leckband SG, Stoner CP, et al. Randomized double-blind study comparing the efficacy of gabapentin with amitriptyline on diabetic peripheral neuropathy. Arch Int Med 1999; 159:1931–1937.

25. Mattia C, Coluzzi F. Tramadol: focus on musculoskeletal and neuropathic pain. Minerva Anestesiol 2005; 71:565–584.

26. Sindrup SH, Jensen TS. Efficacy of pharmacological treatments of neuropathic pain: an update and effect related to mechanism of drug action. Pain 1999; 83:389–400.

27. Sindrup SH, Jensen TS. Pharmacological treatment of pain in polyneuropathy. Neurology 2000; 55:915–920.

28. Rowbotham M, Harden N, Stacey B, et al. Gabapentin for the treatment of postherpetic neuralgia. A randomized controlled trial. JAMA 280:1837–1842.

29. Beydoun A, Uthman BM, Sackellares JC. Gabapentin: pharmacokinetics, efficacy, and safety. Clin Neuropharmacol 1995; 18:469–481.

30. Zareba G. Pregabalin: a new agent for the treatment of neuropathic pain. Drugs Today Barc 2005; 41(8):509–516.

31. Pfizer Inc. Pregabalin (Lyrica) package insert. New York: Pfizer, 2006.

32. Pregabalin Monograph. National PBM Drug Monograph. May, 2007. VHA Pharmacy Benefits Management Strategic Healthcare Group and the Medical Advisory Panel. www.phm.va.gov/monograph/Pregabalin.pdf. Accessed February 27, 2009.

33. Dooley DJ, Taylor CP, Donevan S, et al. Ca^{2+} channel $\alpha 2\delta$ ligands: novel modulators of neurotransmission. Trends Phramacol Sci 2007; 28:75–82.

34. Freynhagen R, Stojek K, Griesing T, et al. Efficacy of pregabalin in neuropathic pain evaluated in a 12-week, randomized, double-blind, multicenter, placebo-controlled trial of flexible- and fixed-dose regimens. Pain 2005; 115(3):254–263.
35. Lesser H, Sharma U, LaMoreaux L, et al. Pregabalin relieves symptoms of painful diabetic neuropathy: a randomized controlled trial. Neurology 2004; 63(11):2104–2110.
36. Richter RW, Portenoy R, Sharma U, et al. Relief of painful diabetic peripheral neuropathy with pregabalin: a randomized, placebo-controlled trial. J Pain 2005; 6(4):253–260.
37. Frampton JE, Scott LJ. Pregabalin: in the treatment of painful diabetic peripheral neuropathy. Drugs 2004; 64(24):2813–2820.
38. Rosenstock J, Tuchman M, LaMoreaux L, et al. Pregabalin for the treatment of painful diabetic peripheral neuropathy: a double-blind, placebo controlled trial. Pain 2004; 110(3):628–638.
39. Hadj Tahar A. Pregabalin for peripheral neuropathic pain. Issues Emerg Health Technol 2005; 67:1–4.
40. Mechcatie, E. Pregabalin is first drug approved for fibromyalgia. Pain Medicine (Lyrica from Pfizer Inc.). Clinical Psychiatry News. International Medical News Group. 2007. *HighBeam Research.* http://www.highbeam.com. Accessed July 10, 2009.
41. Crofford JL, MEase PJ, Simpson SL, et al. Fibromyalgia relapse evaluation and efficacy for durability of meaningful relief (FREEDOM): a 6-month, double-blind, placebo-controlled trial with pregabalin. Pain 2008; 136(3):419–431.
42. Food and Drug Administration. Statistical review and evaluation: antiepileptic drugs and suicidality. www.fda.gov/ohrms/dockets/ac/o8/briefing/2008-4372b1-01-FDA.pdf. Accessed May 23, 2008.
43. Food and Drug Administration. Suicidal behavior and ideation and antiepileptic drugs. FDA Alert, Information for Healthcare Professionals, updated December 16, 2008. www.fda.gov/cder/drug/infopage/antiepileptics/default.htm. Accessed January 31, 2008.

21 Migraine Medications

Gary W. Jay

Clinical Disease Area Expert-Pain, Pfizer, Inc., New London, Connecticut, U.S.A.

The treatment of headache has been varied over the last four or five decades. The purpose of this chapter is to look at the FDA-approved medications for the abortive and prophylactic treatment of migraine and cluster headache.

Migraine is a chronic and apparently progressive disorder characterized by, for the most part, unilateral throbbing headache, aura (most commonly visual, but not always), and other associated symptoms (1,2).

The prevalence of migraine in US population studies is approximately 18% in women and 6% in men (3,4). Overall, migraine affects 12% of adults in occidental countries (4–6). An estimated 28 million Americans are thought to have migraine; this is only considered to be part, possibly half, of the total number of migraineurs (7).

The majority of migraineurs, 90% or more, have moderate-to-severe pain which is associated, in three-quarters of these patients, with a reduction in the ability to function during the ictal period (8).

The triptans, all selective serotonin receptor agonists, were the first major treatment breakthrough in abortive migraine treatment in decades, the first being approved in December of 1992 (injectable sumatriptan) (9).

The triptans are also significant because they target specific serotonin receptor subtypes, 1B and 1D. Ergots, the prior abortive that received the most use, were considered "dirty drugs" as they hit multiple receptors and multiple receptor subtypes.

The mechanism of action of the triptans is best understood when one has a good grasp of the current theories of the pain of migraine (3,10–16): (*i*) activation of the trigeminal nucleus caudalis, either a primary (first) event or secondary to cortical events, possibly including cortical spreading depression (spreading depression of Leaõ). Activation of this area increases the nociceptive ability at the time with a predisposition to pain, along with triggering several concurrent events. (*ii*) Dilation of intracranial blood vessels via CGRP and neurokinins stored within meningeal afferents, and activation of perivascular trigeminal afferent sensory nerves. (*iii*) A sterile inflammation, secondary to the release of proinflammatory neuropeptides released as an efferent function from the trigeminal sensory nerves. (*iv*) The activated trigeminal sensory nerves relay nociceptive impulses to second-order neurons within the trigeminal nuclei in the caudal brain stem as well as the upper cervical spinal cord (C1 and C2 along with the trigeminocervical complex). (*v*) Sensitization of the central trigeminal sensory neurons occurs. (*vi*) Transmission of nociceptive signals to third-order sensory neurons in the thalamus—via the quintothalamic tract and from there to higher cortical centers, registering the migrainous pain.

This information, more of which is understood now than in 1992, helped in the definition of the disorder, as well as acute and prophylactic treatments.

As they created the greatest paradigm shift in the field of headache medicine, we'll begin with the triptans.

THE TRIPTANS

There are seven triptans in the Headache Medicine Armamentarium. As noted above, they are serotonergic agonists that have two common sites of action: the vasoconstrictor 5-hydroxytryptamine (5-HT)$_{1B}$ receptors on the meningeal vasculature, with vasoconstrictive activity, and the 5-HT$_{1D}$ receptors on trigeminal nerve terminals both peripherally and centrally, which inhibit neurogenic inflammation (3,17).

Many are now recognized to also be 5-HT$_{1F}$ agonists (18). A stimulation of this receptor, in guinea pigs, blocks neurogenic plasma protein extravasation in the rat dura mater (19). These receptors are found in the trigeminal nucleus as well as the trigeminal ganglion, and 5-HT$_{1F}$ activation in the rat trigeminal nucleus is inhibitory in both cats and rats. These receptors are not vasoconstrictive (20–24).

As further background, recall that the heterogeneous serotonin receptors have been regrouped within seven different families: 5-HT1 to 5-HT7. All except 5-HT3 (a ligand-gated ion channel) are G-protein–coupled receptors (24).

The triptan pharmacokinetics (PK) is listed in Table 1. Table 2 notes triptan doses and the route of administration as well as migraine recurrence rate.

The triptans have been studied and have apparent issues with both agreement and disagreement; nonetheless, they are effective. The seven triptans are available in different formulations and have been studied individually as well as in head-to-head trials and have good supporting evidence. Table 1 shows that there are different pharmacological profiles for PK.

In terms of research, the triptans were the first drugs tested that looked at migraine headache pain after two hours.

Sumatriptan

Sumatriptan was the first triptan available and was approved in 1992, at that time it was available in a subcutaneous formulation. It was shown to be effective in 14 placebo-controlled trials (26). It was then approved as an oral tablet and then as a nasal spray. It is available in 15 other countries as a suppository.

The subcutaneous form of sumatriptan has the best PK profile, with a T_{max} of 10 minutes and 96% bioavailability. It was found to have a two-hour response rate of 76% (three of three attacks) and 48% of patients were pain free in 60 minutes (27).

The oral formulation had only 14% bioavailability, with a minimally effective dose of 25 mg. The highest dose of 100 mg was found to have more effectiveness when taken at the mild pain level in early migraine (28).

The sumatriptan nasal spray produces a faster onset of action than the tablet, but also a similar headache response at two hours (29). Patients either like the nasal spray for the earlier onset of effect or dislike it secondary to the nasal route of administration and bad taste, among other reasons (25).

As with all triptans, the doses used (Table 2) can be repeated in two hours if needed, with a maximum oral dose of 200 mg/day in the United States.

TABLE 1 Pharmacokinetics of the Triptans (3,25)

	T_{max} (hr)	Half-life (hr)	Bioavailability (%)	Lipophilicity	Metabolism
Sumatriptan		2		Low	Hepatic, MAO-A, 60% renal
50 mg tablet	2.5		14		
20 mg nasal	2		17		
6 mg SC	0.2		19		
Zolmitriptan				Moderate	Hepatic, Cyp-MAO-A
2.5 mg tablet	2	2.5–3.0	40–48		
2.5 mg ZMT (OTD)	3.3	2.5–3.0	40–48		
2.5 mg nasal	2	2.82	42		
Rizatriptan	1.2 tablet 1,6–2.5 ODT	2.0–3.0	45	Moderate	Hepatic MAO-A; renal excretion 30%
Naratriptan	2–3 tablet	2.0–3.0	63 (men) 74 (women)	High	Renal excretion 70%; CYP; not MAO-A
Almotriptan	1.4–3.8	3.2–3.7	80	Unknown	Hepatic; CYP/.MAO-A; renal excretion 35%
Eletriptan	1.0–2.0 tablet	3.6–5.5	50	High	Hepatic CYP3A4; not MAO-A
Frovatriptan	2.0–4.0 tablet	25	24–30	Low	Hepatic; CYP/MAO-A; renal excretion 35%

TABLE 2 Clinical Aspects of the Triptans (3,25)

Generic name	Brand name	Formulation	Doses (mg)	Maximum daily dose (mg)	Headache recurrence rate (%)
Sumatriptan	Imitrex	Tablets	25, 50, 100	200	32
		Nasal spray	5, 20	40	32–34
		SC injection	4, 6	12	34–38
Zolmitriptan	Zomig	Tablets	2.5, 5	10	30
	Zomig-ZNT	ODT	2.5, 5	10	30
	Zomig	Nasal spray	2.5, 10	10	30
Rizatriptan	Maxalt	Tablets	5, 10	30	30
	Maxalt-MLT	ODT	5, 10	30	30–47
Naratriptan	Amerge	Tablets	1, 2.5	5	17–28
Almotriptan	Axert	Tablets	6.25, 12.5	25	18
Frovatriptan	Frova	Tablets	2.5	7.5	25
Eletriptan	Relpax	Tablets	20, 40	80	19–23

Zolmitriptan

Zolmitriptan is more lipophilic than sumatriptan and is centrally active as it is more rapidly absorbed than sumatriptan (30). Four RCTs reviewed in the guidelines found both doses of zolmitriptan, 2.5 or 5 mg, significantly more effective than placebo (26). One trial looked at both doses, and found them to be essentially equivalent at two-hour efficacy (31). Three trials favorably compared zolmitriptan ODT (orally disintegrating tablet) to placebo (32–34), while two studies found efficacy rates for zolmitriptan 2.5 mg ODT *versus* oral were 59% for the 5 mg tablet and placebo rates of 22% and 30.6%, respectively (33,34).

One trial found zolmitriptan 2.5 mg had a similar two-hour efficacy as eletriptan 40 mg (35). When compared to sumatriptan, one trial found zolmitriptan 2.5 and 5 mg to be at least as effective as sumatriptan 50 mg, while another trial found them to more effective than either sumatriptan 25 or 50 mg (36,37).

Of interest is the fact that the absorption of zolmitriptan nasal spray has been demonstrated by PET scan (25).

Naratriptan

The third triptan to be introduced into the United States for the acute treatment of migraine, oral naratriptan was found to differ from sumatriptan with a much longer half-life (six hours) as well as a longer T_{max} of two hours and higher bioavailability (70%) (38).

Two class 1 RCTs, as reported in the guidelines, showed that naratriptan 1 and 2.5 mg was effective in achieving headache relief at four hours, but not two hours (26). In a comparative trial, the two-hour headache response rate for naratriptan 2.5 mg was higher than placebo (48.4% *vs.* 22.4%) but lower than rizatriptan 10 mg (68.7%; $p < 0.001$) (39).

Headache recurrence with naratriptan after four-hour headache response was low (17–28%) and when compared with sumatriptan and rizatriptan, naratriptan showed a lower recurrence rate (40). The need for rescue medication after one dose of naratriptan was low and found to be similar to dihydroergotamine (40).

Rizatriptan

A meta-analysis of four double-blind trials (RCTs) and a total of seven clinical trials noted to 1998, 41% of patients received pain relief at 1 hour, and 71% within 2 hours, with benefits above placebo found from 30 minutes in some patients. The study also found that while both rizatriptan 5 and 10 mg were effective when comparing the efficacy, the 10-mg dose was superior on most measures, making 10 mg the standard dose for most patients (41).

A rizatriptan ODT formulation was found to have a comparable efficacy to the tablets (42).

Almotriptan

Almotriptan is a $5\text{-}HT_{1B,1D,1F}$ agonist (43). It was not reviewed in the guidelines (26). Three RCTs have been published, with doses ranging from 2 to 25 mg, with the 12.5-mg dose in all three studies (44–46). Sumatriptan 100 mg was the active comparator in one of these trials and no differences were seen between zolmitriptan 12.5 and 25 mg (46).

Almotriptan appears to be superior to sumatriptan when tolerability is evaluated specifically with lower numbers of adverse events (AEs), such as chest pain which compared in one study (43,47,48). It must be noted that the chest pain symptoms are rarely cardiac in origin (25).

Eletriptan

While eletriptan has a relatively short T_{max} of 1 to 2 hours, it has a relatively long half-life of 3.6 to 5.5 hours.

Since the guidelines were published, eletriptan was tested in four class 1 RCTs in dosages of 20, 40, and 80 mg (49–52). The 80-mg dosage is not approved in the United States (3).

The studies showed a dose-related headache response at two hours, with eletriptan 20 mg having headache response between 47% and 54%; eletriptan 40 mg having responses between 62% and 65%, and eletriptan 80 mg having responses between 59% and 77% *versus* placebo responses from 19% to 24% at two hours. Eletriptan 40 mg was more effective than eletriptan 20 mg and had fewer side effects than the 80-mg dose (3).

One trial had a sumatriptan 100 mg comparator arm, and eletriptan 80 mg statistically separated over sumatriptan 100 ($p < 0.001$) in the primary end point (49).

Eletriptan inhibits the CYP3A4 enzymatic pathways and may therefore interact with other compounds that are metabolized by this P-450 system, as this could cause an increase in the eletriptan plasma levels (3,25,53). In the United States, it is recommended that eletriptan not be used within 72 hours of treatment with such medications. The medications in question would include macrolide antibiotics (e.g., erythromycin, clarithromycin), antifungals (e.g., fluconazole), and some antivirals (e.g., ritonavir and nelfinavir) (3,25). Pfizer evaluated these issues and noted, from two long-term studies, that the incidence of AEs was similar whether patients took CYP 3A4 inhibitors or not in the presence of eletriptan 40 or 80 mg (25). It was also noted that the concomitant use of CYP 3A4 inhibitors did not influence the incidence of reported AEs in these studies (53).

Frovatriptan

Three RCTs have been reported for frovatriptan utilizing dosages between 0.5 and 40 mg. While 2.5 mg dosages were statistically significant in achieving headache relief in 2 hours (38–40%) *versus* placebo (23–25%), with a $p < 0.05$, doses under 2.5 mg did not differentiate from placebo and doses between 5 and 40 mg demonstrated 38% and 48% headache response rates but did not show a clear dose–response curve. All doses of frovatriptan were superior to placebo at four hours (54,55). Two of the studies in question were reported by Rapaport et al. (54).

Of interest, grade B evidence-based medicine recommendations exist for the use of frovatriptan 2.5 mg twice daily for mini-prophylaxis of menstrual migraine (56,57).

Conclusions

Triptan tablets show, essentially, when broadly evaluated, a comparable efficacy (58). Sumatriptan, rizatriptan, almotriptan, and eletriptan all show a relatively rapid (30 minute) onset of action and good two-hour efficacy (58). Zolmitriptan shows a good 2-hour efficacy and a 45-minute onset of action (58). Naratriptan and frovatriptan show a two-hour onset of action and lower efficacy (two hours after administration) when compared to the other triptans in tablet form, but they do have the longest half-lives (58).

While the subcutaneous sumatriptan (the only SQ triptan formulation) has the fastest onset of action, the sumatriptan and zolmitriptan nasal sprays also have onsets of action that are faster than the oral tablets. See Table 1 for more information.

The most appropriate route of administration of a triptan during a migraine attack, secondary to gastrointestinal dysmotility may be a triptan injection, or in the EU, a suppository may be preferred (59).

Contraindications for triptans, generally, may include uncontrolled hypertension; a family history of coronary artery disease or myocardial infarction; history of stroke, history of myocardial infarction; risk factors for coronary artery disease, uncontrolled diabetes; and high cholesterol levels (9).

As triptans cause vascular constriction secondary to agonism of the 5-HT1B receptors, they can cause constriction of the coronary arteries, as well as an even greater effect on cranial arteries (threefold greater) (60,61).

There have been published reports of acute myocardial infarction with triptan use (62).

Migraine headache can be associated with endothelial dysfunction that can cause via inflammation and abnormal vascular reactivity, ischemic injury to the heart or brain, as well as an association with ST-segment and T-wave abnormalities on electrocardiogram during migraine attacks (63–65).

A Triptan Cardiovascular Safety Expert Panel was convened and concluded that triptan use did not correlate with an increase in the frequency of serious cardiovascular AEs in patients without known or suspected coronary artery disease (66).

The reliability of treatment response to triptans taken orally is surprisingly low (59). Oral therapy with a triptan provides pain relief in only some of the attacks, but the within-patient consistency of triptan response for three of three attacks has been found to occur in only about 40% of patients treated with an oral triptan (67). Within-patient response consistency is poor, with response rates in three of three attacks ranging from 32% to 50% (68).

Good responders, defined as those who responded to the last two migraine headaches with pain relief at two hours, were more likely to respond to treatment during the third attack in a better percentage of patients (58–81%) *versus* those who did not respond to the prior two headaches (69). The probability of a good response to an oral triptan in any individual migraine appears to be related to whether the individual responded to the same treatment on a previous migraine attack (67).

Cutaneous allodynia associated with migraine has been found to have a prevalence ranging from 30% to almost 90% (70). Migraineurs with aura have a higher prevalence of cutaneous allodynia than those with migraine without aura (71). It was found that approximately 50% of migraineurs develop cutaneous allodynia within an hour of migraine onset and approximately 75% within four hours (72). Most pertinent is that the response to treatment with a triptan was poorer after the development of cutaneous allodynia (73).

The key to appropriate treatment is to take the triptan as soon as possible, when migraine pain is just beginning, and within an hour of onset of symptoms. It is also important to note that the use of a mixed cyclooxygenase-1 and cyclooxygenase-2 inhibitor helps to suppress ongoing sensitization inducing allodynia in the central trigeminovascular neurons (74).

A combination medication, consisting of oral sumatriptan 85 mg and naproxen 500 mg has been approved by the FDA for the treatment of acute migraine headache, and may be beneficial in this regard (75,76).

OTHER MEDICATION TREATMENTS

The US Headache Consortium published recommendations for the treatment of migraine in 2000 (26). Under "Specific migraine treatments," it listed the triptans, and then ergot and its derivatives.

Ergotamine–caffeine (Cafergot) tablets remain helpful to those patients who are unresponsive to triptans. Ergotamine, unlike the triptans, has a much more promiscuous receptor profile, including serotonerigic, dopaminergic, and adrenergic receptors (77).

Dihydroergotamine-45 (DHE) can be used SQ, intramuscularly (IM), intravenously (IV) or intranasally (IN) for severe migraine attacks. It may be appropriate to also use an antiemetic. It should be contraindicated in patients with known cardiovascular and peripheral vascular disease (26).

NONSPECIFIC PHARMACOLOGICAL TREATMENT (26)

These medications include

1. Antiemetics
   a. Chlorpromazine (IV/IM)
   b. Prochlorperazine [IV/IM/per rectum (PR)]
   c. Metoclopramide (IV/IM/PR)
2. NSAIDS and nonnarcotic analgesics
   a. Ketorolac (IM/IV);
   b. Oral NSAIDS: aspirin, naproxen, diclofenac, ibuprofen, etc.—for mild migraine
3. Combination analgesics
   a. Aspirin, caffeine—for mild migraine
   b. Butalbital, aspirin, caffeine (inconsistent in migraine, also used for tension-type headache)
   c. Isometheptene mucate, acetaminophen, dichloralphenazone
4. Opiate analgesics—must be used with great reserve, for acute, severe attacks not responsive to abortive agents
   a. Butorphanol IN
   b. Acetaminophen with codeine, hydrocodone, hydromorphone
   c. Oral transmucosal fentanyl citrate
5. Nonopiate analgesics
   a. Tizanidine
   b. Tramadol
6. Miscellaneous medications
   a. Steroids
      i. Methylprednisolone dose pack
      ii. Dexamethasone
   b. Lidocaine IN (better for cluster HA)
   c. Valproaic acid (IV)
   d. Propfol (IV).

PREVENTATIVE MIGRAINE TREATMENT

US evidence-based guidelines for preventive treatment of migraine include (77)

1. Recurring migraine that significantly interferes with a patient's daily routine despite acute treatment (e.g., two or more attacks a month that produce disability that lasts three or more days, headache attacks that are infrequent but produce profound disability).
2. Failure or contraindication to or significant side effects from acute medications.
3. Overuse of acute medications.
4. Special circumstances, i.e., hemiplegic migraine or attacks that may lead to a permanent neurologic injury.
5. Frequent headaches (more than two a week) or a pattern of increasing attacks over time, associated with the risk of developing medication overuse headache (MOH).
6. Patient preference or the desire to have as few acute attacks as possible.

Migraine prophylactic medication (MPM) is used only infrequently, as only 13% of all diagnosed migraineurs use MPM (78). The American Migraine Prevalence and Prevention (AMPP) study noted that 38.8% of all migraine patients should be considered for MPM (13.1%) or offered MPM (25.7%) (79).

There are various types of medications that have been used as an MPM, but the FDA-approved medications for migraine prophylaxis are anticonvulsants (See chap. 20).

When using prophylactic medications, expect a wait: it may take up to three months or more to see a significant change in the number of migraine headaches, which, at the present time, appears to be a 50% reduction in the number of migraine headaches.

Anticonvulsants

Topiramate is approved by the FDA as an MPM. The dosage is typically 50 to 100 mg given twice a day. Start low and go slow—begin patients on 15 or 25 mg given at bedtime, and increase by the same dosages weekly. The most common AEs include paresthesia, fatigue, decreased appetite, nausea, diarrhea, weight decrease, taste perversion/changes, hypoesthesia, and abdominal pain. Common central nervous system (CNS) AEs include somnolence, insomnia, mood problems, anxiety, memory difficulty, language problems, and difficulty with concentration. There is a small incidence of renal calculi (80).

The efficacy and safety of topiramate was evaluated in two large, pivotal, multicenter RCTs (50, 100, and 200 mg/day) in migraine prevention. The first trial showed a responder rate (patients with $\geq$ 50% reduction in monthly migraine frequency) of 52% with topiramate 200 mg/day ($p < 0.001$); 54% with topiramate 100 mg/day ($p < 0.001$); and 35% with topiramate 50 mg/day ($p = 0.039$), as compared to placebo with 23% (81). The second pivotal trial demonstrated more patients with at least a 50% reduction in mean monthly migraines with all dosages of topiramate, and a response rate in a range of 39% to 49%. The response rate for the 200 mg/day dosage was 47% (82). The third RCT (83) compared the 100 mg/day and 200 mg/day dosages of topiramate, with placebo and propranolol (160 mg/day) arms. The 100 mg/day dosage of topiramate was superior to placebo (37% responder rate) when one looked at the reduction in the monthly migraine frequency, with an overall 50% responder rate, a reduction in monthly migraine days, and a reduction in the rate of daily rescue medication usage. The topiramate 100 mg/day and propranolol groups were similar with respect to reductions in the migraine frequency, responder rate, migraine days, and daily rescue medication usage. Topiramate 100 mg/day was better tolerated than the 200 mg/day dosage and was generally comparable to propranolol. Similar efficacy profiles were noted in the topiramate 100 mg/day and propranolol 160 mg/day groups.

Divalproex sodium (a combination of valproic acid and sodium valproate) was the first FDA-approved MPM. The dose to try to achieve is 500 to 1500 mg/day, starting at 250 to 500 mg/day and slowly increasing. Common AEs include nausea, vomiting, and gastrointestinal distress, but these AEs decrease over six months. Tremor and alopecia can occur. CNS effects are minor, including little effect on cognition and rare sedation. Other rare AEs include hepatitis and pancreatitis. Other AEs include hyperandrogenism, ovarian cysts, and weight gain. Contraindications include pregnancy and a history of pancreatitis or a hepatic disorder, thrombocytopenia, pancytopenia, and bleeding disorders. It is helpful to monitor serum levels (84–86).

There are a number of studies, supporting this medication, beginning with a RCT in 1992 which showed it to be effective in preventing migraine or reducing the frequency, and severity and duration of attacks in 86% of 29 patients. Their attacks were reduced from 15.6 to 8.8 a month (87). The second trial evaluated the medication in 43 patients in a triple-blind, crossover trial of the slow-release sodium valproate. In the valproate group, 50% of the patients had a reduction in the migraine frequency of 50% or less, compared with 18% for placebo (88). These results were further confirmed in other RCTs which found responder rates ranging between 43% and 48% and dosages which ranged from 500 to 1500 mg/day (88,89).

β-Adrenergic Blockers

Still widely used, they are also about 50% effective in producing a greater than 50% reduction in the attack frequency. Evidence has shown that propranolol, a nonselective β-blocker, is most consistent. The typical dose is 40 to 400/day. The short-acting form taken twice or three times a day can be used, as can the long-acting form, on a daily or twice daily basis. The significant AEs include drowsiness, fatigue, lethargy, sleep disorders, nightmares, depression, disturbances in memory, and hallucinations. Other AEs include GI complaints, decreased exercise tolerance, bradycardia, orthostatic hypotension, and impotence (7,77).

Propranolol, the most useful β-adrenergic blocker, has had its efficacy demonstrated numerous times (26,90–94).

Calcium Channel Antagonists

Verapamil, a phenylalkylamine, has been evaluated for prophylactic treatment of migraine. Three double-blind, placebo-controlled trials were done but they were very small: with 10 of 12 patients, 8 of 14 patients, and 20 of 23 patients showing improvement, and the 320 mg/day dosage better than the 240 mg/day dosage (95). On the other hand, multiple other authors indicated that verapamil may be useful in migraine prophylaxis (96–98).

The most common AEs include weight gain, somnolence, dry mouth, dizziness, hypotension, occasional extrapyramidal reactions, and depression (7).

It should be noted that flunarizine, widely used in the European Union, but not available in the United States, may be effective in migraine prophylaxis (99).

Antidepressant Medications

The only member of the class of tricyclic antidepressant (TCA) medications that has proven efficacy in migraine prophylaxis is amitriptyline (100,101). Amitriptyline, while helping with migraine, did not affect depression (102,103).

AEs from the antimuscarinic effects of the TCAs include dry mouth, constipation, dizziness, mental confusion, tachycardia, palpitations, blurred vision, urinary retention, and weight gain. Older patients may become confused or develop delirium. While amitriptyline and doxepin are sedating, they should be given at night, starting at 10 to 25 mg at night, with effective dosages being 25 to 200 mg/day. Nortriptyline, a secondary amine, with less sedation, can be used, staring at 10 to 25 mg at night, with dose ranges being 10 to 150 mg at bedtime. Protriptyline is another secondary amine that is more energizing and should be given in the morning, beginning with 5 mg/day, with the dose ranging from 5 to 60 mg/day.

There is no good evidence that any of the selective serotonin reuptake inhibitors (SSRIs) have efficacy in migraine prophylaxis (26).

Venlafaxine, a selective serotonin and norepinephrine reuptake inhibitor (SNRI) has been found to be effective in several open-label studies with instant release and controlled release formulations (104,105); venlafaxine was also found to be more effective than placebo in a RCT (106).

In a study comparing venlafaxine to amitriptyline, venlafaxine had a low number of AEs (nausea and vomiting in one patient) in a randomized, double-blind crossover study. Both medications were equally effective, with amitriptyline having more AEs and patient dropouts secondary to AEs (107).

The typical AEs for venlafaxine include insomnia, nervousness, mydriasis, and seizures. The possibility exists that the mixture of this medication with others can precipitate the serotonin syndrome (108).

Other Medications

Botulinum toxin type A (25 or 75U) has not convincingly been shown to be effective for the prophylaxis of migraine. An early placebo-controlled trial showed the 25U dose to be effective, with no efficacy at the higher dose (109).

A meta-analysis of eight randomized, double-blind, placebo-controlled trials evaluating the efficacy of the prophylaxis of migraine with botulinum toxin A found a high placebo effect and concluded that BotA was no better than placebo for the prophylactic treatment of episodic migraine, either clinically or statistically (110).

In a recent RCT, it was found that subjects treated with BotA demonstrated improvements from baseline as compared to placebo treatment, but the BotA-treated subjects did not differ from placebo-treated subjects in measures of headache frequency and severity (111).

Angiotensin-Converting Enzyme Inhibitors and Angiotensin II Receptor Agonists

Lisinopril, an angiotensin-converting enzyme inhibitor, was evaluated in a double-blind, placebo-controlled crossover trial in migraine prophylaxis at a dosage of 10 mg one (for one week) and two a day (for 11 weeks). There were 47 subjects, and hours with headache, days with headache, days with migraine, and the headache severity index were reduced by 20%, 17%, 21%, and 20% respectively as compared to placebo. Days with migraine were reduced by at least 50% in 14 participants *versus* placebo and 17 patients for active treatment *versus* the run-in period. It was concluded that lisinopril had a clinically important prophylactic effect on migraine (112).

An open-label study using lisinopril 5 mg/day was performed in 21 subjects. The authors found the attack frequency of migraine to be significantly reduced ($p < 0.0005$). Three patients dropped out because of intolerable cough (113).

Another group looked at the angiotensin II receptor blocker candesartan (16 mg/day) in a randomized, double-blind, placebo-controlled crossover study in 60 patients with migraine having two to six attacks a month. The mean number of headache days was 18.5 with placebo *versus* 13.6 days with candesartan ($p = 0.001$) in the intent-to-treat group. The number of drug responders (reduction of $\geq 50\%$ compared with placebo) was 18 (31.6%) of 57 patients for days with headache and 23 (40.4%) of 57 for days with migraine. It was felt that candesartan provided effective migraine prophylaxis and had a tolerability profile comparable to that of the placebo group (114).

Candesartan was given to eight hypertensive patients and reduced both the incidence and the severity of headache, with a reduction in the Migraine Disability Assessment score from 29.4 to 9 points. Blood pressure also decreased from 154.9/90.4 to 129.5/81.9. It was felt that candesartan was a unique but good choice for a migraine prophylactic agent in migraine complicated by hypertension (115).

Herbs and Vitamins

Feverfew (*Tanacetum parthenium*) has questionable effectiveness in migraine prophylaxis at 50 to 82 mg/day (116,117). Riboflavin (400 mg) was effective in one placebo-controlled double-blind trial, with greater than 50% of the patients responding (118). When high-dose riboflavin was used in a RCT for children (at 200 mg/day), there were no differences between riboflavin and placebo (119).

Butterbur root (*Petasites hybridus*) was used (75 mg administered twice daily) and separated from placebo in one study (120). A systematic review shows only moderate evidence of effectiveness for the prophylaxis of migraine (121).

Coenzyme Q10 was found to be efficacious and well tolerated in a RCT for migraine prophylaxis, given 100 mg three times a day (122).

CONCLUSION

In several articles, it was noted that the drugs of first choice for migraine prophylaxis include valproic acid and topiramate, amitriptyline (in the United States), β-blockers, and flunarizine (in the EU). Second-tier drugs, with less efficacy, or poorer evidence, included venlafaxine, gabapentin, naproxen, butterbur root, vitamin B(2), and magnesium (123,124). Propranolol and flunarizine were recommended for children (124).

In the relatively near future, one should not be surprised to see another paradigm shift in the treatment of migraine with calcitonin gene-related peptide (CGRP) used for aborting acute migraine (125,126).

REFERENCES

1. Headache Classification Committee of the International Headache Society. The International Classification of Headache Disorders. 2nd ed. Cephalalgia 2004; 24: 1–149.
2. Lipton RB, Bigal ME. The epidemiology of migraine. Am J Med 2005; 118(Suppl 1):3S–10S.
3. Bigal ME, Krymchantowski V, Hargreaves R. The triptans. Expert Rev Neurother 2009; 9(5):649–659.
4. Bigal ME, Lipton RB. The epidemiology, burden, and comorbidities of migraine. Neurol Clin 2009; 27(2):321–334.
5. Stovner I, Hagen K, Jensen R, et al. The global burden of headache: a documentation of headache prevalence and disability worldwide. Cephalalgia 2007; 27: 193–210.
6. Lipton RB, Diamond S, Reed M, et al. Migraine diagnosis and treatment: results from the American Migraine Study II. Headache 2001; 41:638–645.
7. Jay GW. The Headache Handbook: Diagnosis and Treatment. New York: CRC Press, 2000:17–32.
8. Edmeads J, Mackell JA. The economic impact of migraine: an analysis of direct and indirect costs. Headache 2002; 42:501–509.
9. http://headaches.about.com./cs/druginfo/a/triptan_over.htm?p = 1, updated May 28, 2006, content reviewed by the Medical Review Board, accessed July 3, 2009.
10. Messlinger K. Migraine: where and how does the pain generate? Exp Brain Res 2009; 196:179–193.
11. Bolay H, Moskowitz MA. The emerging importance of cortical spreading depression in migraine headache. Rev Neurol (Paris) 2005; 161(6–7):655–657.
12. Dalkkara T, Zervas NT, Moskowitz MA. From spreading depression to the trigeminovascular system. Neurol Sci 2006; 27(Suppl 2):S86–S90.
13. Moskowitz MA. Defining a pathway to discovery from bench to bedside: the trigeminovascular system and sensitization. Headache 2008; 48(5):688–690.
14. Moskowitz MA. Genes, proteases, cortical spreading depression and migraine: impact on pathophysiology and treatment. Funct Neurol 2007; 22:133–136.
15. Moskowitz MA, Currer FM. Sumatriptan: a receptor targeted treatment for migraine. Annu Rev Med 1993; 44:145–154.
16. Burstein R, Levy D, Jakubowski M. Effects of sensitization of trigeminovascular neurons to triptan therapy during migraine. Rev Neurol (Paris) 2005; 161:658–660.
17. Humphries PP, Feniuk W. Mode of action of the anti-migraine drug sumatriptan. Trends Pharmacol Sci 1991; 12:444–446.
18. Goadsby PJ. Post-triptan era for the treatment of acute migraine. Curr Pain Headache Rep 2004; 8:393–398.
19. Johnson KIW, Schaus JM, Durkin MM, et al. 5-HT1F receptor agonists inhibit neurogenic dural inflammation in guinea pigs. Neuroreport 1997; 8:2237–2240.
20. Fugelli A, Moret C, Fillon G. Autoradiographic localization of 5-HT1E and 5-HT1F binding sites in rat brain: effect of serotonergic lesioning. J Recept Signal Transduct Res 1997; 17:L631–L645.
21. Castro ME, Pascual J, Romon T, et al. Differential distribution of [3H]sumatriptan binding sites (5-HT1B, 5-HT1D and 5-HT1F receptors) in human brain: focus on brain stem and spinal cord. Neuropharmacology 1997; 36:535–542.
22. Goadsby PJ, Classey JD. Evidence for serotonin (5-HT) 1B, 5-HT1D and 5-HT1F receptor inhibitory effects on trigeminal neurons with craniovascular input. Neuroscience 2003; 122(2):491–498.
23. Ramadan NM, Skljarevski V, Phebus LA, et al. 5-HT1F receptor agonists in acute migraine treatment: a hypothesis. Cephalalgia 2003; 23(8):776–785.
24. Hamel E. The biology of serotonin receptors: focus on migraine pathophysiology and treatment. Can J Neurol Sci 1999; 26(Suppl 3):S2–S6.
25. Bigal ME, Bordini CA, Antoniazzi AL, Speciali JG. The triptan formulations: A critical evaluation. Arq Neuropsiquiatr 2003; 61(2-A): 313–320.

26. Silberstein SD. Practice parameter: evidence-based guidelines for migraine headache (an evidence based review): report of the Quality Standards Subcommittee of the American Academy of Neurology. Neurology 2000; 55:754–762.

27. Fowler PA, Lacey LF, Thomas et al. The clinical pharmacology, pharmacokinetics and metabolism of sumatriptan. Eur Neurol 1991; 31:291–294.

28. Halpern MT, Lipton RB, Cady RK, et al. Cost-effectiveness of sumatriptan therapy early vs. delayed treatment. Cephalalgia 2001; 21:336.

29. Ryan R, Elkind A, Baker CC, et al. Sumatriptan nasal spray for the acute treatment of migraine: results of two clinical studies. Neurology 1997; 49:1225–1230.

30. Torres G. Zolmitriptan offers doctors and patients choices for effective treatment of migraine. In: Humphrey P, Ferrari M, Olesen J, eds. The Triptans: Novel Drugs for Migraine. New York: Oxford University Press, 2001:190–198.

31. Rappaport AM, Ramadan NM, Adelman JU, et al.; the 017 Clinical Trial Study Group. Optimizing the dose of zolmitriptan (Zomig), 311C90) for the acute treatment of migraine. A multicenter, double-blind, placebo-controlled dose range-finding trial. Neurology 1997; 49:1210–1218.

32. Loder EW, Dowson AJ, Spierings EL. Part II: clinical efficacy and tolerability of zolmitriptan orally disintegrating tablets in the acute treatment of migraine. Curr Med Res Opin 2005; 21(Suppl 3):S8–S12.

33. Dowson AJ, MacGregor EA, Purdy RA, et al. Zolmitriptan orally disintegrating tablet is effective in the acute treatment of migraine. Cephalalgia 2002; 22: 101–106.

34. Spierings EL, Rapoport AM, Dodick DW, et al. Acute treatment of migraine with zolmitriptan 5 mg orally disintegrating tablet. CNS Drugs 2004; 18:1133–1141.

35. Steiner TJ, Diener HC, MacGregor EA, et al. Comparative efficacy of eletriptan and zolmitriptan in the acute treatment of migraine. Cephalalgia 2003; 23:942–952.

36. Gruffyd-Jones K, Kies B, Middlegton A, et al. Zolmitriptan versus sumatriptan for the acute oral treatment of migraine: a randomized, double-blind, international study. Eur J Neurol 2001; 8:237–245.

37. Gallagher RM, Dennish G, Spierings EI, et al. A comparative trial of zolmitriptan and sumatriptan for the acute oral treatment of migraine. Headache 2000; 40: 119–128.

38. Salonen R. Naratriptan: the gentle triptan. In: Humphrey P, Ferreri M, Olesen J, eds. The Triptans: Novel Drugs for Migraine. New York: Oxford University Press, 2001:228–235.

39. Bomhof M, Paz J, Legg N, et al. Comparison of rizatriptan 10 mg vs. naratriptan 2.5 mg in migraine. Eur Neurol 1999; 42:173–179.

40. Dahlof C, Winter P, Whitehouse H, et al. Randomized double-blind, placebo-controlled comparison of oral naratriptan and oral sumatriptan in the acute treatment of migraine. Neurology 1997; 48 (Suppl 3): S85–S86.

41. Ferrari MD. Rizatriptan: a new milestone in migraine treatment. Introduction. Cedphalalgia 2000; 20(Suppl 1): 1.

42. Ahrens SP, Farmer MV, Williams DL, et al.; Rizatriptan Wafer Protocol 049 Study Group. Efficacy and safety for the rizatriptan wafer for the acute treatment of migraine. Cephalalgia 1999; 19:525–530.

43. Pascual J. Almotriptan. In: Humphrey P, Ferreri M, Olesen J, eds. The Triptans: Novel Drugs for Migraine. New York: Oxford University Press, 2001:199–205.

44. Pascual J, Falk RM, Piessens F, et al. Consistent efficacy and tolerability of almotriptan in the acute treatment of multiple migraine attacks: results of a large, randomized, double-blind, placebo-controlled study. Cephalalgia 2000; 20:588–596.

45. Dahlof C, Tfelt-Hansen P, Massiou H, et al. Dose finding, placebo-controlled study of oral almotriptan in the acute treatment of migraine. Neurology 2001; 57: 1811–1817.

46. Dowson AJ, Massiou H, Láinez JM, et al. Almotriptan is an effective and well-tolerated treatment for migraine pain: results of a randomized, double-blind, placebo-controlled clinical trial. Cephalalgia 2002; 22:453–461.

47. Cabarrocas X, Zayas JM, Suris M. Equivalent efficacy of oral almotriptan. A new 5-HT agonist, compared with sumatriptan 100 mg. Headache 1998; 38:377–337.
48. Fernandes FJ, Jansat JM, Cabarrocas X, et al. Absolute bioavailability of oral and subcutaneous almotriptan. Cephalalgia 1999; 23:363.
49. Goadsby PJ, Ferrari MD, Olesen J, et al. Eletriptan in acute migraine: a double-blind, placebo-controlled comparison to sumatriptan. Eletriptan Steering Committee. Neurology 2000; 54:156–163.
50. Stark R, Dahlof C, Haughie S, et al. Efficacy, safety and tolerability of oral eletriptan in the acute treatment of migraine: results of a phase III, multicentre, placebo-controlled study across three attacks. Cephalalgia 2002; 22:23–32.
51. Sheftell F, Ryan RE, Pitman V. Efficacy, safety, and tolerability of oral eletriptan for treatment of acute migraine: a multicenter, double-blind, placebo-controlled study conducted in the United States. Headache 2003; 43:202–213.
52. Sakai F, Diener HC, Ryan R, et al. Eletriptan for the acute treatment of migraine: results of bridging a Japanese study to western clinical trials. Curr Med Res Opin 2004; 20:269–277.
53. Gupta P, Napler CM, Purdy J, et al. In vitro profile of eletriptan, a new 5-HT1D-like receptor partial agonist. Cephalalgia 1996; 16:368.
54. Rapaport A, Ryan R, Goldstein J, et al. Dose range-finding studies with frovatriptan in the acute treatment of migraine. Headache 2002; 42(Suppl 2):S74–S83.
55. Goldstein J, Keywood C. Frovatriptan for the acute treatment of migraine: a dose finding study. Headache 2002; 42:41–48.
56. Kelman L. Review of frovatriptan in the treatment of migraine. Neuropsyuchiatr Dis Treat 2008; 4(1):49–54.
57. Taylor FR. Clinical aspects of premenstrual headaches. Curr Pain Headache Rep 2009; 13(1):75–81.
58. Salonen R, Scott A. Triptans: do they differ? Curr Pain Headache Rep 2002; 6:133–139.
59. Dahlof CG. Non-oral formulations of triptans and their use in acute migraine. Curr Pain Headache Rep 2005; 9(3):206–212.
60. Nilsson T, Longmore J, Shaw D, et al. Contractile 5-HT1B receptors on human cerebral arteries: pharmacological characterization and localization with immunocytochemistry. Br J Pharacol 1999; 128:1133–1140.
61. Edvinsson L, Uddman E, Wackenfors A, et al. Triptan-induced contractile (5-HT1B receptor) responses in human cerebral and coronary arteries: relationship to clinical effect. Clin Sci (Lond) 2005; 109:335–342.
62. Chalaupka FD. Acute myocardial infarction with sumatriptan: a case report and review of the literature. Headache 2009; 49(5):762–764.
63. Fulton GC, Brown MM, Mo J, et al. Triptans in migraine: the risks of stroke, cardiovascular disease and death in practice. Neurology 2004; 62:563–568.
64. Tietjen EG. Migraine and ischemic heart disease and stroke: potential mechanisms and treatment implications. Cephalalgia 2007; 27:981–987.
65. Melek IM, Seyfeli E, Duru M, et al. Autonomic dysfunction and cardiac repolarization abnormalities in patients with migraine attacks. Med Sci Monit. 2007; 13:RA47–RA49.
66. Dodick D, Lipton RB, Martin V, et al.; the Triptan Cardiovascular Safety Expert Panel. Consensus statement: cardiovascular safety profile of triptans (5-HT1B/1D agonists) in the acute treatment of migraine. Headache 2004; 44:414–425.
67. Dahlof CG. Cutaneous allodynia and migraine: another view. Curr Pain Headache Rep 2006; 10:231–238.
68. Dahlof CG, Lipton RB, Lines CR, et al. Consistency of pain relief over multiple migraine attacks following treatment with rizatriptan. In: Olesen J, Ferrari M, Humphrey PP, eds. Frontiers in Headache Research. The Triptans: Novel Drugs for Migraine. Oxford: Oxford University Press, 2001:222–227.
69. Dahlof CG, Jomes M, Davis K, et al. A comparison of preference for and efficacy of tablet formulations of sumatriptan (50 mg and 100 mg), naratriptan (2.5 mg),

rizatriptan (10 mg), and zolmitriptan (2.5 mg) in the acute treatment of migraine. J Headache Pain 2004; 5:115–122.

70. Burstein R, Yarnitsky D, Goor-Aryeh I, et al. An association between migraine and cutaneous allodynia. Ann Neurol 2000; 47:614–624.

71. Jakubowski M, Silberstein S, Ashkenazi A, et al. Can allodynic migraine patients be identified interictally using a questionnaire? Neurology 2005; 65:1419–1422.

72. Burstein R, Cutrer MF, Yarnitsky D. The development of cutaneous allodynia during a migraine attack: clinical evidence for the sequential recruitment of spinal and supraspinal nociceptive neurons in migraine. Brain 2000; 123: 1703–1709.

73. Burstein R, Collins B, Jakubowski M. Defeating migraine pain with triptans: a race against the development of cutaneous allodynia. Ann Neurol 2004; 55:19–26.

74. Jakubowski M, Levy D, Goor-Aryeh I, et al. Terminating migraine with allodynia and ongoing central sensitization using parenteral administration of COX1/COX2 inhibitors. Headache 2005; 45:850–861.

75. Silberstein SD, Mannix LK, Goldstein J, et al. Multimechanistic (sumatriptan-naproxen) early intervention for the acute treatment of migraine. Neurology 2008; 71(2):114–121.

76. Lipton RB, Dodick DW, Adelman JU, et al. Consistency of response to sumatriptan/naproxen sodium in a placebo-controlled, crossover study. Cephalalgia 2009; 28(8):826–836.

77. Silberstein SD. Preventive migraine treatment. Neurol Clin 2009; 27:429–443.

78. Lipton RB, Diamond M, Freitag F, et al. Migraine prevention patterns in a community sample: results from the American Migraine Prevalence and Prevention (AMPP) study. Headache 2005; 45:792–793 (Abstract).

79. Lipton RB, Bigal MD, Diamond M, et al., on behalf of the AMPP Advisory Group. Migraine prevalence, disease burden and the need for preventive therapy. Neurology 2007; 68:343–349.

80. Sachedo RC, Reife RA, Lim P, et al. Topiramate monotherapy for partial onset seizures. Epilepsia 1997; 38:294–300.

81. Silberstein SD, Neto W, Schmitt J, et al., for the MIGR-001 Study Group. Topiramate in the prevention of migraine headache: a randomized, double blind placebo-controlled, multiple-dose study. Arch Neurol 2004; 61:490–495.

82. Brandes JL, Saper JR, Diamond M, et al. Topiramate for migraine prevention: a randomized controlled trial. JAMA 2004; 291:965–973.

83. Deiner HC, Tfelt-Hensen P, Dahlof C, et al. Topiramate in migraine prophylaxis—results from a placebo-controlled trial with propranolol as an active control. J Neurol 2004; 251:943–950.

84. Silberstein SD. Divalproex sodium in headache-literature review and clinical guidelines. Headache 1996; 36:547–555.

85. Pellock JM, Willmore LJ. A rational guide to routine blood monitoring in patients receiving antiepileptic drugs. Neurology 1991; 41:961–964.

86. Vainionpaa LK, Rattya J, Knip M, et al. Valproate-induced hyperandrogenism during pubertal maturation in girls with epilepsy. Ann Neurol 1999; 45:444–450.

87. Hering R, Kuritzky A. Sodium valproate in the prophylactic treatment of migraine: a double-blind study versus placebo. Cephalalgia 1992; 12:81–84.

88. Jensen R, Brinck T, Olesen J. Sodium valproate has prophylactic effect in migraine without aura, a triple blind, plaeco-controlled crossover study. Neurology 1994; 44:241–244.

89. Mathew NT, Saper JR, Silberstein SD, et al. migraine prophylaxis with divalproex. Arch Neurol 1995; 52:281–286.

90. Cortelli P, Sacquegna T, Albani F, et al. Propranolol plasma levels and relief of migraine. Arch Neurol 1985; 42:46–48.

91. Koella WP. CNS-related (side-) effects of beta blockers with special reference to mechanisms of action. Eur J Clin Pharacol 1985; 28:55–63.

92. Ramadan NM. Prophylactice migraine therapy: mechanism and evidence. Curr Pain Headache Rep 2004; 8:91–95.

93. Ryan RE. Comparative study of nadolol and propranolol in prophylactic treatment of migraine. Am Heart J 1984; 108:1156–1159.
94. Olerud B, Gustavsson CL, Furberg B. Nadolol and propranolol in migraine management. Headache 1986; 26:490–493.
95. Solomon GD. Verapamil in migraine prophyulaxis—a five-year review. Headache 1989; 29(7):425–427.
96. Schuler ME, Goldman MP, Munger MA. The role of calcium channel blocking agents in the prevention of migraine. Drug Intell Clin Pharm 1988; 22(3):187–191.
97. Diamond S, Freitag FG. Treatment of headache. Clin J Pain 1989; 5(Suppl 2):S7–S16.
98. Greenberg DA. Calcium channel antagonists and the treatment of migraine. Clin Neuropharmacol 1986; 9(4):311–328.
99. Wauquier A, Ashton D, Marranes R. The effects of flunarizine in experimental models related to the pathogenesis of migraine. Cephalalgia 1985; 5:119–120.
100. Gomersall JD, Stuart A. Amitriptyline in migraine prophylaxis. Changes in pattern of attacks during a controlled clinical trial. J Neurol Neurosurg Psychiatry 1973; 36(4):684–690.
101. Couch JR, Aiegler DK, Hassanein RS. Evaluation of amitriptyline in migraine prophylaxis. Trans Am Neurol Assoc 1974; 99:94–98.
102. Couch JR, Ziegler DK, Hassanein R. Amitriptyline in the prophylaxis of migraine. Effectiveness and relationship of antimigraine and antidepressant effects. Neurology 1976; 26(2):121–127.
103. Couch JR, Hassanein RS. Amitriptyline in migraine prophylaxis. Arch Neurol 1979; 36(11):695–699.
104. Nascimento ED. Prophylaxis of migraine: open study with venlafaxine in 42 patients. Arq Neuropsiquiatr 1998; 56(4):744–746.
105. Adelman LC, Adelman JU, Von Seggern R, et al. Venlafaxine extended release (XR) for the prophylaxis of migraine and tension-type headache: a retrospective study in a clinical setting. Headache 2000; 40(7):572–580.
106. Ozyalcin SN, Talu GK, Kiziltan E, et al. The efficacy and safety of venlafaxine in the prophylaxis of migraine. Headache 2005; 45(2):144–152.
107. Bulut S, Berilgen MS, Baran A, et al. Venlafaxine versus amitriptyline in the prophylactic treatment of migraine: randomized, double-blind, crossover study. Clin Neurol Neurosurg 2004; 107(1):44–48.
108. Diamond S, Pepper BJ, Diamond ML, et al. Serotonin syndrome induced by transition from phenelzine to venlafaxine: four patient reports. Neurology 1998; 51(1): 274–276.
109. Silberstein SD, Mathew N, Saper J, et al. Botulinum toxin type A as a migraine preventive treatment. Headache 2000; 40:445–450.
110. Shuhendler AJ, Lee S, Siu M, et al. Efficacy of botulinum toxin type A for the prophylaxis of episodic migraine headaches: a meta-analysis of randomized, double-blind, placebo-controlled trials. Pharmacotherapy 2009; 29(7):784–791.
111. Cady R, Schreiber C. Botulinum toxin type A as a migraine preventive treatment in patients previously failing oral prophylactic treatment due to compliance issues. Headache 2008; 48(6):900–913.
112. Schrader H, Stovner LJ, Helde G, et al. Prophylactic treatment of migraine with angiotensin converting enzyme inhibitor (lisinopril): randomized, placebo-controlled crossover study. BMJ 2001; 322(7277):19–22.
113. Schuh-Hofer S, Flach U, Meisel A, et al. Efficacy of lisinopril in migraine prophylaxis—an open label study. Eur J Neurol 2007; 14(6):701–703.
114. Tronvik E, Stovner LJ, Helde G, et al. Prophylactic treatment of migraine with an angiotensin II receptor blocker: a randomized controlled trial. JAMA 2003; 289(1): 65–69.
115. Owada K. Efficacy of candesartan in the treatment of migraine in hypertensive patients. Hypertens Res 2004; 27(6):441–446.
116. Pfaffenrath V, Diener HC, Fischer M, et al. The efficacy and safety of *Tanacetum parthenium* (feverfew) in migraine prophylaxis—a double-blind, multicenter, randomized, placebo-controlled dose-response study. Cephalalgia 2002; 22(7):523–532.

117. Vogler BK, Pittler MH, Ernst E. Feverfew as a preventive treatment for migraine: a systematic review. Cephalalgia 1998; 18:704–724.
118. Schoenen J, Jacquy J, Lenaerts M. Effectiveness of high-dose riboflavin in migraine prophylaxis. A randomized controlled trial. Neurology 1998; 50:466–470.
119. MacLennan SC, Wade FM, Forrest KM, et al. High-dose riboflavin for migraine prophylaxis in children: a double-blind, randomized, placebo controlled trial. J Child Neurol 2008; 23(11):1300–1304.
120. Lipton RB, Gobel H, Wilks K, et al. Efficacy of petasites (an extract from Petasites rhizome) 50 and 70 mg for prophylaxis of migraine: results of a randomized double-blind, placebo-controlled study. Neurology 2002; 58:A472 (Abstract).
121. Agosti R, Duke RK, Chrubasik JE, et al. Effectiveness of *Petasites hybridus* preparations in the prophylaxis of migraine: a systematic review. Phytomedicine 2006; 13(9–10):743–746.
122. Sandor PS, Di Clemente L, Coppola G, et al. Efficacy of coenzyme Q10 in migraine prophylaxis: a randomized controlled study. Neurology 2005; 64(4):713–715.
123. Evers S. Treatment of migraine with prophylactic drugs. Expert Opin Pharacother 2008; 9(15):2565–2573.
124. Evers S. Alternatives to beta blockers in preventive migraine treatment. Nervenarzt 2008; 79(10):1135–1136, 1138–1140, 1142–1143.
125. Durham PL. Inhibition of calcitonin gene-related peptide function: a promising strategy for treating migraine. Headache 2008; 48(8):1269–1275.
126. Edvinsson L. CGRP blockers in migraine therapy: where do they act? Br J Pharmacol 2008; 155(7):967–969.

Index

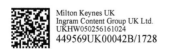

9 781138 116733